19742

THE ELISA: ENZYME-LINKED IMMUNOSORBENT ASSAY IN VETERINARY RESEARCH AND DIAGNOSIS

CURRENT TOPICS IN VETERINARY MEDICINE AND ANIMAL SCIENCE

VOLUME 22

Other titles in this series

Series ISBN: 90-247-2429-5

THE ELISA: ENZYME-LINKED IMMUNOSORBENT ASSAY IN VETERINARY RESEARCH AND DIAGNOSIS

Proceedings of a meeting held at the
University of Surrey, Guildford, UK
September 15-17, 1981

edited by

R.C. Wardley
J.R. Crowther
Animal Virus Resarch Institute
Pirbright
Surrey
UK

1982
MARTINUS NIJHOFF PUBLISHERS
THE HAGUE / BOSTON / LONDON

for

THE COMMISSION OF THE EUROPEAN COMMUNITIES

Distributors

for the United States and Canada
Kluwer Boston, Inc.
190 Old Derby Street
Hingham, MA 02043
USA

for all other countries
Kluwer Academic Publishers Group
Distribution Center
P.O. Box 322
3300 AH Dordrecht
The Netherlands

Library of Congress Cataloging in Publication Data

Main entry under title:

The ELISA.

    (Current topics in veterinary medicine and animal
science ; v. 22)
    1. Veterinary microbiology--Technique--Congresses.
2. Enzyme-linked immunosorbent assay--Congresses.
3. Micro-organisms, Pathogenic--Identification--
Congresses. 4. Veterinary medicine--Diagnosis--
Congresses. 5. Diagnosis, Laboratory--Congresses.
I. Wardley, R. C. II. Crowther, J. R. III. Series.
SF780.2.E44 1982   636.89'69250756   82-18831
ISBN 90-247-2769-3

ISBN 90-247-2769-3 (this volume)
ISBN 90-247-2429-5 (series)

Publication arranged by:
Commission of the European Communities,
Directorate-General Information Market and Innovation

EUR 8074 EN

LEGAL NOTICE

Neither the Commission of the European Communities nor any person acting on behalf of the
Commission is responsible for the use which might be made of the following information.

PRINTED IN THE NETHERLANDS

CONTENTS

VI

INTRODUCTION

The idea behind this meeting was to bring together workers applying enzyme immunoassays to veterinary problems. Groups working in Europe were contacted as to their possible interest and this met with a good response.

Enzyme immunoassays are usually compared favourably with radio immunoassays since they offer the same versatility of testing without the handling and counting problems associated with radioisotopes. This is well illustrated in the papers, where sensitive immunoassays have been made available to laboratories who perhaps would not have pursued radioimmunoassay methods. The diversity of the applications reported serves to emphasise the versatility of such assays to suit the exact needs of experimenters.

ACKNOWLEDGEMENTS

We would like to thank Dr R.F. Sellers, Director, Animal Virus Research Institute, Pirbright, UK for his interest in the meeting; Penny Scott and Pam Hildred for their invaluable administrative assistance, and Mr B. Carpenter and Mr M. Denyer for their general help in running the meeting. The Commission of the European Communities, Directorate General for Agriculture, assisted by financing the participation of some delegates from its budget for coordinating agricultural research.

PART I: FUNDAMENTAL ASPECTS OF ELISA TECHNOLOGY

ELISA METHODOLOGY: VARIATIONS IN TECHNICAL PROCEDURES

C. Burrells and A. McL. Dawson

Moredun Research Institute, 408 Gilmerton Road, Edinburgh EH17 7JH.

ABSTRACT

Areas in which ELISA techniques can vary are:- the type of solid phase employed, conditions for adsorption to the solid phase, wash solutions and washing procedures, conditions during specific reaction steps and methods by which assays are read and results expressed. Each of these is discussed briefly with reference to available literature and to methods currently used at the Moredun Research Institute.

INTRODUCTION

Since the introduction of the enzyme-linked immunosorbent assay (ELISA) (Engvall and Perlmann, 1972) the mass of published work in which the technique is employed is evidence of its broad applicability and potential. It is simple to perform, convenient, economical, reliable, highly sensitive and compares favourably with other assay systems. That the system is also flexible is apparent by the innumerable variations in methodology employed in basic ELISA procedures. This brief review is intended to bring together some of the technical variations which have been applied to the assay.

VARIABLE ASPECTS OF METHODOLOGY

Procedural variations can be illustrated using as an example the indirect ELISA, the main stages of which are:-

1. Adsorption of antigen to the solid phase

2. Wash

3. Addition of antibody - incubation

4. Wash

5. Addition of enzyme-labelled anti-globulin - incubation

6. Wash

7. Addition of enzyme substrate

8. Determination and expression of results.

Manual or Automatic

In general, all procedures are carried out manually or semi-automatically. However, there is available commercially a fully automated ELISA system which utilises racks of polystyrene cuvettes (Gilford Instruments Ltd., Teddington, Middlesex, England). A fully mechanised system has also been described which uses blocks of 9 plastic tubes as the solid phase (Ruitenberg et al, 1977). At this time, we are not aware of any system yet available for a fully automatic system based on microplates as the solid phase.

The Solid Phase

Polystyrene is the most suitable and most widely used material as an antigen carrier (Denmark and Chessum, 1978). Other materials which have been shown to be suitable carriers such as particles of cellulose, polyacrylamide, cross-linked dextrans, silicone rubber and micro-crystalline glass and plastic have the disadvantage of requiring centrifugation during the washing steps. Polystyrene has been used in many forms such as beads or spheres (Guisdon, Thierry and Avrameas, 1978), test-tubes (Bruggman et al, 1977), cuvettes (Ellens and de Leeuw, 1977), dip-sticks (Felgner, 1977) and 96-well microplates (Voller and Bidwell, 1975). Flat-bottomed microplates appear to be employed more widely than round-bottomed plates only because of the unsuitability of round-bottomed plates when reading results with a "through-the-plate" colorimeter. Other materials like cellulose nitrate tubes (Hermann and Collins, 1976) and poly-vinyl chloride plates have been used, but these are less sensitive (McLaren, Lillywhite and Au, 1981).

Adsorption to the Solid Phase

There appears to be uniform agreement that the buffer used for adsorption to the solid phase is a 0.05M carbonate buffer pH 9.6. Everything else associated with solid phase sensitisation is eminently variable. The reported volume of reagents added to microplate wells starts at 50μl (Poxton, 1979), ranges through 100 μl (Ruitenberg, Steerenberg and Brosi, 1975), 150 μl (Lambre and Kasturi, 1979), 200 μl (Voller, Bidwell and Bartlett, 1979), 250 μl (Ellens et al, 1978) to 300 μl (Voller and Bidwell, 1975). With tubes and cuvettes the volume generally used is 1 ml.

Techniques of adsorption vary from incubation at 4°C overnight (Voller, Bidwell and Bartlett, 1979), room temperature overnight (Engvall and Ljungstrom, 1975), 37°C overnight (Halle, Dasch and Weiss, 1977), 37°C for 3 h for tubes (Bruggman et al, 1977) and plates (Ruitenberg, Steerenberg and Brosi, 1975) and 37°C for 30 min (Berg Jorgensen and Thode Jensen, 1978). Incubations carried out at 37°C are usually performed using some form of shaking or rotation. Increased adsorption of some soluble antigens can be achieved when the plastic surface is pre-coated or pre-treated prior to addition of antigens using poly-1-lysine (Kelsoe and Weller, 1978). Foetal bovine serum at 2.5% has been used for this purpose (Saunders and Clinard, 1976) and is allowed to air dry in the wells prior to fixation with glutaraldehyde. When similarly used, 1% bovine serum albumin is allowed to dry in air in the wells without fixation and is followed by antigen which is also allowed to dry in air (Vestergaard, Grauballe and Spanggaard, 1977). A further method of ensuring antigen binding to the solid phase is the pre-coating of wells or tubes with antigen-specific antibody as for a direct ELISA (Yolken et al, 1977).

Once coated or sensitised, solid carriers can be used immediately or they can be satisfactorily stored prior to use by freezing at -20°C (Ellens et al, 1978) or by washing and drying prior to storage at -20°C or -70°C. Dried plates stored in watertight containers show no loss of activity after 1 year even at $+4^{\circ}$C (Voller, Bidwell ad Bartlett, 1979).

Washing

This can be done in many ways, but it is essential that washing completely removes any unadsorbed or unabsorbable reagents which would interfere with subsequent assay procedures. Commercial washers designed specifically for microplates are available (Dynatech Laboratories, Billingshurst, Sussex, England). Washing by immersion is not guaranteed to provide such an efficient "flush" as small jets of wash fluid from a washing machine. A "home-made" washer comprising a microtitre plate from which the well bottoms have been removed has been described (Henriksen, 1979). Plastic pipette tips fitted over the wells then correspond in position to the wells of a test microplates.

Fitted to a reservoir, this can then wash 96 wells simultaneously. Satisfactory plate washing can also be achieved by gentle pressure applied to the plunger of a 50 ml syringe to ensure proper flushing of the wells. Fluids used for washing vary from tap water (Ruitenberg, Steerenberg and Brosi, 1975), distilled water (Ellens and de Leeuw, 1977), deionised water (Ellens et al, 1978), saline (WHO Collaborative Study, 1976), phosphate buffered saline (Voller, Bidwell and Bartlett, 1979) and 0.2M tris buffer (Wolters et al, 1976). Most of these usually incorporate Tween 20 at a concentration of 0.05%, and in some cases Tween 80 is used (Ellens and de Leeuw, 1977). Buffers used during the specific incubations can also vary. They can be the same ionic salt solutions or buffers used as washes or they can incorporate a small amount of protein to avoid any non-specific binding to the plastic of subsequent reagents. The protein can be bovine albumin (Lambre and Kasturi, 1979), egg albumin (Maiolini et al, 1978) or 0.1% chicken plasma (Maiolini and Masseyeff, 1975). Another buffer which is reputed to increase the amount of specific reaction is a high salt (2%) plus Tween 80 buffer (Houwers, personal communication).

Assay procedure

Samples can be assayed in 2 ways. They can either be serially diluted (Ruitenberg, Steerenberg and Brosi, 1975) or they can be tested at a pre-determined optimal dilution and test results compared with a standard curve (Burrells, Wells and Dawson, 1979).

Conditions for the specific reactions

For the indirect ELISA, these are the incubation steps associated with the antigen-antibody reaction, the binding of the labelled antiglobulin to bound antibody and the degradation of the enzyme substrate. Variation in this area is mainly associated with temperature and time (Table 1). Specific reactions are usually carried out either at room temperature (Voller, Bidwell ad Bartlett, 1979) or at 37°C (Leinikki et al, 1978).

Table 1.   Variations in temperature and duration of ELISA incubations

Temp	Antigen/ Antibody Reaction	Anti-Globulin/ Antibody Reaction	Enzyme/Substrate Reaction	
R.T.	2 hours	3 hours	$\frac{1}{2}$-1 hour	(Voller, Bidwell and Bartlett, 1979)
37°C	1 hour	1 hour	1 "	(Rissing et al, 1980)
R.T.	6 hours	overnight	$\frac{1}{2}$-1 "	(Engvall and Ljungstrom, 1975)
R.T.	4 hours	overnight	1 "	(Poxton, 1979)
37°C	1$\frac{1}{2}$ hours	1$\frac{1}{2}$ hours	$\frac{1}{2}$ "	(Leinikki et al, (1978)
37°C	$\frac{1}{2}$ hour	$\frac{1}{2}$ hour	1 "	(Ruitenberg, Steerenberg and Brosi, 1975) (Berg Jorgensen and Thode Jensen, 1978).

In a direct assay for the detection of antigen it was found that if
plates were incubated in a shaker at 37°C, reaction times could be cut
to 10 min each (Yolken and Leister, 1981). Although this resulted in a
10-fold drop in sensitivity over incubation times of 2 hours, the assay
was still sufficiently sensitive for a rapid result to be obtained.
Higher reaction temperatures reduce the reaction times needed, but a
moist chamber should be used for incubations at 37°C to avoid local
evaporation at the edges of the plates. Further variability is
illustrated by an indirect ELISA which is being used at present to
detect antibody in the supernatant fluids from lymphocyte hybridoma
cultures. When standard incubation times of 2 hours for the antigen-
antibody reaction and 3 hours for the conjugate incubation are used at
room temperature, it is found necessary to incubate test plates
overnight at 4°C for sufficient colour reaction to develop (Burrells,
unpublished observations). The same colour might be achieved in a
shorter time if the times and temperatures of the other 2 steps were
changed. This, however, would necessitate adjustment of reagent
concentrations as working dilutions of reagents are determined under
standard conditions of time and temperature, the more dilute the
reagents, the longer the reaction times will be (Voller, Bidwell and
Bartlett, 1979).

6

Reading test reactions

Results of ELISA tests can either be read by eye (Ruitenberg, Steerenberg and Brosi, 1975) or by spectrophotometer. Specially designed spectrophotometers are commercially available which read through microplate wells either singly (Yolken et al, 1977) or in rows (Titertek Multiskan - Flow Laboratories, Irvine, Ayrshire, Scotland). However, these are expensive and standard photometers can be used. Samples can either be transferred to cuvettes and the optical density measured or alternatively, the assay can be carried out in cuvettes (Ellens and de Leeuw, 1977) thus avoiding the transfer of test fluids. There is also a commercially available photometer for use with microplates which aspirates singly the contents of individual wells into a flow-through colorimeter cuvette (MSE Scientific Instruments, Crawley, England). A standard photometer has also been used in conjunction with a continuous flow-line (Burrells, Wells and Dawson, 1979). In this semi-automatic system, samples are aspirated from wells using a manual probe connected via a peristaltic pump. Samples are separated from each other by a diluent wash and the stream segmented with air bubbles. The test fluids pass through a micro-flow-through cuvette and optical densities are recorded by hand or as peaks on a chart-recorder.

Expression of results

Test results can be expressed in a variety of ways (Voller, Bidwell and Bartlett, 1979).

1. End-point titre. This is the only method in which the samples to be assayed are serially diluted as for other serological assays. If a colorimeter is unavailable, then this is the best method for quatitative enzyme immunoassays as end-point titres can be read visually.

2. Positive or negative. This visual method is useful for purely qualitative purposes.

3. Absorbance value. This is merely an expression of the result in terms of optical density. The observed optical density of the test sample is usually compared with the optical density of a known positive sample included in each test.

4.   Ratio. Using this method, the optical density of a test sample is divided by the mean optical density of a group of known negative samples.   A ratio above a pre-set value e.g. 2 or 3 is considered to be positive.

5.   Comparison with a standard curve. In this method, a set of standards of known value are included along with the samples at one pre-determined dilution. A standard curve is obtained from the optical density values of the standards, and the values of the test samples are obtained by reference to the standard curve.

If tests are read in automatic ELISA readers, calculations, especially those involved in comparison with a standard curve, can be facilitated by linking the colorimeter to a computer. The colorimeter can be linked either with a bench-top computer for direct processing of data, or a tape-punch whereby data can be stored on tape and subsequently subjected to computer processing.

CONCLUSION

Variations in technical manipulations are innumerable but it is not suggested that any one modification is superior to others. It is evident that once optimal concentrations of reagents have been determined which give standard optical densities under standard conditions using adequate standard controls, then the main factors governing test procedures are the quality and volume of reagents, the availability of ancillary equipment, the importance of rapid results, and the ability of the test system, or part of it, to fit into a normal working time span. What is illustrated is the adaptability of the ELISA technique to suit varying conditions and individual laboratory requirements.

8

REFERENCES

Berg Jorgensen, J. and Thode Jensen, P. 1978. Enzyme-linked immunosorbent assay (ELISA) for detection of Mycobacterium paratuberculosis in cattle. Acta. Vet. Scand., 19, 310-312.

Bruggman, S., Keller, H., Bertshinger, H.V. and Engberg, B. 1977. Quantitative detection of antibodies to Mycoplasma suipneumoniae in pigs' sera by an enzyme-linked immunosorbent assay. Vet. Record, 101, 109-111.

Burrells, C., Wells, P.W. and Dawson, A.McL. 1979. The quantitative estimation of antibody to Pasteurella haemolytica in sheep sera using a micro-enzyme linked immnosorbent assay (ELISA). Vet. Microbiol., 3, 291-301.

Denmark, J.R. and Chessum, B.S. 1978. Standardisation of enzyme-linked immunosorbent assay (ELISA) and the detection of Toxoplasma antibody. Med. Lab. Science, 35, 227-232.

Ellens, D.J. and de Leeuw, P.W. 1977. Enzyme-linked immunosorbent assay for diagnosis of Rotavirus infections in calves. J. Clin. Micro. , 530-532.

Ellens, D.J., de Leeuw, P.W., Straver, P.J. and van Balken, J.A.M. 1978. Comparison of five diagnostic methods for the detection of Rotavirus antigens in calf faeces. Med. Microbiol. Immunol. 166, 157-163.

Engvall, E. and Ljungstrom, I. 1975. Detection of human antibodies to Trichinella spiralis by enzyme-linked immunosorbent assay, ELISA. Acta Path. Microbiol. Scand. Sect. C., 83, 231-237.

Engvall, E. and Perlmann, P. 1972. Enzyyme-linked immunosorbent assay, ELISA. III Quantitation of specific antibodies by enzyme-labelled anti-immunoglobulin in antigen coated tubes. J. Immunol. 109, 129-135.

Felgner, P. 1977. Serological diagnosis of extraintestinal amebiasis: a comparison of stick-ELISA and other immunological tests. Tropenmed. Parasit. 23, 491-493.

Guisdon, J.L., Thierry, R. and Avrameas, S. 1978. Magnetic enzyme immunoassay for measuring human IgE. J. Allergy Clin. Immunol. 6, 23-27.

Halle, S., Dasch, G.A. and Weiss, E. 1977. Sensitive enzyme-linked immunosorbent assay for detection of antibodies against thyphus rickettsiae, Rickettsia prowazeki and Rickettsia typhi. J. Clin. Micro. 6, 101-110.

Henriksen, S.V. 1979. A simple washing unit for micro-ELISA. Acta. Vet. Scand. 20, 598-600.

Herrman, J.E. and Collins, M.F. 1976. Quantitation of immunoglobulin adsorption to plastics. J. Immunol. 10, 363-366.

Kelsoe, G.H. and Weller, T.H. 1978. Immunodiagnosis of infection with S. mansoni: ELISA for the detection of antibody to circulating antigen. Proc. Natl. Acad. Sci. USA., 75, 5715-5717.

Lambre, C. and Kasturi, K.N. 1979. A microplate immunoenzyme assay for anti-influenza antibodies. J. Immunol. Methods, 26, 61-67.

Leinikki, P.O., Shekarchi, I., Dorsett, P. and Sever, J.L. 1978. Determination of virus-specific IgM antibodies by using ELISA: elimination of false-positive results with protein A sepharose absorption and subsequent IgM antibody assay. J. Lab. Clin. Med.,92, 849-857.

Maiolini, R and Masseyeff, R. 1975. A sandwich method of enzyme-immunoassay. 1. Application to rat and human alpha-fetoprotein. J. Immunol. Methods, 8, 223-234.

McLaren, M., Lillywhite, J.E. and Au, A.C.S. 1981. Indirect enzyme-linked immunosorbent assay (ELISA): practical aspects of standardization and quality control. Med. Lab. Sci. 38, 245-251.

Poxton, I.R. 1979. Serological identification of Bacteroides species by an enzyme-linked immunosorbent assay. J. Clin. Path., 32, 294-298.

Rissing, J.P., Buxton, T.B., Talledo, R.A. and Sprinkle, T.J. 1980. Comarison of two enzyme-linked immunosorbent assays for antigen quantitation: direct competition and antibody inhibition. Inf. and Imm., 27, 405-410.

Ruitenberg, E.J., van Amstel, J.A., Brosi, B.J.M. and Steerenberg, P.A. 1977. Mechanization of the enzyme-linked immunosorbent assay (ELISA) for large scale screening of sera. J. Immunol. Methods 16, 354-359.

Ruitenberg, E.J., Steerenberg, P.A. and Brosi, B.J.M. 1975. Micro-system for the application of ELISA (enzyme-linked immunosorbent assay) for the serodiagnosis of Trichinella spiralis infections. Medikon Nederland, 4, 30-31.

Saunders, G.C. and Clinard, E.H. 1976. Rapid micromethod of screening for antibodies to disease agents using the indirect enzyme-labelled antibody test. J. Clin. Micro., 3, 604-608.

Vestergaard, B.F., Grauballe, P.C. and Spanggaard, H. 1977. Titration of Herpes simplex virus antibodies in human sera by the enzyme-linked immunosorbent assay (ELISA). Acta. Path. Microbiol. Scand. Sect. B, 85, 466-468.

Voller, A. and Bidwell, D.E. 1975. A simple method for detecting antibodies to Rubella. Brit. J. Exp. Path., 56, 338-339.

Voller, A., Bidwell, D.E. and Bartlett, A. 1979. The enzyme-linked immunosorbent assay (ELISA). A guide with abstracts of microplate applications. Dynatech Europe, Guernsey.

World Health Organisation. 1976. Parallel evaluation of serological tests applied in African Trypanosomiasis: a WHO collaborative study. Bull. World Health Org. 54, 141-147.

Wolters, G., Kuijpers, L., Kacaki, J. and Schuurs, A. 1976. Solid phase enzyme-immunoassay for detection of hepatitis B surface antigen. J Clin. Path. 29, 873-879.

Yolken, R.H. and Leister, F.J. 1981. Investigation of enzyme immunoassay time courses: development of rapid assay systems. J. Clin. Micro. 13, 738-741.

Yolken, R.H., Kim, H.W., Clem, T., Wyatt, R.G., Kalica, A.R., Chanock, R.M. and Kapikian, A.Z. 1977. Enzyme-linked immunosorbent assay (ELISA) for detection of human Reovirus-like agent of infantile gastroenteritis. Lancet, ii, 263-267.

CHEMICAL CROSS-LINKING AND THE PREPARATION OF CONJUGATES FOR ELISA

T.R. Doel, T. Collen

Vaccine Research Department
The Animal Virus Research Institute
Pirbright, Woking, Surrey, England

ABSTRACT

Various aspects of the preparation of conjugates for ELISA are described. Special reference is made to experimental variables which influence the rates of reaction between reagents and proteins. Finally, a
number of different conjugation procedures are discussed including glutaraldehyde and periodate oxidation.

INTRODUCTION

An important feature of ELISA is the use of a colorimetric enzyme assay
to detect the reaction between antibody and antigen or antibody and a molecule such as protein A. In its usual form an enzyme molecule is covalently
linked to an antibody molecule. The strength of the bond formed during the
linking reaction, often referred to as 'conjugation', is crucial to the
performance of the ELISA test. Thus, with weakly bonded conjugates there
would be a tendency for uncontrolled leaching of the enzyme both during the
test and subsequent storage of the conjugate. It should be mentioned that
a number of immunoassays based on strong, but nevertheless non-covalent,
interactions between molecules such as biotin and avidin have been developed (Guesdon et al., 1979).

Numerous methods have been used to prepare conjugates with the minimum
necessary amount of denaturation and modification to either the enzyme or
the antibody molecule. In this we owe much to the protein chemists who,
over the last thirty years, have investigated the reactivity of amino acid
side chains and the means whereby they might modify the reactivity of those
side chains. From their work, we can summarise those amino acid residues
which have reactive groups protruding from the polypeptide backbone
(Table 1).

One amino acid is of particular significance in the context of conjugate preparation, namely lysine and its reactive ε-amino group.

TABLE 1

Reactive Group	Amino Acid
AMIDE	ASPARAGINE, GLUTAMINE
AMINO, IMINO	ARGININE, HISTIDINE, LYSINE, TRYPTOPHAN
PHENYL	PHENYLALANINE, TRYPTOPHAN, TYROSINE
CARBOXYL	ASPARTIC ACID, GLUTAMIC ACID
HYDROXYL	SERINE, THREONINE
PHENOLIC	TYROSINE
THIOL	CYSTEINE

In addition to amino acid side chains, a number of proteins, for example horseradish peroxidase (HRPO), possess potentially reactive oligosaccharide groups. These groups are often attached via an amino sugar to the side chains of serine, threonine or aspartic acid and invariably terminate in sialic acid.

The preparation of conjugates usually requires the use of a reagent with two or more distinct and well separated reactive groups which are capable of bridging the gap between the amino acid side chains of the two proteins of interest. Particular reagents will be discussed more fully elsewhere in this paper.

FACTORS WHICH INFLUENCE CONJUGATION

The reaction between a reagent and a protein or mixture of proteins is critically dependent on a number of factors, which may be summarised as follows:

1) The rates of reaction of the reagent with the solvent, usually water, and with the proteins are particularly important with reagents such as imidoesters which are readily destroyed by hydrolysis and, consequently, have a relatively short time in which to react with the proteins. The choice of buffer may also be critical. For example, primary and secondary amine buffers must be avoided with those reagents which react with α and ε-amino groups, otherwise the buffer amino groups will monopolise the available reagent. Tertiary amine buffers such as triethanolamine or non-amine buffers such as sodium bicarbonate are therefore chosen.

2) The relative rates of reaction of the reagent with the proteins is a complex aspect of conjugation and may be considered in terms of a) the

number of particular amino acid side chains in each protein. In its most
simple form, some proteins may contain relatively few residues of a particular amino acid. An interesting version of this situation is seen with
horseradish peroxidase (HRPO) which, because of the natural occurrence of
allyl isothiocyanate in horseradishes, contains relatively few unblocked
amino groups (Nakane et al., 1966) and, therefore, reacts much less readily
with glutaraldehyde than IgG. b) the degree of exposure of particular
amino acid side chains. Clearly, side chains which are buried or obscured
will not participate in cross-linking reactions. One of the probable
advantages of exploiting carbohydrate side chains is that they are often
bulky and easily accessible for reaction. c) the size of the reagent.
The dimensions of the reagent and/or the relative positions of the reactive
groups may not permit reaction with both amino acid side chains for steric
reasons. For example, bifunctional imidoesters such as dimethylsuberimi-
date react optimally with amino groups separated by a distance of 11$\overset{o}{A}$
(Peters and Richards, 1977). One of the probable reasons for the success
of glutaraldehyde is the heterogeneous nature of even the best commercial
preparations. Thus, the simultaneous presence of a large number of different types and lengths of molecule in glutaraldehyde solutions facilitates
cross-linking (Peters and Richards, 1977).

3) The relative and absolute concentrations of the proteins influence the
degree of cross-linking. Intermolecular cross-linking is favoured by high
protein concentrations and, equally, intramolecular cross-linking by the
converse. This holds true regardless of whether or not a single protein or
mixture of proteins is treated with a bifunctional reagent (Wold, 1972).
Grossly different quantities of each of the two proteins in a mixture will
lead to an unbalanced conjugate, for example large complexes of IgG with
relatively few enzyme molecules attached. In our laboratory we prepare
conjugates with equimolar concentrations of the two proteins, although
experience with IgG - HRPO conjugates indicates that the relative concentrations are not particularly critical.

4) Other important factors include temperature and pH of reaction and rate
of addition of reagent. Modesto and Pesce (1971) observed that more moles
of DFDNDPS (difluoro-dinitro-diphenyl sulphone) bound to HRPO or IgG when
added incrementally rather than as a single dose. Peters and Richards(1977)
reported similar findings with bifunctional imidoesters. Although it is
difficult to generalise with regard to temperature of reaction, conjugation

is often carried out at room temperature. Modesto and Pesce (1971) reported that double the number of moles of DFDNDPS bound to HRPO at 25°C than at
4°C. With regard to pH, the conditions are dictated very much by the
nature of the reagent and the amino acid side chains destined to be linked.
Although pH values of 8 to 9.5 are commonly used for reactions involving
ε-amino groups of lysine, glutaraldehyde conjugates are usually prepared
at pH 6.8 (Avrameas, 1969).

ONE-STAGE AND TWO-STAGE REACTION PROCEDURES

One of the most common problems associated with the simple one-stage
reaction in which the reagent is added to a mixture of the proteins to be
conjugated is the selective polymerisation of one of the proteins to the
exclusion of the other. This is particularly the case with conjugates prepared by glutaraldehyde treatment of HRPO and IgG mixtures because of the
low reactivity of HRPO with glutaraldehyde (Kennedy et al., 1976). Nakane
and Kawaoi (1974) reported that only about 2% of the added HRPO was conjugated to IgG in a number of different one-stage reaction procedures. Otto
et al. (1973) reported that glutaraldehyde conjugates of ferritin and IgG
prepared by a one-stage reaction were less stable and less soluble than
conjugates prepared by a two-stage procedure.

In the simplest form of the two-stage reaction procedure, a bifunction
-al reagent is used with one of the proteins under optimum conditions,
excess bifunctional reagent removed by dialysis or filtration through
Sephadex G-25 (Pharmacia Ltd, Uxbridge, England) and the second protein
added. The two-stage reaction may be further improved by selective blocking of particular amino acids.

COUPLING REAGENTS AND PROCEDURES

Before discussing in detail two commonly used methods, it is appropriate to review briefly some of the many published conjugation procedures.

1) Di-isocyanates

The reactivity of isocyanates with hydroxyl, thiol and amino functional
groups has led to the application of di-isocyanates and, in particular, aryl
di-isocyanates for protein-protein coupling (Kennedy et al., 1976). Fig. 1
shows the reaction of toluene di-isocyanate (TDIC) with the ε-amino group of
lysine. At neutral to alkaline pH, the reaction is predominantly with amino
groups yielding urea derivatives (Wold, 1972). Because of the differential

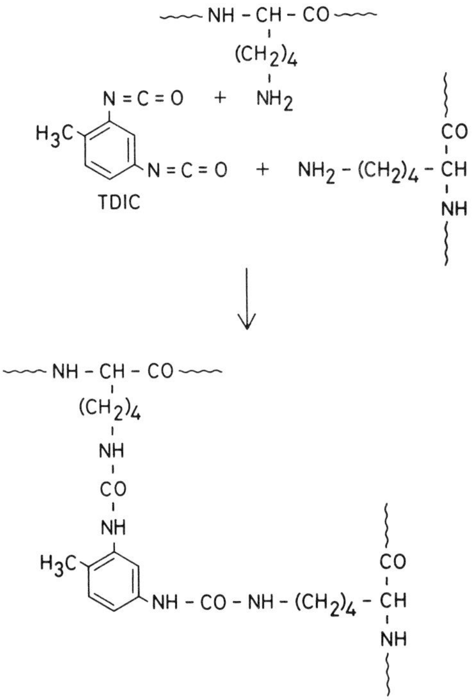

14

~~~ NH – CH – CO ~~~
|
(CH$_2$)$_4$
|
N = C = O   +   NH$_2$

H$_3$C

N = C = O   +   NH$_2$ – (CH$_2$)$_4$ – CH

TDIC

CO
|
CH
|
NH

↓

~~~ NH – CH – CO ~~~
|
(CH$_2$)$_4$
|
NH
|
CO
|
NH

H$_3$C

NH – CO – NH – (CH$_2$)$_4$ – CH

CO
|
CH
|
NH

Fig. 1   Reaction of toluene di-isocyanate (TDIC) with Ɛ-amino groups
of lysine.

reactivity of the isocyanate groups, TDIC has been used in a two-stage
reaction procedure. Thus one of the proteins may be reacted with TDIC close
to neutrality, the excess TDIC removed and the conjugation achieved by
addition of the second protein and adjustment of the pH to 9.5 (Wold, 1972).

2) Halonitrobenzenes

Halonitrobenzenes such as 1,5-difluoro-2,4-dinitrobenzene (DFDNB) have
also been used in two-stage conjugation reactions because of the unequal
reactivity of the two fluorine atoms. At alkaline pH the reaction is mainly
with tyrosine phenolic groups and Ɛ-amino groups of lysine (Kennedy et al.,
1976). Wold (1972) reported 50% yields of IgG-ferritin conjugate with a 40%
loss of IgG activity.

3) Imidoesters

Although the bifunctional imidoesters have not been used extensively for the preparation of conjugates, they represent an interesting group of substances, being relatively mild in terms of their effect on antigenic determinants. Imidoesters react exclusively with amino groups, as shown in Fig. 2.

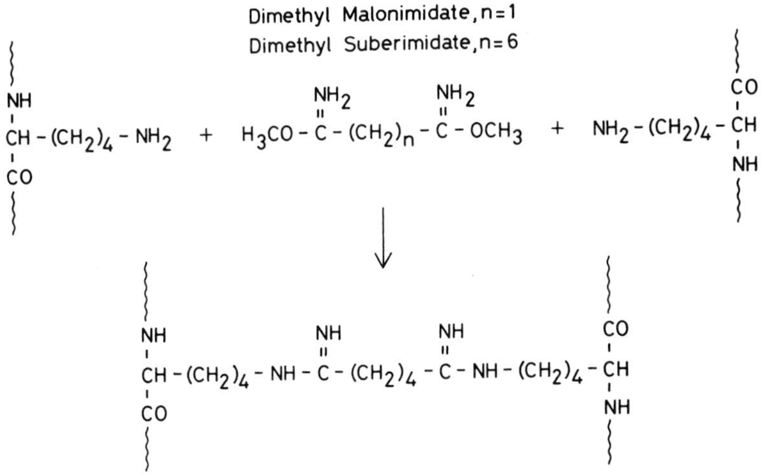

Fig. 2   Reaction of bifunctional imidoesters with ε-amino groups of lysine.

Although the reaction involves the positively charged amino group of lysine, the net charge of the protein remains the same because of the amino functions on the imidoester. Hence this mild and specific modification is accompanied by little change in physical or biological properties of the protein. Thus dimethyl malonimidate reacts with 85% of free lysines of IgG without destroying antigenic determinants (Wold, 1972). Yields of 10 to 20% were obtained when the same reagent was used to cross-link BSA and IgG (Wold, 1972).

4) Glutaraldehyde Conjugation

Glutaraldehyde has been widely used for the preparation of protein conjugates (Avrameas, 1969; Avrameas et al., 1978). The reaction of

glutaraldehyde with proteins is complex and is still the subject of much
debate (Kabakoff, 1980). It is known that the composition of commercial
glutaraldehyde solutions is pH dependent and that 25% solutions contain in
addition to water, 3% glutaraldehyde and 18% derivatives of higher molecular weight which can be broken down to glutaraldehyde (Peters and Richards,
1977). When cross-linking is performed at pH 3.0, the predominant reaction
probably involves the formation of Schiff base linkages with lysine residues. This reaction generates acid unstable products in contrast to the
products of conjugation under neutral to alkaline conditions. The reason
for this difference could be due to the fact that, under alkaline conditions, glutaraldehyde forms variable chainlength α, β unsaturated aldehydes
which also take part in Schiff base linkages but between amino groups and
aldehyde groups in conjugation with double bonds (Fig. 3).

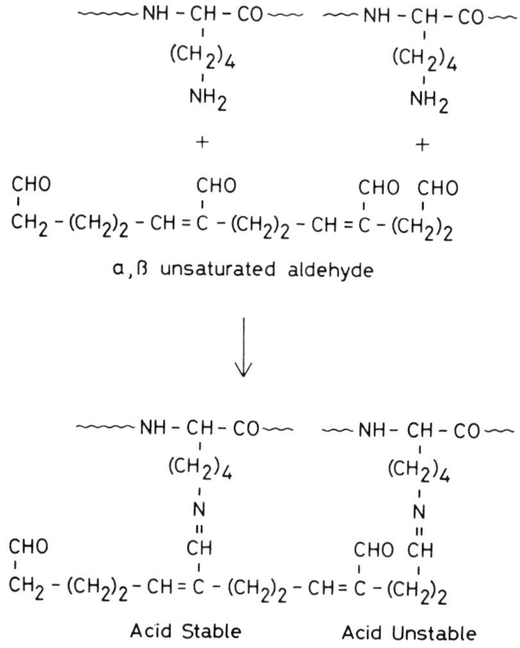

Fig. 3   Reaction of α, β unsaturated aldehyde derivatives of glutaraldehyde with ϵ-amino groups of lysine.

Thus, stable Schiff base linkages are formed with all but the terminal
aldehyde groups of the polymeric derivatives of glutaraldehyde. To what

extent α, β unsaturated aldehydes are involved in conjugation reactions at pH 6.8 is still a matter of conjecture (Kabakoff, 1980). The considerable success of glutaraldehyde is probably attributable to the large number of different types of molecule present simultaneously under normal cross-linking conditions.

Although the one-stage glutaraldehyde procedure may be used to produce adequate enzyme/antibody conjugates, the products are of high molecular weight and heterogeneous in nature. Avrameas et al. (1978) cited values of 5% of HRPO and 100% of lactoperoxidase coupled to antibody. The enzyme activity after coupling was found to be 60 to 70% of the initial activity. The immunological activities of these conjugates were difficult to assess because of the heterogeneous nature of the conjugate population.

Higher activity conjugates may be produced by first reacting antibody with glutaraldehyde, followed by dialysis or chromatography to remove unreacted glutaraldehyde and, finally, addition of enzyme. A conjugate of HRPO and IgG prepared in this manner was shown to be composed of a homogeneous derivative of 90,000 mol. wt. The immunological and enzymatic activities were 50% and 50% to 75% of the initial activities respectively (cited by Avrameas et al., 1978).

Unreacted aldehyde groups may be blocked by treating the conjugate with low mol. wt. amines such as glycine.

Periodate-Schiffs Base Procedure

Numerous attempts have been made to produce high quality HRPO/immunoglobulin conjugates. This is due in part to the relatively low cost of HRPO compared with alkaline phosphatase and the fact that a wide range of substrates is available for HRPO. Some of these substrates, for example O-phenylenediamine, offer the possibility of reading the end point in microtitre plates without recourse to photometry. However, most of the conjugation procedures have been less than successful because of the large number of blocked amino groups in HRPO.

Nakane and Kawaoi (1974) developed a conjugation procedure based on the carbohydrate moieties of HRPO. They cited evidence by Theorell that oxidation of HRPO yielded HRPO-aldehyde without significant loss of activity. The procedure developed by these workers is as follows:

Residual amino and hydroxyl groups are blocked by briefly reacting with fluorodinitrobenzene (FDNB). Periodate oxidation is then used to generate aldehyde groups from vicinal hydroxyl groups throughout the oligosaccharide

side chains and the excess periodate neutralised after 30 minutes reaction
by the addition of ethylene glycol. Following thorough dialysis against
sodium carbonate buffer, pH 9.5, to remove excess reagents and in particular HF which inhibits HRPO activity, conjugation is achieved by reaction
with IgG and sodium borohydride ($NaBH_4$). The essential features of the
reaction are shown in Fig. 4 (Kabakoff, 1980).

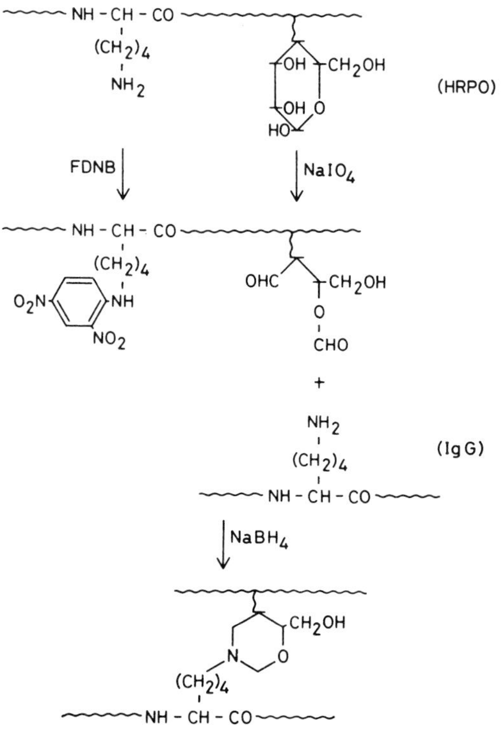

Fig. 4   Conjugation of horseradish peroxidase (HRPO) to an immunoglobulin (Ig) molecule by the procedure of Nakane and Kawaoi (1974).

Relatively few steps in the procedure are particularly critical. For
example, excellent conjugates may be prepared by the modified procedure of
Wilson and Nakane (1978) in which the FDNB step is omitted. Periodate
oxidation must be carefully controlled to avoid progressive inactivation of
HRPO. Following oxidation for 30 minutes, excess periodate should be
quenched with ethylene glycol or glycerol. Although conjugation is not
dependent on the use of sodium borohydride, this reagent serves to stabilise

the Schiff base. There is reasonable latitude with borohydride concentrations, but we err on the side of safety by using 1 mg per mg of HRPO. Finally, there is the aspect of relative amounts of HRPO and the protein to be conjugated. Nakane and Kawaoi (1974) recommended levels of the order of 2 moles of HRPO per mole IgG, i.e. on a weight for weight basis 0.5 mg HRPO to 1.0 mg IgG. We have prepared IgG-HRPO conjugates ranging from equimolar concentrations to 4 moles HRPO to 1 mole IgG. Equimolar HRPO conjugates appear to be at least as good as those which contain higher ratios of HRPO and are, of course, exceptionally economical to produce. The Nakane and Kawaoi procedure is also excellent for the production of HRPO-Protein A conjugates using equimolar concentrations of the two proteins. The resultant conjugates may be of a sufficiently high titre and quality to be used even for the detection and measurement of bovine IgG. This is in spite of the fact that of various species of IgG tested with protein A, bovine IgG reacts relatively poorly (Crowther and Abu Elzein, 1980).

CONCLUSIONS

The aim of all procedures for the preparation of conjugates for ELISA is the maximum retention of antigenic and enzymatic activities. While the glutaraldehyde procedure, among others, has often been criticised because of the tendency to form inactive homopolymers, there is little doubt that it performs perfectly adequately in the hands of many investigators. Indeed, commercial conjugates prepared by a glutaraldehyde procedure have proved satisfactory in our laboratory. We retain the Nakane and Kawaoi method for the preparation of unusual or expensive conjugates involving reagents such as Protein A.

REFERENCES

Avrameas, S. 1969. Coupling of enzymes to proteins with glutaraldehyde. Use of the conjugates for the detection of antigens and antibodies. Immunochemistry, 6, 43.
Avrameas, S., Ternynck, T. and Guesdon, J.L. 1978. Coupling of enzymes to antibodies and antigens. Scand. J. Immunol., 8, Suppl.7, 7.
Crowther, J.R. and Abu Elzein, E.M.E. 1980. Detection of antibodies against foot-and-mouth disease virus using purified Staphylococcus A protein conjugated with alkaline phosphatase. J. Immunol. Methods, 34, 261.
Guesdon, J.L., Ternynck, T. and Avrameas, S. 1979. The use of avidin-biotin interaction in immunoenzymatic techniques. J. Histochem. Cytochem., 27, 1131.
Kabakoff, D.S. 1980. Chemical aspects of enzyme-immunoassay: in: Enzyme Immunoassay. E.T. Maggio (Ed). CRC Press Inc., Florida.

Kennedy, J.H., Kricka, L.J. and Wilding, P. 1976. Protein-protein coupling reactions and the applications of protein conjugates. Clin. Chim. Acta 70, 1.

Modesto, R.R. and Pesce, A.J. 1971. The reaction of 4,4'-difluoro-3,3'-dinitro-diphenyl sulphone with γ-globulin and horseradish peroxidase. Biochim. Biophys. Acta 229, 384.

Nakane, P.K., Sri Ram, J. and Pierce, G.B. 1966. Enzyme labeled antibodies for light and electron microscopic localisation of antigens. J. Histo-chem. Cytochem., 14, 789.

Nakane, P.K. and Kawaoi, A. 1974. Peroxidase-labelled antibody. A new method of conjugation. J. Histochem. Cytochem., 22, 1084.

Otto, H., Takamiya, H. and Vogt, A. 1973. A two-stage method for cross-linking antibody globulin to ferritin by glutaraldehyde. Comparison between the one-stage and the two-stage method. J. Immunol. Methods, 3, 137.

Peters, K. and Richards, F.M. 1977. Chemical cross-linking reagents and problems in studies of membrane structure. Ann. Rev. Biochem., 46, 523.

Wilson, M.B. and Nakane, P.K. 1978. in: Immunofluorescence and related staining techniques. W. Knapp, K. Holubar and G. Wick (Eds). Elsevier Press, Amsterdam.

Wold, F. 1972. Bifunctional reagents: in: Methods in Enzymology XXV; enzyme structure; Part B. C.H.W. Hirs and Serge N. Timasheff (Eds). Academic Press, New York and London.

A COMPUTERISED MICRO-ELISA SYSTEM FOR THE ANALYSIS OF IN VIVO AND IN VITRO ANTIBODY PRODUCTION

A.M. Smithyman, G.L. Kampfner, J.H. Platt and G.T. Layton

Imperial Chemical Industries PLC, Pharmaceuticals Division, Mereside, Alderley Park, Macclesfield, Cheshire.

ABSTRACT

A computerised micro-ELISA system is described in which calculations are performed by a Commodore Pet desk computer interfaced with a Titertek Multiskan micro-ELISA plate reader. Up to 1200 analyses per day can be performed by one person. Its application to the measurement of both in vivo and in vitro antibody production is illustrated here with reference to (a) the IgG antibody response in mice to Sendai virus vaccine and (b) the synthesis of specific antibody to a hapten (DNP) by lymphocytes cultured in vitro.

KEY WORDS: ELISA, Computer, Parainfluenza, Sendai.

INTRODUCTION

The use of ELISA for the measurement of antibody in a variety of biological fluids is now well documented (1-6). One of the main advantages of the technique is that the equipment necessary to carry out basic assays can be both simple and cheap, with end points that may be read semi-quantitatively by eye. In order to increase the sensitivity and accuracy of the assay, however, a spectrophotometer must be used to measure the optical density of the coloured enzyme reaction products. Initially single channel spectrophotometers of the type common to most laboratories were used but more recently the introduction of single or multiple channel photometers for through-the-plate reading of microtitre plates has greatly facilitated the assay procedure (7,8). The calculation and translation of results from the raw optical density data can still be very time consuming though, and in order to overcome this problem and in response to a greatly increased sample load we have attempted to devise a computer linked micro-ELISA system in which the reading, calculation and translation steps are combined.

The system has been developed for the analysis of total and antigen specific immunoglobulins to a wide variety of viral, bacterial and pure protein antigens but will be illustrated here with reference to the detection of specific IgG class antibodies to Sendai virus in the serum of vaccinated mice and the measurement of IgA anti-DNP antibody in lymphocyte cell culture supernatants

MATERIALS AND METHODS

Antigens

1) Concentrated parainfluenza type 1 Sendai (D/52 strain) antigen was prepared by ultracentrifugation of infected egg allantoic fluid (200ml) at 27,000g for 1 hour. The virus concentrates were washed twice with saline (2 x 200ml), reconstituted in 5ml of phosphate buffered saline (P.B.S.) and then dispersed by ultrasonicating for 30 seconds. The preparation had a haemagglutination titer of 1/20,000 (per 0.025ml). Control antigen was prepared in the same way but using non-infected allantoic fluid.

2) Sheep red blood cells (SRBC) were washed three times in phosphate-buffered saline (P.B.S.) and conjugated to trinitrobenzene sulphonic acid (TNP-SRBC) by the method of Rittenberg and Pratt (9).

3) DNP-HSA was prepared by the method of Hudson and Hay (10) at a concentration of 1.46mg/ml with a molar ratio of 6:1 DNP:HSA.

Immunisation Procedures

1) Sendai Virus

Swiss White mice (Alderley Park strain) were immunised intra-muscularly with 0.1ml of a Sendai virus vaccine (M.A. Bioproducts, Walkersville, Maryland).

2) TNP-SRBC

CBA mice were immunised intra-peritoneally (IP) with 5' x 10^8 TNP-SRBC in 0.5ml PBS.

Cell Cultures

Cells obtained from both spleen and Peyer's Patches from 5 day TNP-SRBC primed CBA mice were cultured at a concentration of 2 x 10^6 cells/ml in a standard Mishell-Dutton system using RPMI-1640 medium (Gibco Labs) buffered with 25mM Hepes. The cells were incubated at 37°C in a 5% CO_2 gas chamber for 7 days. The method was slightly modified in that a mitogen, E.coli lipopolysaccharide (LPS) was added to the medium (at a concentration of 25μg/ml) to stimulate antibody production in vitro.

Samples

Sera and secretions from Swiss white mice (Alderley Park strain) or supernatants from lymphocyte cell cultures were stored in 'special' poly-styrene tubes in a transfer tube strip holder (Flow Labs, Irvine, Scotland).

Eighty-eight samples are stored on the equivalent of one microtitre plate in this way. Stock dilutions (if required) were made by transferring a small volume of sample into 250µl of diluent (PBS/0.05% Tween 20) in a microtitration plate. A 12 channel variable volume micropipette (5-50µl, Flow Labs) was used to transfer each row of samples. Stock dilutions and sample plates were sealed with adhesive tape or cap strips (Flow Labs) and stored at -20°C.

Standards

(a) Sendai-virus specific immunoglobulins

Mouse sera having an antibody titre of greater than 1/50,000, previously determined by ELISA were pooled, dispensed in 0.5ml aliquots, lyophilised and stored at -20°C.

(b) IgA anti-DNP

IgA anti-DNP antibody was purified by affinity chromatography from the supernatant of the mouse myeloma cell line, MOPC 315, grown in continuous culture (I. Willshire, ICI Research Labs).

Antisera and Conjugates

Rabbit antiserum to mouse IgG and Goat anti-rabbit (GAR) IgG peroxidase-labelled antiserum were obtained commercially (Nordic Imm., Maidenhead, Berks., Meloy Labs.). Rabbit antiserum to mouse IgA was a gift from Dr. H. Gregory.

Substrate

0-phenylene diamine (OPD) (0.4mg/ml)/urea peroxide (0.23mg/ml) was freshly prepared in PBS/Tween.

Enzyme-linked Immunosorbent Assay (ELISA)

Microelisa plates (Greiner M 129 B, Dynatech Labs Ltd., Billingshurst, Sussex) were coated with either Sendai virus antigen or DNP-HSA diluted 1/2000 in coating buffer (0.05M carbonate - bicarbonate buffer pH 9.6). 250µl of the appropriate antigen was placed into each well and left overnight at +4°C. Plates were washed by total immersion in a bath of tap water for 2 minutes (10). A continuous stream of fresh water was supplied to the bath and excess water was allowed to overflow to waste. The plates were manually agitated for 5 seconds to remove all air bubbles. We have compared this method with standard washing procedures (5) and have found no evidence of non-specific adsorption. Washed plates may be stored at +4°C after thorough drying.

Transfer of diluted samples onto pre-coated plates was facilitated by the use of the 12-channel micro-pipette. All dilutions were made in PBS/ Tween. Duplicate samples were analysed at a single dilution.

A standard curve was prepared by making serial dilutions of the appropriate standard and transferring 200µl volumes into the wells on row 12 of each plate. Optimum results for serum antibody were obtained with a standard curve constructed using five-fold dilution steps whereas a two-fold dilution step was found to be more accurate for the much narrower range of antibody found in cell culture supernatants. The plates were then left for two hours at room temperature in a humid box.

After another washing step, 200µl of the appropriate diluted rabbit antiserum was added and incubated for one hour at room temperature in a humidified chamber. After a further washing step GAR IgG enzyme con-jugated antiserum (200µl at 1/2000 dilution) was added and again incubated for one hour at room temperature in a humidified chamber.

After a final washing step, 200µl of freshly prepared 0-phenylene diamine substrate was added to each well. The resulting colour reaction was allowed to develop in the dark for 45 minutes. The enzymatic activity was then inhibited by the addition of 50µl of 25% sulphuric acid and the plates were agitated for 30 seconds on a microtitre shaker.

Optimum dilutions of all antigens and antisera used were determined using checkerboard type assays on positive and negative samples (5,6).

Reading and Calculations

Optical density determinations at 492nm and calculation of results were carried out automatically using a Titertek Multiskan reader (Flow Labs) interfaced with a Commodore Pet desk computer and printer (Cytek UK Ltd., Old Trafford, Manchester), using a Titertek Multiskan interface (Flow Labs) and an RS 232C serial interface type B (Small Systems Engineer-ing Ltd.) (Figs. 1 and 2). The plate reader is first blanked using sub-strate/acid solution (250µl). Information concerning experimental details is typed into the computer in response to pre-programmed questions dis-played on the visual display unit (VDU). The plate is then read auto-matically and optical densities and information are printed out.

The computer programme which was designed and written by the authors fits data from the standard curve to a second degree polynomial equation

(12). The standard curve computer plot is displayed on the VDU and printed on the results sheet (see Fig. 5). Optical density versus concentration of standard, or reciprocal of dilution of standard is used in the
equation:

$$y = a + b \, (\log x) + c \, (\log x)^2$$

where y = optical density and x = concentration of standard or reciprocal
of dilution of standard.

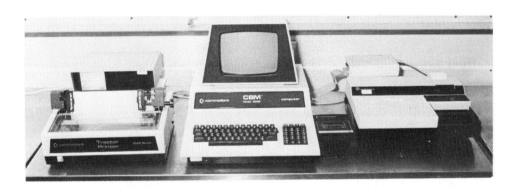

Fig. 1   Computer-linked micro-ELISA system. The Multiskan ELISA
         reader (right) is seen connected to a Pet micro-computer
         (centre) and printer (left).

Sample immunoglobulin concentrations are determined directly from the
equation. Antibody titres are determined by comparing the optical density
of the sample to the standard curve and extrapolating to predict an end
point titre (that is the dilution of the sample giving an optical density
of 0.1).

RESULTS

Reproducibility of Computer Predicted Values

To assess the reproducibility and precision of the method different
dilutions of the standard serum pool were analysed several times on one
microtitration plate for Sendai virus IgG antibody (Table 1). One of these
sets of analyses was taken as a standard (Column 6, Table 1) and used to
calculate the others. End point titres (Table 2) were predicted by the
computer using this standard curve (Fig. 3). The results compare favourably with the titre of 1/289,500 determined from the serial dilution of the
standard. The coefficient of variation for the predicted titres was 3.7%
over the range of optical densities from 0.078 to 1.84.

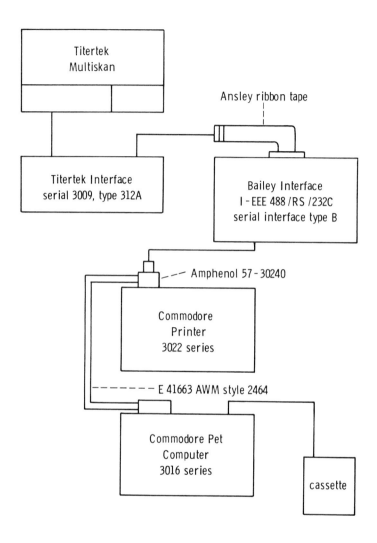

Figure 2. INTERFACING of TITERTEK MULTISKAN with COMMODORE PET COMPUTER and PRINTER.

TABLE 1.

OPTICAL DENSITIES OBTAINED from ELISA ANALYSIS of REPLICATE SERUM STANDARDS for SENDAI VIRUS IgG ANTIBODY.

Serum Dilution	Optical Density				Standards
1/625	1.813	1.819	1.840	1.745	1.788
1/3,125	1.183	1.179	1.200	1.166	1.173
1/15,625	0.592	0.603	0.556	0.547	0.578
1/78,125	0.232	0.240	0.201	0.212	0.263
1/390,625	0.078	0.080	0.087	0.081	0.095
1/1,953,125	0.042	0.030	0.029	0.031	0.044
1/9,765,625	0.013	0.004	0.007	0.012	0.008

TABLE 2.

COMPUTER PREDICTED END POINT TITRES for RESULTS SHOWN in TABLE 1.

Serum Dilution	Predicted End Point Titres			
1/625	295,937	299,750	313,375	255,750
1/3,125	334,687	331,250	350,000	320,000
1/15,625	262,500	275,000	228,198	220,380
1/78,125	234,450	242,265	187,560	203,190
1/390,625	273,525	273,525	312,600	273,525

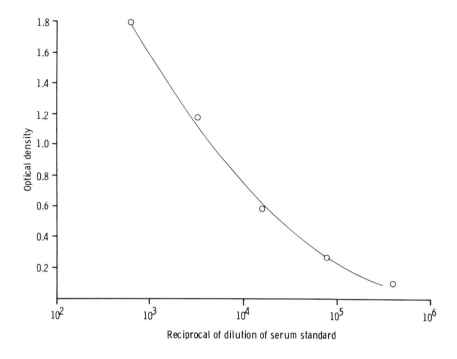

Figure 3. <u>COMPUTER PLOT of ELISA RESULTS for SENDAI VIRUS IgG ANTIBODIES in STANDARD SERUM POOL.</u>
<u>from $y = a + b (\log x) + c (\log x)^2$</u>

The next two sections give examples of the type of rapid screening situation for which the computerised micro-ELISA was designed. The first concerns the analysis of serum antibody levels in Sendai virus vaccinated mice and the second the detection of <u>in vitro</u> antibody synthesis by lymphocytes in culture.

1) <u>Detection of serum antibody levels in mice to Sendai virus</u>

Several hundred serum samples from mice immunised with a commercial Sendai virus vaccine were analysed for IgG antibody levels to the virus. The mice were immunised intra-muscularly with 0.1ml of the vaccine and challenged several weeks later with live virus. The response of the vaccinated mice was compared to that of controls exposed only to live virus challenge. The detailed analysis of this experiment is outwith the scope of this paper but Figure 4 shows the primary and secondary antibody responses as measured by the ELISA system. (13) The titres obtained were

29

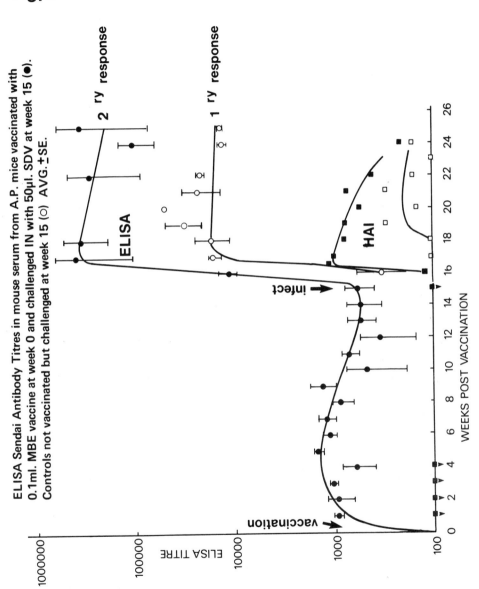

ELISA Sendai Antibody Titres in mouse serum from A.P. mice vaccinated with
0.1ml. MBE vaccine at week 0 and challenged IN with 50µl. SDV at week 15 (●).
Controls not vaccinated but challenged at week 15 (○) AVG.±SE.

Fig.5

considerably higher than those found by a conventional haemagluttination inhibition (HAI) assay. The main advantage however was the considerable saving in time when compared to the manual calculation of results for such a large number of samples.

2) Detection of antibody synthesis in vitro (14)

The computerised micro-ELISA system was also used to analyse the levels of antibody produced in vitro by a high throughput lymphocyte micro culture system in which large numbers of culture supernatants required to be processed at one time. In a closed system such as this the range of antibody likely to be encountered is much narrower than in serum and so the standard curve was constructed on a doubling dilution basis (Fig. 5).

Using this standard curve which was based on purified IgA anti-DNP antibody from the mouse myeloma cell line MOPC 315C it was possible to assess antibody production in vitro by lymphocytes from TNP-SRBC primed mice. The results of one such culture, in which LPS was added to the medium to stimulate antibody production, are shown in Table 3. Cells from both the spleen and Peyer's patches were cultured for periods of 1-10 days and the IgA anti-DNP antibody levels in the supernatants read off the standard curve. The effect of the LPS stimulation is shown quite clearly. Again the time-saving was considerable as was the saving on the very limited sample quantities. One obvious application of this technique which we have used successfully is the rapid screening of hybridoma supernatants for monoclonal antibody production.

DISCUSSION

Reading, calculation and tabulation of results from one plate takes less than two minutes to complete. Using a single dilution of sample stored and analysed as described it is possible for one person to process 14 plates (1200 samples) in one day. The system was designed for use in a high throughput screen but greater precision would be obtained by using replicate points on the standard curve. It should be appreciated that by extrapolating from a pooled serum standard we are assuming that the curves are the same for all sera and secretions. This method does have the advantage that only one dilution of the sample is required yet results are expressed in a linear form covering a large range of values as opposed to optical density measurement alone (15).

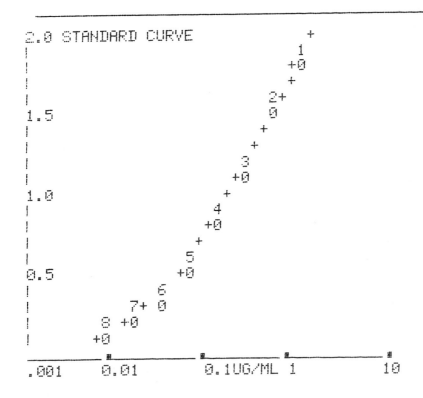

Fig. 5   IgA anti-DNP standard curve as printed by the Pet computer.
The top concentration of IgA in the first well was 1.0µg/ml.

Day	Spleen		Pp	
	IgA anti-DNP (µg/ml)		IgA anti-DNP (µg/ml)	
	+ LPS	- LPS	+ LPS	- LPS
0	< 0.020	< 0.020	< 0.020	< 0.020
2	< 0.020	< 0.020	< 0.020	< 0.020
4	0.114	< 0.020	0.041	0.022
7	0.459	0.021	0.431	0.028
10	0.471	0.023	0.532	0.032

The results represent the means of quadruplicate cultures, and the standard deviation for each result was < 5% from the mean. LPS concentration = 25µg/ml. Cells were cultured at 2 x 10^6/ml.

TABLE 3   The effect of culture duration on IgA anti-DNP production in LPS stimulated, and unstimulated cultures.

Sensitivity of the assay for mouse IgA antibody is of the order of 10ng/ml. The use of a common second antibody which is enzyme conjugated (Goat anti-rabbit peroxidase) means that not only is the sensitivity of the assay increased but also that the system may be easily adapted for a range of antigens. We have used the computerised micro-ELISA system to analyse immune responses to antigens such as human and rat serum albumin, cholera toxin and toxoid, and E.coli outer membrane proteins. Furthermore, the principles employed here may be used for other microtitre based assays which make use of a colorimetric change, for example, the minimal inhibitory concentrations (MIC) test for antibiotics or the colorimetric interferon assay.

The ELISA technique described is now used routinely in our laboratory and we consider that it may represent a logical progression towards a new generation of computerised ELISA systems.

ACKNOWLEDGEMENTS

The authors wish to thank Mr. A. McNab for his help with the statistical evaluation and Mr. A. Shore for his assistance with the reader-computer linkage and programming of the computer. Thanks also to Miss N. Wallace, Miss S. Hinchliffe and Mrs. S. Stringer for their excellent technical assistance and Mr. I. Willshire for the preparation of the mouse IgA anti-DNP antibody. They are indebted to Dr. G.E. Davies for his original suggestions concerning the use of the Pet microcomputer and to M. Bloor for typing the manuscript.

REFERENCES

1. Voller, A., Bidwell, D.E. and Bartlett, A. 1976. Enzyme immunoassays in diagnostic medicine. Bull W.H.O., 54, 55-65.
2. Bidwell, D.E. et al. 1976. The enzyme linked immunosorbent assay (ELISA). Bull W.H.O., 54, 129-139.
3. Engvall, E. and Pexe, A.J. (eds.). 1978. Quantitative enzyme immuno-assay. Scand. J. Immun., Suppl. 7, Blackwell Scientific Publications Ltd.
4. Parker, J.D., O'Bierne, A.J. and Collins, M.J. 1979. Sensitivity of enzyme linked immunosorbent assay; Complement fixation and haemagglutination inhibition serological tests for detection of Sendai virus antibody in laboratory mice. J. Clin. Microbiol., 9, 444-447.
5. Voller, A., Bidwell, D. and Bartlett, A. 1980. Enzyme-linked immuno-sorbent assay. In: Manual of Clinical Immunology, 2nd Edition. (Rose, N., Friedman, H. eds.). Published by American Society for Micro-biology, Washington. Chapter 45, p.359-371.
6. Voller, A., Bidwell, D.E. and Bartlett, A. The enzyme-linked immuno-sorbent assay (ELISA). A guide with abstracts of microplate applica-tions. p. 1-125. Flowline Press, Guernsey.
7. Ruitenberg, E.J., Sekhuis, V.M. and Brosi, B.J.M. 1980. Some characteristics of a new multiple channel photometer for through-the-plate reading of microplates to be used in enzyme-linked immuno-sorbent assay. J. Clin. Microbiol., 11, 132-134.
8. Carlier, Y., Bart, D. and Capron, A. 1979. Automation of Enzyme-linked immunosorbent assay (ELISA). J. Immun. Methods, 31, 237-246.
9. Rittenberg, M.B. and Pratt, K.L. 1969. Antitrinitrophenyl (TNP) Plaque assay. Primary response of Balb/c mice to soluble and particulate immunogen. Proc. Soc. Exp. Biol. Med., 132, 575.
10. Hudson, L. and Hay, F.C. 1980. Practical Immunology, 2nd Edition, Blackwell Scientific Publications. pp. 5-7.
11. Ruitenberg, E.J., Steerenberg, P.A., Brosi, B.J.M. and Buys, J. 1974. Serodiagnosis of Trichinella spiralis infections in pigs by enzyme-linked immunosorbent assays. Bull W.H.O., 51, 108.
12. Carr, S., Outch, K. and Russell, J. 1978. A computer programme for the processing and analysis of both radioimmunoassay (RIA) and enzyme immunoassay (EIA). Data. Pathology, 10, 391.
13. Kampfner, G.L., Atkinson, A., Platt, J.H., Harrison, J.H. and Tucker, M.J. 1980. The efficacy of a commercially available Sendai virus vaccine in common inbred/outbred strains of mice. Abstr. IV Int. Immunology Congress, 17.8.12.

14. Layton, G.T. and Smithyman, A.M. 1982. Antibody Production _in vitro_ by Peyer's Patch lymphocytes. In press.
15. de Savigny, D. and Voller, A. 1980. The communications of ELISA data from laboratory to clinician. J. Immunoassay, <u>1</u>,(1), 105.

PART II: APPLICATION OF ELISA TO THE STUDY OF HELMINTHS

REVIEW OF APPLICATION OF ELISA IN HELMINTHOLOGY

I.J. Sinclair

Central Veterinary Laboratory
Weybridge, England

ABSTRACT

The use that the enzyme-linked immunosorbent assay (ELISA) has been put to in the diagnosis of helminths of veterinary importance is reviewed. The technique has the advantages that it is easy to perform, is normally very sensitive and is capable of being adapted to automated procedures. Although the test has been used on a grand scale only for the diagnosis of *Trichinella spiralis* in pigs (Ruitenberg, 1977), preliminary observations carried out on a considerable number of other animal parasites, including *Fasciola hepatica*, *Taenia saginata* and *Toxocara canis*, suggest that ELISA has a potentiality which has yet to be fully realised. The results which have been reported so far, are too variable to suggest that ELISA will have universal applicability without considerable adaptation to meet the requirements of different host-parasite systems. Among the problems which have been encountered and which require further attention, the main one would appear to be the production of suitable, specific antigens which will increase the sensitivity of the technique and remove or reduce the influence of cross-reacting antibodies and non-specific reactions.

INTRODUCTION

Since the enzyme-linked immunosorbent assay (ELISA) was introduced by Engvall and Perlman (1971), its potential for serodiagnosis has been investigated for a wide spectrum of infections. Its application for human diseases has been reviewed by Voller and his co-workers (1976) and a review has also been made of its veterinary applications (Ruitenberg and Van Knapen, 1977). It could be argued that helminth infections do not receive as much attention as their importance deserves and that, consequently, new techniques make their impact on this discipline long after they were first evolved. However, this is not the case for ELISA. Helminth infections have figured prominently in the development of practical methods for improving the technique. This is at least partly due to its use in the diagnosis of *Trichinella spiralis* infections in pigs and the public health aspects of this disease.

TRICHINELLA SPIRALIS

T.spiralis is an unusual nematode as it spends both its adult and larval life in the same host and that quite a wide variety of mammals, including man are susceptible to an initial infection. All immunologically competent hosts develop resistance to reinfection and this is another unusual feature of this host-parasite system. Many investigations into the immunology of the infection have been conducted and so it is not surprising that this is the most studied system with regard to the application of ELISA for serodiagnosis. It was also the first helminth infection to be studied with ELISA (Ljungström et al., 1974). An alkaline phosphatase conjugate was used and the test was found to correlate well with the passive haemagglutination test and the fluorescent antibody test (FAT). In addition it was shown to be more sensitive and objective than the other serological tests. ELISA was later refined by the introduction of a conjugate incorporating horseradish peroxidase which replaced the alkaline phosphatase and produced a darker colour change in the substrate (Ruitenberg et al., 1975a). This modification detected antibody during the first days of infection and produced no false positive reactions with the sera from pigs infected with *Ascaris suum* or with over 1000 sera collected from commercially reared pigs sent for slaughter. The latter had their uninfected status confirmed by direct examination for cysts by the digestion method. The authors estimated that 4000 sera could be examined daily by the ELISA technique and considered that the test could perhaps be employed at abattoirs for the diagnosis of *T.spiralis* infections.

The same laboratory reported another major development (Ruitenberg et al., 1975b). They adapted the test to a micro-plate system in which the volumes of the reactants were reduced to 0.1ml per well. This made the test much less expensive and also enabled end-point titrations to be carried out more easily. They found that this micro-ELISA was much more sensitive than FAT (Ruitenberg et al., 1976). In an experiment with 34 pigs infected with *T.spiralis* in doses ranging from 50 to 25,000, ELISA detected 27 of the infected animals while the FAT diagnosed only 11. However, this result was obtained from a comparison of the extinction values of serum taken before infection and 28 days after infection. When the extinction values of the post-infection sera were compared with the highest values from a panel of 74 sera from uninfected pigs, the number which ELISA could diagnose with certainty dropped from 27 to 19. They also reported that one animal from a group of ten uninfected pigs had given a false positive reaction.

In a further experiment carried out in conjunction with eight EEC laboratories (van Knapen et al., 1980), the previous results were essentially confirmed by all the participants. In addition, it was observed that, both ELISA and FAT were more sensitive than the direct methods of diagnosis when the pigs were infected with 1500 or less larvae. They concluded that ELISA was probably not a realistic alternative to the direct methods for diagnosis in abattoirs but might be useful for surveys.

Considerable effort has been expended on investigating the reasons why false reactions, particularly false positive reactions, occur. Clinard and his co-workers (1978) reported that 15% of 265 pigs sent for slaughter, gave false positive reactions with ELISA and suggested that the specificity of the test might be increased by fractionation and purification of the antigen used in the test. They also, (Clinard, 1978) fractionated positive and false positive pig sera with DEAE-Cellulose and found that the activity of the positive sera appeared in the first three fractions, which corresponded to the IgG class, while the activity of the false positive sera was to be found in the last three fractions which contained the IgM class. Attempts to identify this false positive serum factor with antibody to gram-negative bacteria were unsuccessful. Further investigations (Clinard, 1979) revealed that pig sera giving false positive reactions contained two immunoglobulin classes, an IgG fraction which could be absorbed with *T.spiralis* larvae and an IgM component which was unaffected by absorption. Neither fraction could be shown to precipitate with *T.spiralis* antigen in the Ouchterlony test or counter-immunoelectrophoresis (CEP). It was also observed that the IgM factor increased with the age of the animal. This was in agreement with the results of a study on the influence of age and husbandry on the extinction values obtained by ELISA for the sera from uninfected pigs (Taylor et al., 1978). It was found that these values increased significantly with age and that specific pathogen free pigs had lower extinction values than commercially reared pigs of a comparable age.

This group continued work on the problem by fractionating the larval antigen on a sephadex (G200) molecular filtration column (Taylor et al., 1980). They obtained a fraction which reduced the extinction values of the false positive sera to a level which approached that of the negative sera. Improvements in the functioning of the test were also obtained by recrystalizing the substrate (5 amino salicylic acid) and by using a more efficient conjugate.

Although there is still a considerable amount of work to be done to increase the efficiency of the test, the outlook appears to hold out a promise of a test which can be used with confidence in the diagnosis of trichinosis in pigs. One interesting line of research which has, as yet, received little attention is the possibility of detecting antigen in the circulation. Garcia and his co-workers (1979) have demonstrated this in the sera of rats infected 48 hours previously and it would be interesting to know whether the same phenomenon occurs in pigs.

FASCIOLA HEPATICA

Although a variety of opinions have been expressed on the degree of resistance engendered by a fluke infection in various species of host, there are many serological tests for demonstrating the resulting antibody. The Ouchterlony test has been used (Kendall et al., 1978) to demonstrate antibody in calves infected with 1000 metacercariae. The antibody appeared within two weeks of infection and remained in the circulation for at least 40 weeks. Similar results were obtained in small animals (Hillyer and de Weil, 1981). The haemagglutination test and the complement fixation test have also been found to give specific results (Tailliez and Korach, 1970). The FAT has demonstrated antibody in lambs infected with 500 metacercariae four weeks after dosing (Movsesijan et al., 1975). Deelder and Pleom (1975) used a variant of FAT, in which the antigen was attached to agarose beads. They found that this technique was more sensitive than the standard FAT which used fluke sections.

The ELISA technique was compared with the standard FAT as a method of diagnosing *F.hepatica* infections in cattle sent for slaughter (Grelck and Horchner, 1977). It was reported that FAT was able to diagnose all of the 153 infected cattle but that only 142 could be diagnosed with ELISA. However, ELISA produced no false positive reactions in uninfected cattle while FAT gave 10% in this category.

Further work on the diagnosis of *F.hepatica* infections in cattle has been carried out by Burden and Hammet (1978). In this investigation five calves were infected daily with 20 metacercariae for a 21 week period and another five calves were infected with 1500 *Ostertagia ostertagi* larvae per day for the same period. The ELISA detected antibodies in the sera of the fluke infected calves from the fifth week of infection and the antibody titre continued to rise throughout the experiment. The extinction values of the *O.ostertagi* infected calves remained at their pre-infection level, so no cross-reactions were demonstrated between those two common infections , when tested with *F.hepatica* antigen. They also reported that the Ouchterlony test detected antibody in only one of the fluke infected calves.

ELISA has also been compared with the CEP technique (Levine et al., 1980) as a means of diagnosing fascioliasis in small animals. With the micro-ELISA technique it was possible to demonstrate antibodies in both rabbits and mice within two weeks on infection and these rose to high levels two weeks later. The CEP showed that precipitating antibodies were also present in mice two weeks after infection (p.i.) but appeared later in rabbits (4-6 weeks p.i.). Both tests showed a drop in antibody levels eight weeks p.i. in mice but remained strongly positive for 34 weeks in rabbits. In rabbits treated with the anthelmintic rafoxamide, the egg counts became negative four weeks after treatment and the precipitating antibodies dropped to a very low level, but the ELISA titre remained high. The same laboratory reported that whole worm antigen cross-reacted with sera taken from animals infected with *Schistosoma mansoni*. However, they were able to remove this cross-reaction by gel filtration of the antigen through Sephadex G200 (Hillyer, 1978).

A further study on various parameters of the test showed that for *F.hepatica* infections in rats and rabbits, the test performed better if it were conducted in polyvinyl rather than in the commonly used polystyrene micro-titre plates and that more antigen adhered if the plates were filled and then left overnight at $4^{o}C$ rather than incubated for three hours at $37^{o}C$ (Hillyer and de Weil, 1979). We have confirmed this finding in our own laboratory but have found that it also increased the extinction values obtained from the uninfected control sera and that the difference between the positive and negative sera was not increased in the cattle - *F.hepatica* system which we were investigating.

TAENIA SAGINATA

Cysticercosis in cattle is responsible for a considerable amount of economic loss which can approach 30% when allowance is made for the loss in the carcass weight and the cost of freezing the infected meat (Pawlowski and Schultz, 1972). This, combined with the danger of infection to persons eating insufficiently cooked meat, has led to considerable research effort being expended upon this parasite. The efficiency of ELISA as a diagnostic tool for cysticercosis was first investigated by Ruitenberg (1977). His preliminary results suggested that the test was of value for diagnosis, although the antibody titre of naturally infected cattle was lower than that found in experimentally infected animals. It was also discovered that the antibody titre decreased during the course of the infection and this was presumed to be the effect of the cysticerci settling in the musculature of the host. Other work on experimental infections (Kassai et al., 1979) showed that animals given 100,000 eggs contained antibody in their circulation on day 10 of the infection and that they reached a peak in their titre on or about day 20. A lyophilised proglottid antigen was used. Walther and Sanitz (1979) also employed experimentally infected calves and found that, in this case, the antibody appeared later (2-5 weeks p.i.) but that the ELISA results were comparable to those obtained with the haemagglutination test. They also reported that an antigen prepared from *T.crassiceps* gave results which were essentially similar to those produced by *T.saginata*.

In an experiment carried out over an extended period, it was found that the antibody titre demonstrated by ELISA increased, in some animals, until week 28 (Albert and Horchner, 1979). The maximum titres ranged from 1/64 to 1/512; thereafter the titres fell one or two doubling dilutions by the end of the experiment. The ELISA demonstrated a non-specific increase in titre in the uninfected control cattle over the period of the experiment and this had reached a value of 1/16 after two years. These findings have been confirmed by Harrison and Sewell (1981). Harrison (1978) has also reported finding *T.saginata* antigen in both experimentally and naturally infected cattle, but the level, as judged by ELISA, remained demonstrable for only 10 to 20 weeks after experimental infection. He used ELISA to search for both antigen and antibody in a group of 19 naturally infected animals. *T.saginata* antigen was found in two animals and antibody in the rest. In addition the test produced one false positive.

The degree of specificity produced by ELISA has received considerable attention in recent years. Ballad and his co-workers (1979) found that the test required an antigen purified of heterologous and cross-reacting components by a multi-step filtration of the cyst extract. Others have shown that, when a crude antigen is used, cross-reactions occurred with the sera of calves harbouring infections of *T.hydatigena, F.hepatica* and even gastro-intestinal nematodes. While clear diagnostic evidence was obtained for experimental infections, the test was not reliable for natural infections particularly when compared with the results obtained from cattle with *F.hepatica* infections. They concluded that ELISA with a crude antigen could not be used as a diagnostic tool, but might prove useful as an indicator of the prevalence of *T.saginata* infections within a group or a herd (Craig and Rickard, 1980).

Geerts and his co-workers (1981) have been more successful. They used a *T.crassiceps* metacestode antigen which had been lyophilised and delipidised with ethanol. Although the antigen reacted with sera from *Cysticercus tenuicollis* infections, it did not cross-react with sera from cattle with

F.hepatica or *Echinococcus granulosus*. Their results also showed that the ELISA titre for cattle infected with more than 100 metacestodes, was directly proportional to the metacestode burden. Below this figure, ELISA did not provide an effective diagnosis, and this applied in particular to a group of naturally infected animals which were examined. These animals carried a light infection which had been contracted a considerable time previously, since it was shown that the majority of the metacestodes had degenerated. Only 9 out of 24 of these cattle had detectable antibody titres.

On the basis of these reports, it would seem that further work is necessary before ELISA can be used with confidence in the diagnosis of light infections, particularly in older cattle which have higher extinction values for normal serum than calves.

TAENIA INFECTIONS IN SHEEP

T.hydatigena, T.ovis and to a lesser extent *T.multiceps* can cause considerable economic losses in sheep. ELISA has been used to detect anti-oncospheral antibodies in the sera of lambs given primary or challenge infections of *T.ovis* or *T.hydatigena* (Craig and Rickard, 1981). These antibodies reached a peak 3-4 weeks after a primary infection or 1-3 weeks after challenge. However, they decreased quickly and within 8-12 weeks had returned to the levels of the uninfected animals. Detection of antibodies to strobilar or cystic fluid extracts showed a different pattern and also persisted for much longer than the antibodies to oncospheres, which, although they appeared to be stage specific were not species specific.

ELISA has also been used to test the sera of lambs sent for slaughter (Hackett et al., 1981) the antigen used was cystic fluid of *T.hydatigena*. Nine lambs, from a group of 29 which had their infected status confirmed, were shown to have elevated ELISA responses while the rest gave false negative reactions. The results of the indirect haemagglutination test were even less satisfactory. This gave a few false positive reactions as well as false negatives. It may be that in naturally infected animals the antibodies are of a transient nature and no serological test will diagnose more than the small proportion of infected animals which are tested shortly after they picked up the disease.

SCHISTOSOME INFECTIONS

A study of the work done on schistosome infections is outside the scope of this review, as the main effort of the research has been directed towards the species of medical rather than veterinary importance and no work has yet been carried out on *S.bovis*. However it is worth mentioning some of the developments which have occurred in this field. An investigation into the presence of antibodies to DNA in mice infected with *S.mansoni* showed that these antibodies appeared six weeks p.i., remained high until the end of the experiment 12 weeks later and reached a titre of 1/512 (Hillyer and Rossy, 1980). There were two sharp falls in titre at weeks 9 and 11 and it is postulated that these were due to the appearance of DNA-anti DNA complexes in the serum of the mice. Schistosome DNA has been found in the serum of infected hamsters (Hillyer, 1971), and it is to be hoped that the effectiveness of ELISA in measuring this material will soon be tested.

ELISA has also been used to detect the presence of polysaccharide and protein antigens of *S.mansoni* in the sera of mice harbouring bisexual and unisexual infections. Antisera specific for these worm components were prepared in sheep and conjugated with horseradish peroxidase. This test was able to detect as little as 6 mμg/ml of the protein antigen and half this amount of the polysaccharide antigen (Ferreira et al., 1979).

DIROFILARIA IMMITIS

Weil and his co-workers (1981) have carried out an investigation of the antibodies produced in dogs in response to infection with *D.immitis*, the dog heart worm. They used the micro-ELISA with a saline extract of adult worms to detect antibody in 22 experimentally infected animals. The test discriminated well between infected and uninfected dogs. The infected group had titres ranging from 1/320 to something in excess of 1/5000, while the controls had titres of 1/160 or less. However they found that there was no correlation between these titres and the dose given or the number of adult worms recovered at *post mortem* examination. They concluded that ELISA was probably more sensitive than the complement fixation test and might be of value as a diagnostic test since 8 out of the 22 dogs were amicrofilaremic and would therefore be classed as uninfected if a non-serological test was used. No attempt was made to gauge the specificity of the test and this should be done before it is used for diagnosis since it has been shown that there are extensive cross-reactions between *D.immitis*, *Ascaris* spp. and *Litomosoides carinii* (Bagai et al., 1968).

TOXOCARA CANIS

Ruitenberg and van Knapen (1977) extended the use of ELISA to diagnose infections of *T.canis* in monkeys and concluded that it could be used as an additional serological tool for the detection of this disease. However other workers (Scharzhuber, 1978; Weiland and Scharzhuber, 1978) were unable to obtain a satisfactory diagnosis of visceral larva migrans using ELISA. Mice infected with *T.canis* and dogs infected with *T.canis* or *Toxascaris leonina* or *Ancylostoma caninum* were examined. Both the experimentally infected mice and dogs had demonstrably higher antibody titres than the controls but the naturally infected dogs had titres from 0–1/160 compared with the uninfected control dogs which showed titres of 1/20. Various water–soluble extracts of whole adult females of *T.canis* and *A.suum* were used and these gave similar results. They also found cross–reactions between these antigens and the sera of dogs infected with *Ancylostoma caninum* and *Uncinaria stenocephala,* the dog hookworms. From these results it would seem that there is still a great deal of work to be done on the specificity of the antigen used in this system, not only in the form that the fractionation takes but in the methods which are employed to prepare the antigenic extract. Barriga (1981) has compared homogenisation, ultra–sonication, extrusion, lyophilisation and freezing and thawing as means of preparing antigens from the larvae of *Trichinella spiralis*. He found that these methods produced quite different materials as judged by their reactions to hyperimmune sera in electrophoresis in polyacrylamide gel, immunoelectrophoresis and the Ouchterlony test. The methods also gave different total amounts of material and varied in their protein/carbohydrate ratios.

REFERENCES

Albert, H. and Horchner, F. 1979. Zur Bekampfung und Diagnostik der Rind-
    erfinnen II. Serologische Untersuchungen mit dem ELISA. Berliner and
    Munchener Tierarztliche Wochenschrift 92,189–193.
Bagai, R.C., Subrahmanyan, D. and Singh, V.B. 1968. Immunochemical studies
    with filarial antigens. Indian J. Med. Res., 56, 1064–1073.
Ballad, N.E., Gavrilova, E.M. and Zorikhina, V.I. 1979. Effective use of
    the immuno-enzyme method (ELISA) for the diagnosis of unilocular and
    multilocular hydatidosis related to the degree of purification of the
    antigen. Meditsinskaya Parazitologiya i Parazitarnye Bolezni 48, 70–
    76.
Barriga, O.O. 1981. Influence of routine extraction procedures in the com-
    position of *Trichinella spiralis* extracts. J. Parasitol., 67, 120–123.
Burden, D.J. and Hammet, N.C. 1978. Microplate enzyme linked immunosorbent
    assay for antibody to *Fasciola hepatica* in cattle. Vet. Rec., 103, 158.
Clinard, E.H. 1978. Serum fractions associated with positive and false posi-
    tive reactions in the ELA test for trichinellosis in swine. Proc. 4th

44

Int. Conf. on Trichinellosis (Ed. C.W. Kim and Z.S. Powlowski) (University Press of New England) p509-517.

Clinard, E.H. 1979. Identification and distribution of swine serum immunoglobulins that react with *Trichinella spiralis* antigens and may interfere with the enzyme labelled antibody test for trichinosis. Am. J. Vet. Res., 40, 1558-1563.

Clinard, E.H., Saunders, G.C., Leighly, J.C. 1978. Prospects for use of the ELA test in the control of trichinellosis in swine. Proc. 4th Int. Conf. on Trichinellosis (Ed. C.W. Kim and Z.S. Pawlowski) (University Press of New England) p501-507.

Craig, P.S. and Rickard, M.D. 1980. Evaluation of "crude" antigen prepared from *Taenia saginata* for the serological diagnosis of *T.saginata* cysticercosis in cattle using the enzyme-linked immunosorbent assay (ELISA). Zeitschrift fur Parasitenkunde. 61, 287-297.

Craig, P.S. and Rickard, M.D. 1981. Anti-oncospheral antibodies in the serum of lambs experimentally infected with either *Taenia ovis* or *Taenia hydatigena*. Zeitschrift fur Parasitenkunde. 64, 169-177.

Deelder, A.M. and Ploem, J.S. 1975. An immunofluorescence reaction for *Fasciola hepatica* using the defined antigen substrate spheres (DASS) system. Exptl. Parasitol.,37, 173-178.

Engvall, E. and Perlmann, P. 1971. Enzyme-linked immunosorbent assay (ELISA). Quantitative assay of Immunoglobulin G. Immunochemistry. 8, 871-873.

Ferreira, A.W., Caldini, A.L.M., Hoshino-Shimizu, S. and Camargo, M.E. 1979. Immuno-enzyme assay for the detection of *Schistosoma mansoni* antigens in the serum of mice harbouring bisexual or unisexual light worm infections. J. Helminth., 53, 189-194.

Garcia, V.G., Osorio, M.R., Castro, J.G. 1979. Application de la tecnica micro-ELISA de dobles anticuerpos en la investigacion de antigenos en la triquinosis experimental de la rata. Revista Iberica de Parasitologia., 39, 55-63.

Geerts, S., Kumar, V., Ceulemans, F. and Mortelmans, J. 1981. Serodiagnosis of *Taenia saginata* cystercosis in experimentally and naturally infected cattle by enzyme-linked immunosorbent assay. Res. Vet. Sci., 30, 288-293.

Grelck, H. and Horchner, F. 1977. Vergleichende Untersuchungen zur Serodiagnostik der Rinderfasziolose mit dem indirekten immunofluoreszenz – und immunoperoxidasetest (ELISA). Berliner und Munchener Tierarztliche Wochenschrift, 90, 332-335.

Hackett, F., Willis, J.M., Herbert, I.V., and Edwards, G.T. 1981. Micro-ELISA and indirect haemagglutination tests in the diagnosis of *Taenia hydatigena* metacestode infections in lambs. Vet. Parasit., 8, 137-142.

Harrison, L.J.S. 1978. Detection of *Taenia saginata* infection in cattle by the enzyme-linked immunosorbent assay (ELISA). Trans. Roy. Soc. Trop. Med. Hyg., 72, 642.

Harrison, L.J.S. and Sewell, M.M.H. 1981. A comparison of the enzyme-linked immunosorbent assay and the indirect haemagglutination technique applied to sera from cattle experimentally infected with *Taenia saginata*. Vet. Immunol. Immunopath., 2, 67-73.

Hillyer, G.V. 1971. Deoxyribonucleic acid (DNA) and antibodies to DNA in the serum of hamsters and man infected with schistosomes. Proc. Soc. Exp. Biol. Med., 136, 880-883.

Hillyer, G.V. 1978. Immunodiagnosis of fascioliasis in experimental animals and man. Proc. IV Int. Cong. Parasit, Warsaw Sect C p89.

Hillyer, G.V. and de Weil, N.S. 1979. Use of immunologic techniques to detect chemotherapeutic success in infections with *Fasciola hepatica* II. The enzyme-linked immunosorbent assay in infected rats and rabbits. J.

Parasit., 65, 680-684.

Hillyer, G.V. and Rossy, M. 1980. The enzyme-linked immunosorbent assay (ELISA) for the detection of antibodies to DNA. Studies with New Zealand mice and murine *Schistosomiasis mansoni*. Am. J. Trop. Med. Hyg., 29, 411-415.

Hillyer, G.V. and de Weil, N.S. 1981. Serodiagnosis of experimental fascioliasis by immunoprecipitation tests. Int. J. Parasit., 11, 71-78.

Kassai, T., Balla, E., Redl, P. and Nagy, M.C. 1979. The detection of bovine cysticercosis by the enzyme-linked immunosorbent assay. xxi Wld. Vet. Cong., Moscow (Moscow, USSR), 2, Sect III, 48-49.

Kendall, S.B., Sinclair, I.J., Everett, G. and Parfitt, J.W. 1978. Resistance to *Fasciola hepatica* in cattle. I. Parasitological and serological observations. J. Comp. Path., 88, 115-122.

van Knapen, F., Franchimont, J.H., Ruitenberg, E.J., Baldelli, B., Bradley, J., Gibson, T.E., Cottal, C., Henriksen, S.A., Kohler, G., Skovgaard, N., Soule, C. and Taylor, S.M. 1980. Comparison of the enzyme-linked immunosorbent assay (ELISA) with three other methods for the detection of *Trichinella spiralis* infections in pigs. Vet. Parasit., 7, 109-121.

Levine, D.M., Hillyer, G.V. and Flores, S.I. 1980. Comparison of counterelectrophoresis, the enzyme-linked immunosorbent assay, and Kato fecal examination for the diagnosis of fascioliasis in infected mice and rabbits. Am. J. Trop. Med. Hyg., 29, 602-608.

Ljungstrom, I., Engvall, E. and Ruitenberg, E.J. 1974. ELISA, enzyme-linked immunosorbent assay - a new technique for sero-diagnosis of trichinosis. Parasitology, 69, Proc. Br. Soc. xxiv.

Movsesijan, M., Jovanovic, B., Aalund, O. and Nansen, O. 1975. Immune response of sheep to *Fasciola hepatica* infection. Res. vet. Sci., 18 171-174.

Pawlowski, Z. and Schultz, M.G. 1972. Taeniasis and Cysticercosis (*Taenia saginata*). Adv. Parasit., 10, 269-343.

Ruitenberg, E.J. 1977. Serological diagnosis of trichinosis in pigs and cysticercosis in cattle. Tijdschrift voor Diergeneeskunde, 102, 826.

Ruitenberg, E.J., Steerenberg, P.A., Brosi, B.J.M. and Buys, J. 1975a. ELISA (enzyme-linked immunosorbent assay) as preventive and repressive control method for the detection of *Trichinella spiralis* infections in slaughter pigs. Wiadomosci Parazytologiczme, 21, 747-751.

Ruitenberg, E.J., Steerenberg, P.A. and Brosi, B.J.M. 1975b. Micro system for the application of ELISA (enzyme-linked immunosorbent assay) in the serodiagnosis of *Trichinella spiralis* infections. Medikon, Netherland, 4, 30-31.

Ruitenberg, E.J., Steerenberg, P.A., Brosi, B.J.M. and Buys, J. 1976. Reliability of the enzyme-linked immunosorbent assay (ELISA) for the serodiagnosis of *Trichinella spiralis* infections in conventionally raised pigs. J. Immunol. Meth., 10, 67-83.

Ruitenberg, E.J. and van Knapen, F. 1977. The enzyme-linked immunosorbent assay and its application to parasitic infections. J. Inf. Dis., 136, (supplement) S267-S273.

Schwarzhuber, A. 1978. Untersuchungen uber die Moglichkeit des serologischen Nachweises von larva migrans visceralis mit dem Peroxydase-Test. Inaugural Dissertation, Fachbereich Tiermedizin, Munchen.

Tailliez, R. and Korach, S. 1970. Les antigenes de *Fasciola hepatica* ii. Etude immunologique et localisation in situ d'un antigene specifique du genre.Annls. Inst. Pasteur, 118, 330-339.

Taylor, S.M., Kilpatrick, D. and Kenny, J. 1978. The influence of age and husbandry of pigs on evaluation of the enzyme-linked immunosorbent assay (ELISA) for *Trichinella spiralis* infection. Zentralblatt fur veterinarmedizin, 25b, 282-289.

Taylor, S.M., Kenny, J., Mallon, T. and Davidson, W.B. 1980. The micro-ELISA for antibodies to *Trichinella spiralis:* Elimination of false positive reactions by antigen fractionation and technical improvements. Zentralblatt fur Veterinarmedizin, 27b, 764-772.

Voller, A., Bartlett, A. and Bidwell, D.E. 1976. Enzyme immunoassays for parasite diseases. Trans. R. Soc. Trop. Med. Hyg., 70, 98-106.

Walther, M. and Sanitz, W. 1979. Untersuchungen zur serologischen Feststellung der Zystizerkose des Rindes mit Hilfe des Enzyme-Linked Immunosorbent Assay (ELISA). Berliner und Muchener Tierarztliche Wochenschrift, 92, 131-135.

Weil, G.J., Ottesen, E.A. and Powers, K.G. 1981. *Dirofilaria immitis:* Parasite specific humoral and cellular immune responses in experimentally infected dogs. Exptl. Parasit., 51, 80-86.

Weiland, G. and Schwarzhuber, A. 1978. Untersuchungen Zum Nachweis von larva migrans visceralis mit dem Peroxydase-test (ELISA) und der immunofluoreszenz. Berliner and Muchenen Tierarztliche Wochenschrift, 91, 209-213.

ELISA USED FOR THE DETECTION OF *TAENIA SAGINATA* METACESTODE INFECTION IN CATTLE

L.J.S. Harrison

Centre for Tropical Veterinary Medicine, Easter Bush, Roslin, Midlothian, Scotland

ABSTRACT

The antibody levels in cattle either naturally or experimentally infected with *Taenia saginata* meta-cestodes were measured by the enzyme linked immunosorbent assay (ELISA) using homologous and heter-ologous antigens.

In animals experimentally infected at 3-12 months of age a serum antibody response was detected by 2-4 weeks post infection, rising to a plateau by about 4-6 weeks post infection. The serum antibody levels began to decline by about 30 weeks post infection. The ELISA technique gave comparable results to the indirect haemagglutination technique. Calves experimentally infected at only 2-3 days old also developed an antibody response to infection which was detectable by ELISA. However, when studied individually there was a marked variation in the serum antibody levels of these young cattle, as although some calves gave a relatively strong serological response, others hardly varied from the controls. When the ELISA results from naturally infected cattle were analysed on a herd basis the antibody levels in all but one of these herds were significantly higher than control herds with no history of *T. saginata* infection. At present ELISA is unreliable in detecting individual infected animals in a herd and in detecting lightly infected herds.

INTRODUCTION

Many serological techniques have been used in the diagnosis of *T. saginata* infection in cattle, these have been reviewed. (Geerts et al., 1977). The enzyme-linked immunosorbent assay for the detection of serum antibodies has found wide application in parasitology (WHO, 1976; Voller et al., 1976). ELISA is potentially a very versatile technique, since it may be used either as a simple visual indicator of the presence of serum antibodies or as a very sensitive quantitative technique when the results are read accurately on a spectrophotometer.

The ELISA technique has been used to monitor the response of cattle to experimental infection with *T. saginata* metacestodes. (Van Knapen et al., 1979; Harrison and Sewell, 1981a;Geerts et al., 1981), to monitor the serological response to drug treatment in experimentally infected animals (Albert and Horchner, 1979; Walther and Sanitz, 1979) and to monitor the serological response of cattle in inoculation studies (Gallie and Sewell, 1981). ELISA has also been applied to the detection of cattle naturally infected with *T. saginata* metacestodes (Craig and Rickard, 1980; Geerts et al., 1981; Harrison and Sewell, 1981b).

The purpose of this paper is to outline the various uses made of ELISA with experimentally and naturally infected cattle and to summarise some of the problems associated with its use in detecting naturally infected animals.

MATERIALS AND METHODS

Calves infected at 3 months to 1 year old

Six calves were experimentally infected with between 60,000 and 100,000 *T. saginata* eggs at 3-12 months of age. The serum antibody response to infection was monitored by the enzyme-linked immuno-sorbent assay (ELISA) and the indirect haemagglutination test (IDH). Full details of this experiment were given by Gallie and Sewell (1974a) and Harrison and Sewell (1981a).

Neonatally infected calves

Five calves in each of two groups each received 10,000 *T. saginata* eggs orally at 2-3 days of age. The calves in the first of these groups also received repeated doses of 500 eggs at weekly intervals throughout

48

the experiment. Five calves in a third group were kept as uninfected controls. The serum antibody levels in the cattle were measured by ELISA. Full details of this experiment were given by Gallie and Sewell (1972; 1974b) and Harrison and Sewell (1981a).

Naturally infected calves

ELISA was used to measure the serum antibody levels in serum collected from cattle on seven farms at various locations in Scotland. Four of these farms were known to have suffered a recent outbreak of *T. saginata* metacestode infection in their herds. Samples were also obtained from cattle on a farm with a recent history of clinical disease resulting from *Ostertagia ostertagi* infection and from cattle on two farms with no history of clinical disease resulting from helminth infection. Three different antigens were used to test the sera *T. saginata* somatic extract, *T. saginata* excretory/secretory products and *T. crassiceps* metacestode extract. Full details of this experiment were given by Harrison and Sewell (1981b).

RESULTS

Calves infected at 3 months to 1 year old

Both the ELISA and the IDH technique consistently detected an antibody response to *T. saginata* infection in cattle by 2-4 weeks post infection. In the absence of further infection, the titres usually began to decline by about 30 weeks after infection. In one calf given a second oral infection of 80,000 *T. saginata* eggs, 20 weeks after the original infection the IDH titres and the ELISA values remained high. The response of a typical calf is shown in Fig. 1.

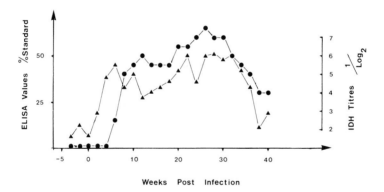

Fig. 1   The serological response of a typical calf to experimental oral infection with *T. saginata* eggs, monitored by the ELISA (▲—▲) and IDH (●—●) techniques using *T. saginata* somatic extract as antigen.

Neonatally infected calves

Regression analysis indicated that between 4 and 14 months after infection the ELISA values of the two experimental groups were not significantly different in slope or height above the x-axis but there was a significant difference between the control and experimental groups (P<.01). When looked at individually however, (Fig. 2) the serological response of the infected calves was very variable. Of the 10 infected calves two gave average post infection ELISA values, close to the mean for the 5 control calves.

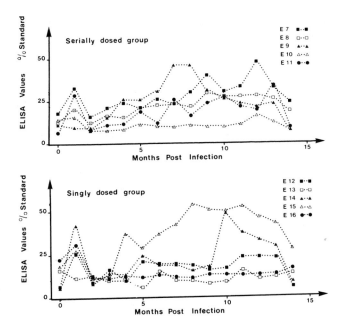

Fig. 2   The serological response of neonate calves to oral infection with *T. saginata* eggs, monitored by the ELISA technique using *T. saginata* somatic extract as antigen.

Naturally infected cattle

The individual results for the three different antigens correlated to a high level of significance (P<.001). The results for each farm with each antigen are shown in Table 1, along with the pooled results from the control farms. The results for each group of cattle were analysed by the Wilcoxon two sample test by comparing the results from each farm against the pooled results from the two control farms. The sera from cattle from the farm with the recent outbreak of ostertagiasis appeared to cross react with *T. saginata* somatic antigen but not with the *T. saginata* excretory/secretory products or the *T. crassiceps* extract.

The sera from cattle on farms 1 to 3 all gave significantly higher titres than the control sera with all three antigens but in no case were the ELISA readings for farm 4 significantly greater than the controls.

TABLE 1   Mean ± SD of the ELISA values obtained with sera from cattle from farms either exposed to natural infection with *T. saginata* or not

Farm	History	Sample size	Ts	E/S	Tc
1	Natural *T. saginata* infection	18	0.38±0.19 (2.16)*	0.57±0.23 (3.73)*	0.24±0.15 (2.00)*
2		21	0.38±0.15 (2.53)*	0.68±0.15 (5.05)*	0.32±0.11 (4.04)*
3		12	0.44±0.15 (3.63)*	0.45±0.18 (2.17)*	0.33±0.13 (3.68)*
4		17	0.32±0.17 (1.5)	0.25±0.13 (0.26)	0.21±0.11 (1.45)
5	*O. ostertagi* infection	22	0.42±0.21 (2.48)*	0.24±0.15 (1.07)	0.16±0.16 (0.40)
6 & 7	No known helminth infection	22	0.24±0.15	0.28±0.17	0.15±0.10

Three different antigens were used. The ELISA values for each group of sera were compared with the control sera using the Wilcoxon two sample test, *t* values are given in brackets
* Significantly greater than the pooled control cattle serum readings   Ts *T. saginata* somatic extract
E/S *T. saginata* metacestode excretory/secretory products   Tc *T. crassiceps* metacestode extract

DISCUSSION

The antibody response of calves orally infected with *T. saginata* eggs at between 3 months and 1 year old was similar when monitored by ELISA or IDH. *T. saginata* metacestodes are not infective until 10–11 weeks post infection (McIntosh and Miller, 1960). In calves orally infected with large numbers of *T. saginata* eggs between 3 months to 1 year old the ELISA technique registers a positive serological response within 2–4 weeks post infection, well before the metacestodes reach the infective stage. These results are in agreement with those published by Walther and Sanitz (1979), Albert and Horchner (1979) and Geerts et al. (1981). The latter authors also found, however, that in cattle in which less than 100 metacestodes were found at *post mortem* the ELISA titres did not rise until 6 weeks post infection and only a slight rise was noted thereafter.

Several of the infective neonates failed to give a good serological response to infection and the extent of the response was not related to the presence or absence of metacestodes in the calves when they were slaughtered (Gallie and Sewell, 1972; 1974b). In this respect this experiment replicated the situation which occurs in areas of high endemicity such as East Africa, where calves with a poor serological response to infection with *T. saginata* may be resistant to reinfection with *T. saginata* eggs but still harbour viable cysts in the musculature. It, therefore, seems unlikely that even sensitive immunological techniques such as ELISA or IDH, used to measure serum antibody levels will afford a reliable diagnosis in calves which have been infected when they are very young.

At present meat inspection is the main control measure against *T. saginata*. Only the statutory meat inspection cuts are made on cattle sold on the open market, therefore, it is not possible to find the exact number of metacestodes present in each animal; in order to do this every animal would have to be totally dissected. For this reason we elected to analyse the results for our naturally infected animals on a herd basis to see if it was possible to detect herds which had been exposed to infection. In three out of four herds this proved to be the case but the sera from the fourth farm did not give results significantly greater than the control farm sera. This may have been because the cattle in this herd were relatively lightly infected; no more than 10 *T. saginata* metacestodes were found when the hearts were totally dissected. Approximately 20 percent of the total cyst burden of an animal may be expected to be found in the heart so a proportion of these animals may have had up to 50 cysts in the whole carcase. ELISA cannot, therefore, be regarded as completely reliable in detecting lightly infected herds. In addition cross reactions were encountered with *O. ostertagi* infected cattle. However, Harrison (1978) found that in a herd of 22 animals with a heavy naturally acquired *T. saginata* infection normal meat inspection procedures detected infection in 15 out of 21 carcasses shown by more thorough dissection to contain cysts. ELISA used to measure serum antibodies detected 18 of these 21. There were 2 false negative reactions and 1 false positive reaction. Craig and Rickard (1980) and Geerts et al. (1981) noted cross reactions in cattle infected with *Fasciola hepatica* and other helminths and found the ELISA to be unreliable in detecting individual infected animals.

ELISA, therefore, is a technique of sensitivity comparable to IDH, useful in monitoring the response of cattle to experimental *T. saginata* infection. A highly sensitive test is needed for the serological detection of *T. saginata* infection as the parasite is highly adapted to its bovine host and does not provoke a strong serological response. This is particularly apparent in the lightly infected animals most commonly found in natural infections in Britain and Europe. There are also the additional complications to diagnosis caused by a possible tolerance and lack of antibody response to the parasite induced in cattle naturally infected within a few days of birth and also non-specificity caused by cross reactions with other helminth parasites. These problems will have to be overcome if the ELISA or any other serological technique can be used with accuracy in the diagnosis of naturally acquired *T. saginata* metacestode infections in cattle.

REFERENCES

Albert, Von H. and Horchner, F. 1979. Zur Bekampfung und Diagnostik der Rinderfinnen II. Serologische

Untersuchungen mit dem ELISA. Berl. Munch. tierartzl. Wschr., *10*, 189-193.

Craig, P.S. and Rickard, M.D. 1980. Evaluation of "Crude" antigen prepared from *Taenia saginata* for the serological diagnosis of *T. saginata* cysticercosis in cattle. Z. ParasitKde., *61*, 287-297.

Gallie, G.J. and Sewell, M.M.H., 1972. The survival of *Cysticercus bovis* in resistant calves. Vet. Rec., *91*, 481-482.

Gallie, G.J. and Sewell, M.M.H. 1974a. The serological response of three month old calves to infection with *Taenia saginata* (*Cysticercus bovis*) and their resistance to reinfection. Trop. Anim. Hlth Prod., *6*, 163-171.

Gallie, G.J. and Sewell, M.M.H. 1974b. The serological response of calves infected neonatally with *Taenia saginata* (*Cysticercus bovis*). Trop. Anim. Hlth Prod., *6*, 173-177.

Gallie, G.J. and Sewell, M.M.H. 1981. Inoculation of calves and adult cattle with oncospheres of *Taenia saginata* and their resistance to challenge infection. Trop. Anim. Hlth Prod., *13*, 147-154.

Geerts, S., Kumar, V. and Vercruysse, J. 1977. *In vivo* diagnosis of bovine cysticercosis. Vet. Bull., *47*, 653-664.

Geerts, S., Kumar, V., Ceulemans, F. and Mortelmans, J. 1981. Serodiagnosis of *Taenia saginata* cysticercosis in experimentally and naturally infected cattle by enzyme linked immunosorbent assay. Res. Vet. Sci., *30*, 288-293.

Harrison, L.J.S. 1978. Detection of *Taenia saginata* infection in cattle by the enzyme linked immunosorbent assay. Trans. R. Soc. trop. Med. Hyg., *72*, 642.

Harrison, L.J.S. and Sewell, M.M.H. 1981a. A comparison of the enzyme linked immunosorbent assay and the indirect haemagglutination technique applied to sera from cattle experimentally infected with *Taenia saginata* (Goeze, 1782). Vet. Immunol. Immunopath., *2*, 67-73.

Harrison, L.J.S. and Sewell, M.M.H. 1981b. Antibody levels in cattle naturally infected with *Taenia saginata* metacestodes in Britain. Res. Vet. Sci., *31*, 62-64.

McIntosh, A. and Miller, D. 1960. Bovine cysticercosis with special reference to the early developmental stages of *Taenia saginata*. Am. J. Vet. Res., *21*, 169-177.

Walther, Von M. and Sanitz, W. 1979. Untersuchungen zur serologischen Feststellung der Zystizerkose des Rindes mit Hilfe des Enzyme-Linked Immunosorbent Assay (ELISA). Berl. Munch. tierarztl. Wschr., *92*, 131-135.

Van Knapen, F., Fridas, S. and Franchimont, J.H. 1979. The serodiagnosis of *Taenia saginata* cysticercosis by means of the enzyme linked immunosorbent assay (ELISA). Report No. 131/79 Path Rijks Institute Voor de Volksgezondheid, Bilthoven, Holland.

Voller, A., Bartlett, A. and Bidwell, D.E. 1976. Enzyme immunoassay for parasitic diseases. Trans. R. Soc. trop. Med. Hyg., *70*, 98-106.

WHO. 1976. The enzyme-linked immunosorbent assay (ELISA). Bull. Wld Hlth Org., *54*, 129-139.

THE USE OF ELISA TO DETECT ANTIGEN RELEASE
FROM JUVENILE FASCIOLA HEPATICA

D. A. Lammas and W. P. H. Duffus

University of Cambridge
Department of Clinical Veterinary Medicine,
Madingley Road,
Cambridge
CB3 0ES

SUMMARY

Freshly excysted <u>Fasciola hepatica</u> pocess an outer glycocalyx which on incubation at 37°C is rapidly shed. This reaction was visualised by using specific antisera to form aggregates of antibody and shed antigen. To detect this parasite antigen an ELISA technique was established by which the release of antigen was shown to be temperature dependent and to occur in normal bovine serum as well as in serum free conditions. However the Elisa failed to detect the antibody-antigen complexes that occurred when flukes were incubated in immune serum. Release of parasite antigen fell slowly with <u>invitro</u> cultured flukes but increased with <u>invivo</u> cultured flukes. Using a fluorescence inhibition assay, antigens with high Elisa titres inhibited surface fluorescence of the parasite suggesting that the Elisa was detecting surface antigens as well as other parasite metabolic products.

INTRODUCTION

Juvenile stages of <u>F. hepatica</u> have a glycoprotein rich layer overlaying the tegument, termed the outer glycocalyx (Threadgold 1976; Hanna, 1978) which is antigenically unique in that it is only found in migrating juveniles (Bennet 1978; Hanna 1978). Fluorescent antibody labelling studies have shown that shedding of this outer glycocalyx layer occurs and is rapidly replaced by exocrine secreations from the tegument below (Hanna 1978; Duffus and Franks, 1981). Recent studies suggest that the functional antigen(s) responsible for the stimulation of a protective response in rats to <u>F. hepatica</u> are those released by juvenile stages (Rajasekariah and Howell; 1979, Howell, 1979; Howell and Sandeman 1979) and that successful vaccination of rats and mice to challenge infections have been reported by Lang (1976) and Lang and Hall (1977) using <u>invitro</u> cultured antigens from juvenile flukes.

To detect and study the release of parasite specific antigen in <u>in vitro</u> cultured <u>F. hepatica</u> juveniles, an Elisa sandwich technique was established together with a surface fluorescence inhibition test in an attempt to demonstrate the presence of specific coat antigen.

MATERIALS AND METHODS

These will be reported in full elsewhere (Lammas and Duffus, submitted for publication).

RESULTS

a) Effect of Temperature

The results confirmed previous fluorescence labelling studies that very little specific antigen is shed by newly excysted juvenile flukes (nej-flukes) at 4°C or below (Fig 1a).

b) Effect of Incubating Medium

Production of 'shed' antigen occured in the presence of both RPMI-1640 medium (MED) and normal bovine serum (NBS) but showed a marked fall with immune bovine serum (Fig 1b)

EFFECT OF TEMPERATURE AND INCUBATION MEDIA ON ELISA
TITRE OF `SHED´ FLUKE ANTIGEN

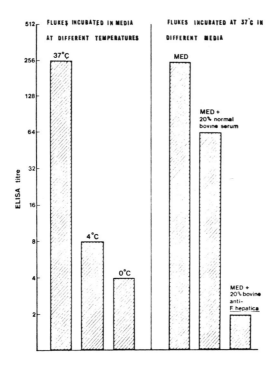

FIG 1a   FIG 1b

54

c) <u>Comparison of in vivo and in vitro cultured flukes</u>

An attempt was made to compare the release of parasite antigen
from juvenile <u>F. hepatica</u> reared by either <u>in vivo</u> or <u>in vitro</u>
culture over a 7-day period. The results demonstrated that the
release of specific antigen rises with time with <u>in vivo</u> cultured
flukes and falls with <u>in vitro</u> cultured flukes (Fig 2). This fall
paralleled an increase in mortality and decrease in motility of
<u>in vitro</u> cultured flukes (Results not shown).

ELISA TITRATION OF ANTIGEN RELEASE FROM <u>IN VIVO</u> AND <u>IN VITRO</u>
CULTURED JUVENILE <u>F.HEPATICA</u>

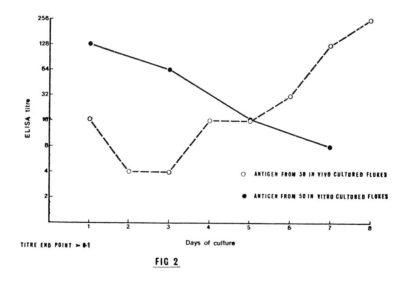

FIG 2

d) <u>Fluorescence Inhibition Test</u>

The results of these experiments show that supernatants with a low
Elisa titre were similar to MED controls in being unable to inhibit
the specific surface fluorescence on nej <u>F. hepatica</u>. (Fig 3)

However an increasing Elisa titre had a parallel effect on the
inhibition of surface fluorescence. i.e. above an Elisa titre of
1:128 there was total inhibition of surface fluorescence (Fig. 3)

COMPARISON OF ELISA TITRE OF FLUKE `SHED` ANTIGEN
AND FLUORESCENCE INHIBITION

100 juvenile F. hepatica incubated at 37°C	ELISA titre	Fluorescence Inhibition Test
Hours 0	8	+++
4	32	+
24	64	±
48	128	--
72	256	--
120	512	--
RPMI medium control (no flukes)	0	++++

FIG 3

DISCUSSION

The Elisa technique was successful in that it was able to detect
juvenile fluke antigen in incubate media, and showed that its release was
temperature dependent. The fall in titre of fluke antigen in the
prescence of immune sera could be attributed to the failure of shed
antigen-antibody complexes to attach to the coated Elisa plates in excess
antibody; as fluorescent studies have clearly shown that the outer
glycocalyx is shed in the prescence of specific antisera (Duffus and

Franks, 1981). Whether the anitgen detected by the Elisa is the 'shed'
outer glycocalyx described by Hanna (1978) or merely fluke metabolic
products is still uncertain; however the results of the fluorescence
inhibition test would suggest that at least some of the antigen(s)
detected was derived from the surface coat of juvenile flukes. The
gradual fall in antigen release with age in blood cultured flukes
supports morphological and fluorescent labelling studies which showed
that although _invitro_ cultured flukes did increase to some extent in
size in culture, their motility and shedding of surface fluorescence
decreased with age. Conversely _invivo_ cultured flukes showed an increase
in antigen release with age which again was supported by morphological
and fluorescent studies which confirmed that the flukes rapidly increased
in size and retained their motility. However an increasing proportion
of this antigen release is likely to be metabolic products rather than
coat antigen.

BIBLIOGRAPHY

Bennett, C.E. 1978. The identification of soluble adult antigen on the
tegumental surface of juvenile _Fasciola hepatica_. Parasitol.
77, 325-331

Duffus, W.P.H. and Franks, D. 1981. The interaction _in vitro_ between
bovine immunoglobulin and juvenile _Fasciola hepatica_. Parasit.,
82, 1-10.

Hanna, R.E.B., 1978. A possible immunological role for the tegument of
Fasciola hepatica. Parasitol. 77 IX.

Howell, M.J. 1979. Vaccination of rats against _Fasciola hepatica_
J. Parasitol. 65 817-819.

Howell, M.J., and Sandeman, R.M. 1979. Fasciola hepatica: some properties
of a precipitate which forms when metacercarie are cultured in
immune rat serum. Int J. Parasit. 9, 41-45.

Lang, B.Z., 1976. Host-parasite relationships of _Fasciola hepatica_ in
the white mouse. VII. Effects of anti-worm incubate sera on
transferred worms and successful vaccination with a crude incubate
antigen. J. Parasitol. 62, 232-236.

Lang, B.Z. and Hall, R.F. 1977. Host-parasite relationships of
Fasciola hepatica in the white mouse. VIII. Succesful vaccination
with culture incubate antigens and antigens from sonic disruption
of immature worms. J. Parasitol. 63 1046-1049.

Rajasekariah, G.R. and Howell, M.J. 1979. _Fasciola hepatica_ in rats:
Transfer of immunity by serum and cells from infected to F. hepatica
naive animals. J. Parasitol. 65 481-487.

Threadgold, L.T. 1976. _Fasciola hepatica_: Ultrastructure and histo-
chemistry of the glycocalyx of the tegument. Expt. parasit.
39, 119-134.

ANTIBODY RESPONSES TO FASCIOLA HEPATICA
ANTIGENS DURING LIVER FLUKE INFECTION OF CATTLE

G. Oldham

Agricultural Research Council
Institute for Research on Animal Diseases,
Compton, Nr. Newbury, Berkshire, England, U.K.

ABSTRACT

An enzyme-linked immunosorbent assay is described for the measurement of antibodies to Fasciola hepatica using a semi-purified antigen prepared by G200 gel chromatography of a crude whole worm extract. Day-to-day reproducibility of the assays was achieved by including in every assay a standard serum given an arbitrary antibody concentration. The intra-assay variation was 9% and the inter-assay variation was 26%.

Anti-F. hepatica antibody titres rose rapidly after infection and were above pre-infection levels by 2 to 3 weeks post-infection. Both IgG and IgM responses were clearly seen with peaks in the responses at 2-4 weeks, 11 weeks and 20 weeks post-infection. IgA antibody levels were much lower than IgG or IgM antibody levels but there appeared to be an IgA response detectable by 8 weeks post-infection.

A large number of false positive results were obtained with sera from cattle raised under normal field conditions. The assay using the Fl antigen preparation would not therefore be a success for immunodiagnosis. These false positive results appeared to be related to the age of the cattle and animals infected with the parasitic nematodes Trichostrongylus colubriformis, Cooperia oncophera or Ostertagia ostertagi did not possess cross-reacting antibodies.

INTRODUCTION

A number of enzyme-linked immunosorbent assays (ELISA) have been described for the measurement of antibodies to F. hepatica (Hillyer and de Weil, 1977; Burden and Hammet, 1978; Farrell, Shen, Wescott and Lang, 1981). However, these assays tend, on the whole, to lack careful standardisation, use complex antigen mixtures and only measure total antibody. In addition non-specific cross-reactions appear to be a problem in measuring antibodies to F. hepatica (Burden, personal communication).

This paper describes an ELISA system for the measurement of antibodies to F. hepatica incorporating a standard serum providing day-to-day reproducibility. A G200 fraction of a crude F. hepatica extract containing a limited number of antigens was used as the test 'antigen' in an attempt to improve specificity. The assay has also been further adapted to make class-specific antibody determinations. Antibody responses in cattle with experimental F. hepatica infection are described and the potential use of the assay as an immunodiagnostic test is investigated.

MATERIALS AND METHODS

Antigen preparation

Adult <u>Fasciola hepatica</u> were collected from the bile ducts of
experimentally infected sheep, goats and cattle. The flukes were washed
in phosphate buffered saline (PBS) pH 7.2 four times for 30 min each wash
(during which time most of the caecal contents were lost), drained and
freeze-dried. The dried flukes were ground to a fine powder with a pestle
and mortar and the powder stored at -20°C until used.

A 4% (w/v) suspension of this powdered material in PBS was homogenised
and allowed to extract at 4°C for 24 h. The suspension was centrifuged at
38,000 x g for 2 h and the supernatant taken. Ten ml of this solution
(20-25 mg protein/ml) was then applied to a G200 (Pharmacia Fine Chemicals
AB, Uppsala, Sweden) column (100 x 2.5 cm) and fractionated in PBS at a
flow rate of 14 ml/h by upward flow. Fractions (5 ml) were collected on
an automated fraction collector and the absorbance of each fraction at

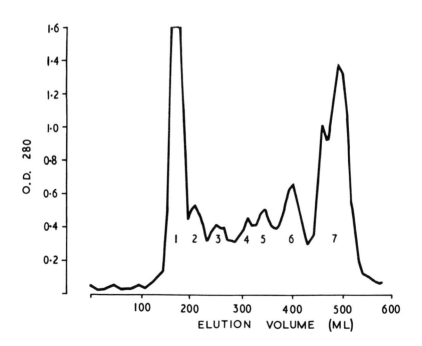

Fig. 1   Fractionation of whole adult antigen extract by G200 gel
chromatography into seven fractions (Fl to F7) (see Materials
and Methods for details).

280 nm measured. This revealed 7 peaks designated F1 to F7 (Fig. 1), F1 being eluted in the void volume. The fractions of each peak were pooled and concentrated back to 10 ml by ultrafiltration (except F7) using a PM10 Diaflo Ultrafilter (Amicon, Mass., U.S.A.) and stored frozen at -20°C until used. The proteins present in fraction 7 passed through the PM10 filter (and therefore had a Mol. wt. <10000) and this fraction was concentrated by lyophilisation and reconstituted with 10 ml of distilled water.

Determination of protein concentrations

The protein concentration of antigen extracts and G200 fractions was assayed by the method of Bradford (1976) using bovine plasma albumin (Miles, Slough, England) as the standard.

Animals

Four calves were experimentally infected with 1000 F. hepatica metacercariae orally at 3 to 4 months of age, two other calves were left uninfected. A further group of 6 calves were experimentally infected with both Trichostrongylus colubriformis and Cooperia oncophera. At 6 months of age these calves received a primary infection of 40,000 T. colubriformis and 80,000 C. oncophera third stage larvae per os. Eight weeks later they received a secondary infection of 6,000 T. colubriformis and 34,000 C. oncophera. A control group of 5 calves was left uninfected.

Serum samples from cows aged from 1 to 12 years which had been reared in F. hepatica free conditions and from calves experimentally infected with Ostertagia ostertagi were kindly provided by Dr. D.J. Burden.

Cattle being slaughtered at a public abattoir provided serum samples for analysis. Along with each sample a record was kept on whether the liver of that animal was condemned for fascioliasis or not. Faeces samples were also taken and examined for F. hepatica eggs. The serum samples and information on liver condemnations and presence of liver fluke eggs were generously provided by Dr. D.J. Burden.

ELISA procedure

Coating of microelisa plates (Dynatech, Sussex, England) with antigen F1 (5 µg/protein/ml, 0.1 ml/well) in coating buffer (0.05 M carbonate buffer pH 9.6) was accomplished at 37°C for 3 h. The plates were then washed three times in ELISA buffer (PBS + 0.05% Tween 20 + 0.02% NaN$_3$) and well drained. All further dilutions of sera and conjugates were made in ELISA buffer. Standard serum at various dilutions or test sera at a dilution of 1/100 (or greater) were added to wells in 0.1 ml volumes and incubated for 3 h at R.T. The plates were then washed three times in ELISA buffer.

To measure total antibody levels a 1/250 dilution of horse radish peroxidase (HRP) conjugated rabbit anti-bovine immunoglobulin (Miles) was added to each well (0.1 ml/well) and incubated at RT for 2 h followed by overnight incubation at 4°C.

For the measurement of class specific antibodies, after incubation of test serum samples and washing of the plate, a 1/400 dilution of swine anti-bovine IgG, IgA or IgM (Biogenes, Middx., England) was added to each well (0.1 ml). The plates were incubated at RT for 2 h and at 4°C overnight and the plates washed. A 1/300 dilution of HRP conjugated goat anti-swine IgG (Miles) was added to each well (0.1 ml) and incubated at RT for 3 h.

After incubation with the conjugate the plates were washed and substrate (o-phenylenediamine) added to each well (0.1 ml). After 10 min the reaction was stopped by addition of 2 N H_2SO_4 (0.1 ml/well). The colour reactions were measured on an automatic plate reader (Titertek Multiskan) at 492 nm. Background readings were automatically subtracted from reading due to antibody by blanking the plate reader with wells that had had all reagents except test or standard sera added.

Standardisation of assays

In order to provide day-to-day reproducibility of the assay, serum from a calf with a 16 week F. hepatica infection was included in every assay. For the measurements of total antibody this serum was given an arbitrary antibody concentration such that a 1/80 dilution contained 100 units per ml of anti-Fl antibodies. A range of dilutions of this serum were included in every assay plate and a graph was plotted of the OD_{492} versus the antibody concentration in Units i.e. the control curve (Fig. 2). From this control curve the antibody concentration of a test serum can be read off from its OD_{492} reading in units - see Fig. 2. Test sera were assayed at a dilution of 1/100 or greater because non-specific binding increased at dilutions less than 1/100. The limit of detection on this assay was approximately 3 units per ml of a 1/100 dilution of serum, this is equivalent to 3×10^2 units per ml of neat serum. By calculating the

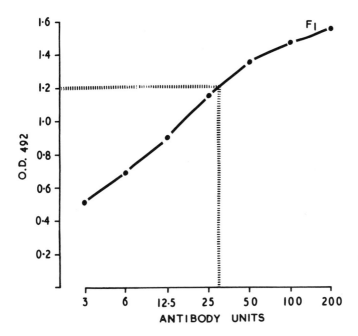

Fig. 2   Control curve for determination of total anti-Fl antibody
levels using a standard serum given an arbitrary antibody concentration.

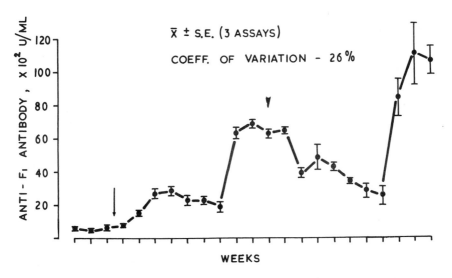

Fig. 3   Analysis of reproducibility of ELISA. Sequential serum
samples from a calf experimentally infected with F. hepatica were
assayed for anti-Fl antibodies on 3 different occasions and the
mean ± S.E. of the 3 assays is shown. The average coefficient
of variation was calculated to be 26%

62

coefficient of variation it was found that the mean intra-assay variation
of duplicate samples was 9% and the mean inter-assay variation for the same
23 sera in 3 assays was 26% (Fig. 3).

In order to ascribe antibody units to the 3 immunoglobulin classes
being considered in the class-specific assays, it was first necessary to
determine the proportions in which they occurred in the standard serum. To
do this doubling dilutions of the standard serum were incubated in Fl-
coated wells and the binding of the different classes determined as
described in ELISA assay procedure. Three curves were then drawn, one for
each Ig class, plotting OD_{492} against dilution of standard serum (Fig. 4).
A horizontal line was drawn across the graph at an OD_{492} value of 0.4,
chosen such that the line would cut all 3 curves near the bottom of the
central linear portion of the sigmoid curve. Reading vertically from the
intersections of this line with the curves 3 dilutions of standard serum
were read off. These 3 dilutions of standard serum, 1/4096, 1/700 and
1/200 for IgG, IgM and IgA anti-Fl antibodies respectively, therefore
contained the same antibody activity and were each given the arbitrary
value of 10 antibody units (see Fig. 4). Standard curves for class specific

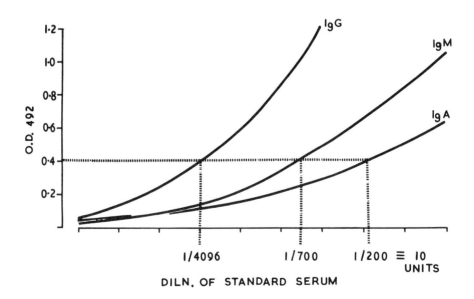

Fig. 4   Determination of the relative proportions of IgG, IgM and IgA
anti-Fl antibodies in the standard serum.

assays were constructed in much the same way as for total antibody levels using dilutions of standard serum having antibody levels from 5 to 160 antibody units per ml.

RESULTS

Assessment of antigenicity of G200 fractions by ELISA

As described in Materials and Methods whole adult antigen extract could be divided into 7 fractions by G200 gel chromatography (Fig. 1). These fractions were coated to the wells of microelisa plates over a range of dilutions at known protein concentrations. Binding by antibodies from F. hepatica infected calf sera to these different fractions was detected using an anti-bovine Ig-HRP conjugate as described in Materials and Methods. The absorbance at 492 nm plotted against the protein concentration (used for coating the wells) of each of the antigen fractions is shown in Fig. 5

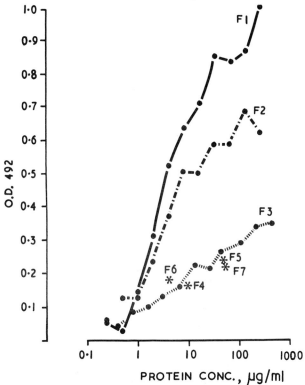

Fig. 5   Antigenicity of G200 fractions F1 to F7 determined by the binding of antibody in serum from a F. hepatica infected calf. Antibody binding (OD_{492}) is plotted against the concentrations of antigens (µg protein/ml) used for coating the wells.

using just one infected serum at a constant dilution (1/100). The curves
for F1, F2 and F3 are shown in entirety but only the maximum OD_{492} readings
are indicated for fractions 4 to 7. It is clear from the results of this
assay that fractions 1 and 2 contain the major portion of the antigenic
material present in the whole adult antigen extract. F1 appeared to be
stronger antigenically than F2 and was used in all further assays for
detecting anti-F. hepatica antibodies.

Antibody responses to F. hepatica antigen F1 during experimental F. hepatica infection

Total antibody responses to F1 antigen were measured in 4 calves
experimentally infected with 1000 F. hepatica metacercariae and in 2
uninfected calves over a 20 to 25 week period (Fig. 6). Antibody levels

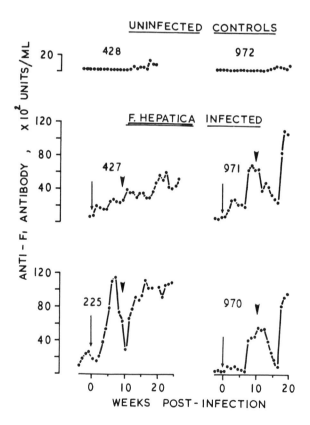

Fig. 6   Total anti-F1 antibody responses in 4 calves infected with
1000 F. hepatica metacercariae as indicated by the arrows (↓) and in
2 uninfected calves. F. hepatica eggs were first found in the
faeces at the time indicated by the arrow heads (▼).

in the sera of the uninfected calves remained below 6×10^2 units per ml for approximately 15 weeks but then began to rise slowly. Pre-infection sera from 3 of the 4 calves to be infected were also equally low though in 1 animal (#225) 4 pre-infection samples had antibody levels ranging from 10 to 28×10^2 units per ml. Two to three weeks following infection a rise in antibody titre could be seen above pre-infection levels. In one animal (#427) the antibody titres increased steadily over the period of infection but in the three other calves a peak in antibody titre was seen 8 to 11 weeks post infection followed by a dramatic fall in serum antibody titre. This peak and fall coincided approximately with the detection of F. hepatica eggs in the faeces of the animals. The fall in antibody levels was only transient and the anti-F1 titre rose steeply again and remained high for the rest of the period of observation.

Class-specific (IgG, IgM and IgA) antibody responses were determined in one of these four infected calves, #971 (Fig. 7). The IgG response

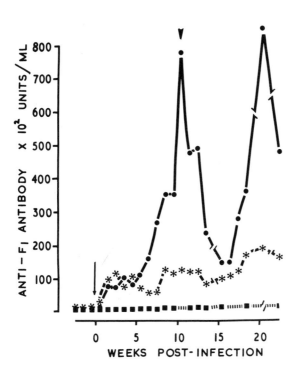

Fig. 7   IgG (●━●), IgM (✳◗◖✳) and IgA (■◗◖■) anti-F1 antibody responses in calf 971 infected with 1000 F. hepatica metacercariae (↓, infected; ▼, eggs first found in faeces).

closely followed the total antibody response already seen in Fig. 6, with two very prominent peaks at weeks 11 and 20 post-infection and the suggestion of an earlier peak at weeks 2 to 4. This early peak is more obvious when the IgM response is examined and is of the same magnitude for both classes. The 11 week- and 20 week-peaks are also present in the IgM response though these were much smaller than those seen in the IgG response. While increases in antibody titres of between 10 and 40 fold above background were seen for IgM and IgG antibody responses respectively the IgA response was much less dramatic. The background IgA level (less than 5×10^2 units/ml) increased to 10×10^2 units/ml by about 8 weeks of infection and by week 20 reached 15×10^2 units/ml. The obvious fall in the IgG antibody levels between weeks 11 and 16 of infection was much less clear for IgM antibody and was not seen at all in the IgA response.

Anti-F1 antibody levels in sera from cattle slaughtered at a local abattoir

Total anti-F1 antibody levels were measured in 146 sera from cattle being slaughtered at an abattoir. The antibody levels were compared with liver condemnations and the presence of F. hepatica eggs in faecal samples (Fig. 8). In the small group of veal calves anti-F1 antibody levels were very low, similar to levels found in calves known not to have been in contact with F. hepatica. None of the livers from these animals were condemned nor were any liver fluke eggs found in their faeces. The large majority of samples came from heifers and steers and as can be seen many animals without signs of liver fluke infestation (i.e. without liver condemnation or liver fluke eggs in their faeces) had antibody levels as high or higher than animals which did have obvious fascioliasis. This was also true of the small group of cows examined. The majority (9 out of 12; 75%) of animals with liver fluke had antibody levels that would have been considered positive (greater than 20×10^2 units/ml) based on levels seen in non-infected calves of 3 to 6 months of age but as already stated many (57 out of 121, 47%) uninfected older cattle would also be considered positive. There were also 3 out of 12 animals (25%) with condemned livers and/or liver fluke eggs in their faeces which would have been considered negative by this assay.

Anti-F.hepatica antibody levels in calves experimentally infected with parasitic nematodes and in cattle of different ages

The findings described above suggest that the assay was not specific for liver fluke particularly when the animal has been subjected to normal field conditions. To test whether this lack of specificity was due to

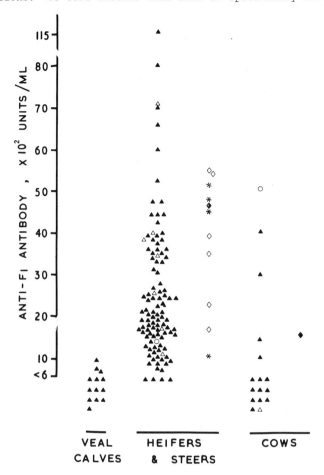

Fig. 8   Anti-F1 antibody levels in sera from 146 cattle at slaughter. ▲, normal liver, no eggs; △, normal liver, no faeces samples; O, cysts (not fascioliasis); ✻, condemned liver and F. hepatica eggs in faeces; ◆, condemned liver, no eggs; ◑, condemned liver, no faeces sample; ◇, F. hepatica eggs only.

cross-reacting antibodies produced against commonly occurring intestinal parasites, sera from 2 groups of calves, one experimentally infected with a mixture of T. colubriformis and C. oncophera and the other infected with O. ostertagi, were assayed for anti-F1 antibodies. In both groups of infected animals there was an increase in anti-F1 titres over the period of infection as can be seen in Fig. 9b where the data on the T. colubriformis and C. oncophera infected group is presented (data from the O. ostertagi group is not shown). However, there was a similar

68

increase in anti-Fl antibody titres in the control non-infected animals over the same period (Fig. 9a).

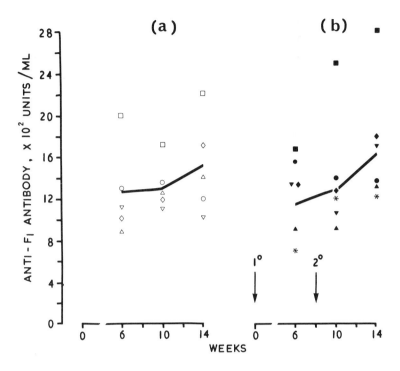

Fig. 9   Anti-Fl antibody levels (a) in uninfected calves and (b) in calves with a mixed infection of T. colubriformis and C. oncophera.

To examine this apparent age effect further anti-Fl antibody levels in calves less than 6 months old, calves 6 to 12 months old and cows greater than 1 year old were compared (Fig. 10). None of these animals had experienced F. hepatica-infection. There was a clear trend of increased anti-Fl antibody with age, increasing from barely detectable levels at less than 6 months of age to a median level of 28×10^2 units in the group of cows.

DISCUSSION

The ELISA technique described in this paper gave consistent results when used to assess responses to experimental F. hepatica infections in young calves. The assay described by Farrell et al (1981) gave no evidence of fluke infection until 4-5 weeks post-infection whereas the assay described here was able to detect antibody responses as early as 2 weeks post-infection. Antibody levels in natural infections were studied by Farrell et al (1981) only in young calves and they did not study the performance of their assay in a true clinical setting where much older animals would need to be tested. When sera from animals (greater than one year old) raised in a conventional farm manner were assayed by the technique described here high antibody titres did not correlate with liver condemnations or F. hepatica eggs in the faeces. In addition, these false positive results did not correlate with the presence of strongylidae eggs or coccidia in the faeces of these animals (D.J. Burden, personal communication). It is possible that these false positive results were due

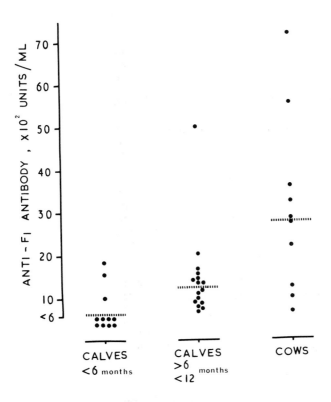

Fig. 10   Anti-Fl antibody levels in calves and cows of various ages raised in fluke-free conditions.

to early (pre-hepatic) F. hepatica infections in the animals, undetectable
at slaughter, but this was considered unlikely. More probably these
findings are due to the presence antibodies raised to some other antigen
but cross-reacting with an antigen in the Fl preparation. Experimental
infection of calves with the common intestinal parasites T. colubriformis,
C. oncophera and O. ostertagi did not induce levels of cross-reacting
antibodies higher than those found in age matched controls. There was
clear evidence however that cross-reacting antibodies began to develop in
fluke-free cattle from approximately 6 months of age. The most likely
source of the stimulus for the production of these antibodies would be
antigens from normal gut flora or even food. The problem of false
positive results may possibly be overcome by further fractionation of the
Fl antigen or the use of antigens extracted under different conditions.

The three peaks seen during the course of the IgG and IgM responses may
indicate either 3 responses to the same antigen or, more likely, responses
to 3 different antigens (present in the Fl preparation) expressed by the
parasite at different stages of infection. If the 3 responses were to the
same antigen the second and third IgM responses would have been expected
to be smaller than they in fact were. These distinct responses raise the
problem that if a single antigen were to be purified from Fl and used in
the assay would this restrict the stage of infection which could be
detected? If a single antigen is to be used it must be able to detect
serologically an infection of up to 10 weeks old (i.e. until the infection
can be detected by faecal egg counts). The peak in antibody titre seen at
week 11 post-infection coincides with the finding of F. hepatica eggs in
the faeces. This peak may represent a response to a new antigen being
expressed by the flukes shortly before they migrate into the bile ducts.
A possible candidate for the source of this antigen could be the T2 granules
described by Bennett and Threadgold (1975) which are seen to be expressed
on the surface of the fluke at this time in infection (Hanna, 1980).
However Hughes, Hanna and Symonds (1981) found that in cattle anti-T2
antibody titres did not fall as this antibody response did. The increase
in IgA antibody also coincides with the time when flukes are starting to
break through into the bile ducts. Fluke antigens passing down the bile
ducts and into the gut may have stimulated an intestinal IgA response of
which this serum IgA is but a small reflection.

In summary, an ELISA technique is described which has been used to
provide information on the immune responses of calves to experimental

infection with F. hepatica. Further development is required however before the assay can be applied to immunodiagnostic purposes.

REFERENCES

Bennett, C.E. and Threadgold, L.T. 1975. Fasciola hepatica: Development of tegument during migration in mouse. Exp. Parasitol., 38, 38-55.
Bradford, M.M. 1976. A rapid and sensitive method for the quantitation of microgram quantities of protein using the principles of protein-dye binding. Analyt. Biochem., 72, 248-254.
Burden, D.J. and Hammet, N.C. 1978. Microplate enzyme-linked immunosorbent assay for antibody to Fasciola hepatica in cattle. Vet. Rec., 103, 158.
Farrell, C.J., Shen, D.T., Westcott, R.B. and Lang, B.Z. 1981. An enzyme-linked immunosorbent assay for diagnosis of Fasciola hepatica infection in cattle. Am. J. Vet. Res., 42, 237-240.
Hanna, R.E.B. 1980. Fasciola hepatica: An immunofluorescent study of antigenic changes in the tegument during development in the rat and the sheep. Exp. Parasitol., 155-170.
Hillyer, G.V. and de Weil, N.S. 1979. Use of immunologic techniques to detect chemotherapeutic success in infections with Fasciola hepatica. II The enzyme-linked immunosorbent assay in infected rats and rabbits. J. Parasitol., 65, 680-684.
Hughes, D.L., Hanna, R.E.B. and Symonds, H.W. 1981. Fasciola hepatica: IgG and IgA levels in the serum and bile of infected cattle. Exp. Parasitol., 52 (in press).

ACKNOWLEDGEMENTS

I am grateful to Dr. D.J. Burden for providing the sera and information on liver condemnations and on faecal egg counts of the slaughterhouse material, for the sera from O. ostertagi infected calves and for useful discussion. I would also like to thank Miss A. Ashford for excellent technical assistance.

PART III: REVIEW OF APPLICATION OF ELISA TO THE STUDY OF PROTOZOA

APPLICATION OF THE ENZYME LINKED IMMUNOSORBENT ASSAY (ELISA) IN VETERINARY PROTOZOOLOGY

W. P. H. DUFFUS

University of Cambridge, Department of Clinical Veterinary
Medicine, Madingley Road, Cambridge CB3 0ES.

INTRODUCTION

During the last ten years there has been a dramatic increase in the amount of research involving specific antibody to pathogens, and the field of protozoology is no exception. All such research requires assays which at some stage involve the recognition of antigen by specific antibody. Immunoglobulins are molecules with two functions, i.e. they recognize antigen and they also initiate a range of secondary phenomena like histamine release from mast cells. It is this second function which has led to the development of traditional serological tests such as complement fixation (CFT). Such assays, as well as those involving other functions like agglutination, precipitation and neutralization rely on secondary biological phenomena resulting from the initial antigen -antibody binding. This apparent drawback has led to the rapid development of immunoassays to measure the level of actual binding occuring between the protozoal antigen and specific antibody.

The two most promising candidates for such tests are the radioimmuno-assay (RIA) and ELISA. Both have their advantages and disadvantages, and there have been comparative trials between both tests for several protozoal diseases, such as trypanosomiasis, toxoplasmosis and malaria (Voller et al, 1977), both assays seem to give essentially the same results.

It is not the intention of this review to exhaustively list all the papers published on the application of the ELISA to protozoology, but more to use the literature to illustrate the areas where the ELISA will be most applicable to protozoal diseases.

Potential Use of ELISA

In the context of protozoal diseases there are three major areas involving an assay such as the ELISA:

1) SERODIAGNOSIS

2) SERO-EPIDEMIOLOGY

3) LABORATORY RESEARCH

Although there is overlap between all three tests as far as needs
and application are concerned, this overlap is especially obvious between
1) and 2).

SERODIAGNOSIS

Two of the major needs of a successful serodiagnostic test are
firstly sensitivity and secondly specificity. With protozoal diseases like
babesiosis and anaplasmosis a state of premunition (i.e. carrier state) is
common and diagnosis often difficult; the ELISA has been used in attempts
to satisfy both conditions. Bidwell et al (1978) compared the ELISA with
the indirect fluorescent antibody test (IFA) and CFT using sera from cattle
experimentally infected with B. divergens or B. major. These authors
found little to choose between the IFA and ELISA, both tests being more
sensitive than the CFT; although the latter did detect specific antibody
at an earlier date during primary infection.

Again with the ELISA Kratzer (1979) used both metabolic and somatic
antigens isolated from B. rodhaini parasitized mouse blood. He found that
the somatic antigen could be used to detect infection due to other species
of babesia in cattle and horses. With the ELISA positive results were
obtained when blood examination proved negative, the latter only reappear-
ing after splenectomy.

Thoen et al (1980) have applied the ELISA to diagnose anaplasmosis in
cattle. They compared the ELISA with CFT and the card test in 97 cattle
from a herd with confirmed anaplasmosis. (All tests proved negative using
clean control herds). Their results confirmed the increased sensitivity
obtained with the ELISA.

Gray et al, (1980) working with the cattle protozoa Theileria parva
and Th. annulata found excellent correlation between the IFA and ELISA
although antisera against either species of Theileria cross reacted
strongly with the heterologous antigen.

Although all this work would seem to indicate the suitability of the
ELISA as a serodiagnostic tool, the work of Gray et al (1980) I have just
mentioned does emphasize a potential drawback: The ELISA IS ONLY AS
SPECIFIC AS THE ANTIGEN ALLOWS.

This problem is further illustrated by work on two protozoa of medical importance, Trypanosoma cruzi and T. rangeli; both these parasites can occur together, the highly pathogenic T. cruzi and the nonpathogenic but common T. rangeli. Using the ELISA, Anthony et al (1979) demonstrated cross reaction between the two species. This is not surprising as Afchain et al (1978) have found common antigen between the two species, and as in so many of the ELISA and RIA work the protozoal antigen is a soluble preparation from the entire parasites with a Pandora's box of antigens. But in wishing to use the ELISA to help to identify foci of disease and to assess the immune status of populations against T. cruzi, Anthony and his co-workers argued that a positive result against both antigens could mean either a dual infection or a single infection with cross reacting antibody. This major problem of specificity is now the main reason preventing the rapid development of sensitive binding assays like the ELISA.

A similar problem occurs in bovine trypanosomiasis where the cosmopolitan T. theileri may be the cause of nonspecificity in the sero-diagnosis of T. brucei, T. congolense and T. vivax. Luckins (1977) using serum samples from T. theileri infected cattle found no cross-reaction with the salivarian trypanosome antigens, but work in our laboratory to some extent contradicts this (Townsend, unpublished results).

Finally, work involving another protozoa, Leishmania, can illustrate the advantages and disadvantages of the ELISA as a diagnostic tool. Roffi et al (1980) used L. tropica major as a source of antigen to serodiagnose cutaneous leishmaniasis in humans. The ELISA proved to be a highly sensitive and repeatable test, but they found cross reaction against the T. brucei group as well as T. cruzi and the more likely L. donovani.

What we desperately need are species specific and even strain specific protozoal antigens, free from contaminating mammalian cell material.

SERO-EPIDEMIOLOGY

The requirements of a serological assay for epidemiological surveys are closely interwoven with straight forward diagnostic tests, and the title should not push us solely to concentrate on the development of simple tests for the field. However, the simplicity of the ELISA, its lack of expensive and temperamental equipment and the relatively long "shelf-life" of its reagents do make it an attractive proposition for field work; utilizing small laboratories.

What exactly do we expect to gain from seroepidemiology research in veterinary protozoology? In the medical field examples are readily available: Bos et al (1980) used the ELISA in a seroepidemiological study of amoebiasis in Surinam. These authors examined nine populations, comparing the ELISA and the precipitinin test, their results were very encouraging: all patients with amoebic liver abscesses were positive, and 50% of symptomless carriers were positive (all these latter group were negative with the precipitinin test), whilst after treatment and with no reinfection there was a gradual _fall_ in the ELISA titre. So with such an assay one is poised to really try and eradicate a pathogen.

The ELISA has also been widely applied to another human protozoal disease, malaria. Spencer et al (1979a) used a crude _Plasmodium falciparum_ antigen found the assay excellent in the laboratory situation, but worried about problems in the field situation where many pathogenic and commensal protozoa coexist with cross reacting antigens; also where antibodies occur against contaminating antigens of mammalian origin in the crude _P. falciparum_ preparation, causing false positives. In separate experiments the same authors (Spencer et al, 1979b) and Voller (1980) found that a drawback of ELISA in malaria sero-epidemiology is a failure to detect all patients with confirmed infection e.g. of 15 individuals +ve on slide examination all 15 were positive with IFA but only 12/15 with the ELISA: the three negatives were all infants, a finding echoed by Voller (1980).

The use of the ELISA in the sero-epidemiology of protozoa of veterinary importance is still in its infancy. One important contribution is by Young and Purnell (1980) who examined the suitability of dried blood on filter paper as a source of antibody to _B. divergens_ in the ELISA. These authors also tested serum samples taken simultaneously and found excellent correlation between the two methods. The use of dried blood samples is likely to be of immeasurable benefit to sero-epidemiologists, especially those working with ruminants.

Special reference should be made to two protozoal zoonoses, Leishmania spp. and _Toxoplasma gondii_. Sero-epidemiology is vital with these pathogens as dogs and cats can act as reservoirs of infection, and accurate diagnosis will play an important part in their eventual control. Roffi et al (1980) have used _L. tropica major_ antigen in the ELISA for both cutaneous and visceral leishmaniasis and Denmark and Clessun (1978) and

Linet et al (1980) have studied toxoplasma with the ELISA.

RESEARCH

The protozoologist, whether a clinician or an epidemiologist, has come to regard serodiagnostic tests with some scepticism. One of the major problems is that parasites possess an armoury of antigens, of which those that actually are responsible for eliciting a functional immune response, and those that are species/strain specific, might well be minor constituents. With the ELISA we now have an assay with the potential to provide the means but we still lack the specificity, i.e. the purified antigen.

This is the area where our research in protozoology should now be directed, towards the isolation of these functional antigens. One of the techniques most likely to produce results is the use of monoclonals. This latter technique, and here I am sure I talk to the converted, can provide immortalized cell lines producing useful amounts of monospecific antibody. Monoclonal antibodies are now being used in conjunction with the ELISA (Polin and Kennett, 1980), to produce sensitive and reliable techniques to detect either specific antigen directly or by using a sandwich technique to detect specific antibody. In the ELISA we have an ideal tool for the rapid testing of potentially positive supernatents from hybridoma fusions.

In veterinary protozoology this problem of antigen is best illustrated by trypanosomiasis. A lot of the initial work on the use of the ELISA with trypanosomes of ruminants has been done by Luckins and his colleagues (Luckins, 1977; Luckins et al, 1978; Luckins and Nehlitz, 1978; Silago et al, 1980). These authors found that in vitro cultured forms of T. brucei gave similar ELISA values to those obtained with blood-stream form antigens (Silago et al, 1980), with the advantage that culture form antigen can more easily be prepared free from host proteins.

One problem that still exists with sero-diagnosis for salivarian trypanosomes is potential interference due to cross-reacting antigen from non-pathogenic species such as T. theileri. Although Luckins (1977) using the ELISA found no evidence of cross-reaction, work in our laboratory also using the ELISA has shown clear evidence of cross-reactivity. For example antisera from T.theileri infected calves when tested against both T. theileri and T. vivax antigen show a response against T. vivax

which follows closely the response against T. theileri, but usually 1 to
2 logs of specific antibody less. As the highest ELISA titre was 1:320
against the T. vivax antigen and Luckins only used the one dilution
of 1:500 this might well explain the different results.

Turning now to the use of the ELISA in research directed towards
the immune status of the host towards protozoa. This must be a two
pronged approach. Firstly to work out the level of specific immunoglobulin class and subclass activity against the relevant antigen in
situations like primary infection, serious fulminating infections,
carrier state, following drug sterilization etc. Following on from this
largely experimental approach, the situation in the field examined to
finally produce the evidence of what a certain combination of specific
immunoglobulins means i.e. the immune status (as far as antibody is
concerned). It will be only binding assays such as the ELISA, in conjunction with specific antigen, that will be able to produce such data.

We must always bear in mind pitfalls with serological tests. It is
interesting to read for instance of results obtained by Van Loon et al
(1980) who compared two commercially available ELISA kits for rubella
antibody with a standard haemagglutination inhibition test and the
author's own laboratory ELISA. Both commercial ELISAs failed to pick
out all positives (one of them picked out only approximately 25%). Big
improvements are still to be looked for in respect to the solid phase
used, storage, and inconsistent selective absorbtion of antigen and
antibody.

REFERENCES

Afchain, D., Fruit, J., Yarzabal, L. and Capron, A. 1978. Purification
of a specific antigen of Trypanosoma cruzi from culture forms.
Am. J. Trop. Med Hyg. 27, 478-482.

Anthony, R.L., Johnson, C.M. and Sousa, O.E. 1979. Use of the micro-
ELISA for quantitating antibody to Trypanosoma cruzi and Trypanosoma
rangeli. Am. J. Trop. Med. Hyg. 28, 969-973.

Bidwell, D.E., Turp, P., Joyner, L.P., Payne, R.C. and Purnell, R.E. 1978
Comparison of serological tests for Babesia in British cattle. Vet.
Rec. 103, 446-449.

Bos, H.J., Schouten, W.J., Noordpool, H., Makbin, M. and Oostbury, B.F.J.
1980. A seroepidemiological study of amebiasis in Surinam by the
ELISA. Am. J. Trop. Med. and Hyg., 29, 358-363.

Denmark, J.R. and Chessum, B.S. 1978. Standardization of enzyme-linked
immunosorbent assay (ELISA) and the detection of Toxoplasma antibody.
Med. Lab. Sc., 35, 227-232.

Gray, M.A., Luckins, A.G., Rae, P.F. and Brown, C.G.D. 1980. Evaluation of an enzyme immunoassay for serodiagnosis of infection with Theileria parva and Theileria annulata. Res.Vet.Sci., 29 360-366.

Kratzer, I., 1979. Die Brauchbarkeit der Babesia rodhaini-antigene zum Nachweis von Babesien-Infecktionen im ELISA. Dissertation, Fachbereich Tiermedizin, Munchen.

Lin, T.M., Halbert, S.P. and O'Connor, G.R. 1980. Standardized quantative enzyme-linked immunoassay for antibodies to Toxoplasma gondii. J.Clin.Microbiol., 11, 675-681.

Luckins, A.G., 1977. Detection of antibodies in trypanosome-infected cattle by means of a microplate enzyme-linked immunosorbent assay. Trop. Anim. Hlth. and Prod., 9, 53-62.

Luckins, A.G., Gray, A.R. and Rae, P. 1978. Comparison of the diagnostic value of serum immunoglobulin levels, on enzyme-linked immunoabsorbent assay and a fluorescent antibody test in experimental infections with Trypanosoma evansi in rabbits. Annals Trop. Med. Parasitol. 72, 429-441.

Luckins, A.G. and Mehlitz, D. 1978. Evaluation of an indirect fluorescent antibody test, enzyme-linked immunosorbent assay and quantification in the diagnosis of bovine trypanosomiasis. Trop. An. Hlth. and Prod. 10, 149-159.

Polin, R.A. and Kennett, R. 1980. Use of monoclonal antibodies in an enzyme immunoassay for rapid identification of group B streptococcus Types II and III. J. Clin. Microbiol. 11, 332-336.

Roffi. J., Dedet, J.P., Desjeux, P. and Garre, M-T. 1980. Detection of circulating antibodies in cutaneous leishmaniasis by ELISA. Am.J. Trop. Med. and Hyg., 29, 183-189.

Silayo, R.S., Gray, A.R. and Luckins, A.G. 1980. Use of antigens of cultured Trypanosoma brucei in tests for bovine trypanosomiasis. Trop. Anim. Hlth. Prod. 12, 127-131.

Spencer, H.C., Collins, W.E., Chin, W. and Skinner, J.C. 1979a. The enzyme linked immunosorbent assay (ELISA) for malaria. I The use of in vitro cultured Plasmodium falciparum as antigen. Am.J.Trop. Med. and Hyg., 28, 929-932.

Spencer, H.C., Collins, W.E. and Skinner, J.C. 1979b. The enzyme linked immunosorbent assay (ELISA) for malaria. II Comparison with the malaria IFA test. Am.J.Trop.Med. and Hyg. 28, 933-936

Thoen, C.O., Blackburn, B., Mills, K., Lomme, J. and Hopkins, M.P. 1980. Enzyme-linked immunosorbent assay for detecting antibodies in cattle in a herd in which anaplasmosis was diagnosed. J.Clin. Microbiol. 11, 499-505.

Van Loon, A.M., Van der Logt, J.Th.M. and Van der Veen, J. 1980. Evaluation of commercial ELISA tests. Lancet, 1980(1) 319.

Voller, A., Bidwell, D.E., Bartlett, A. and Edwards, R. 1977. A comparison of isotopic and enzyme immunoassays for tropical parasitic diseases. Trans. R. Soc. Trop.Med.Hyg., 71, 431-437

Voller, A. 1980. The use of solid phase isotopic and non-isotopic immunoassays in parasitic diseases with special reference to malaria. Int. J.Nucl.Med.Biol. 7, 157-163.

Young, E.R. and Purnell, R.E. 1980. Evaluation of dried blood samples as a source of antibody in the micro ELISA test for Babesia divergens. Vet. Rec., 106, 60-61.

THE IMPORTANCE OF COMPETITIVE BINDING IN THE DETECTION
OF ANTIGEN SPECIFIC BOVINE ISOTYPES AND SUBISOTYPES BY
THE MICRO-ELISA

Jackie Townsend, W.P.H. Duffus and D.A. Lammas

University of Cambridge, Department of Clinical Veterinary Medicine,
Madingley Road, Cambridge, CB3 OES, U.K.

ABSTRACT

An enzyme-linked immunosorbent assay was developed to detect and
quantify the specific bovine immunoglobulin class response to Trypanosoma
theileri, Dictyocaulus viviparus and Infectious bovine rhinotracheitis
virus. Comparative measurement of the specific immunoglobulin classes in
whole serum was achieved using monospecific rabbit anti-bovine IgG_1, IgG_2
and IgM, followed by goat anti-rabbit Ig-enzyme conjugate. Competitive
inhibition between specific immunoglobulins of different isotypes and subisotypes was a major disadvantage. The assay failed to detect specific
IgG_2 against T. theileri antigen in both calf and adult whole serum, which
was the result of competitive inhibition by specific IgG_1. However,
competitive inhibition between specific immunoglobulins was not observed
in either of the other tests systems using D. viviparus and IBR virus
antigens.

INTRODUCTION

The structural heterogeneity of ruminant immunoglobulins has been

established for some while (Butler et al., 1971) although little is known

about the functional properties of the different classes and subclasses.

Bovine IgG_1 and IgG_2 have been shown to fix complement (McGuire, Musoke

and Kurtti, 1979) and mediate antibody-dependent cell-mediated cytotoxicity

(ADCC, Duffus et al., 1978). The cytophilic activity of ruminant IgG sub-

classes has also been investigated (Watson, 1976; McGuire et al., 1979).

A binding assay, such as the ELISA, provides a sensitive and reliable

method by which more information may be obtained about the specific immuno-

globulin class response to immunogens and pathogens. The ELISA was first

used for this purpose by Engvall, Jonsson and Perlmann (1971). Using the

ELISA, there are various methods which may be employed to detect and

quantify the specific immunoglobulin class response. These include:

(1) Direct measurement of specific activity in purified immunoglobulins,

(2) Indirect measurement of specific immunoglobulins in whole serum using

monospecific anti-immunoglobulin class sera conjugated directly to the

enzyme, (3) Indirect measurement of specific immunoglobulins in whole serum

using unconjugated monospecific anti-immunoglobulin class sera followed by either a polyvalent anti-species immunoglobulin conjugated with the enzyme, or a bridging antibody plus an antibody-enzyme complex (the amplified ELISA, Butler et al., 1978).

The ability to directly detect class specific antibodies in whole serum is obviously less time consuming than having to fractionate immunoglobulins. However, competitive binding between antibodies which differ in their avidity or affinity is a potential problem (Butler et al., 1978). We have developed an ELISA assay to quantify the class specific response in whole bovine antiserum against 3 different pathogens, while at the same time the problem of competitive binding was investigated.

MATERIALS AND METHODS

These are described in detail elsewhere (Townsend et al., 1982). Briefly monospecific antisera were prepared against bovine IgG_1, IgG_2 and IgM by inoculating rabbits with purified fractions. Each antiserum was extensively absorbed using Sepharose immunoadsorbents and the two heterologous immunoglobulins.

The optimal concentration of each immunoglobulin was first calculated in the ELISA using dose response curves. Each affinity purified antiserum was then tested against both the homologous and the two heterologous immunoglobulins. Each antiserum had a titre of at least 1:10,000 and the amount of cross-reaction with the heterologous antigen was 1% or less.

The purification of antigen from Trypanosoma theileri, Dictyocaulus viviparus and Infectious bovine rhinotracheitis virus (IBR) is reported elsewhere (Townsend et al., 1982). Each antigen was also titrated in the Elisa to establish the optimal concentration for coating the microplates.

The ELISA technique using Alkaline phosphatase conjugated anti-bovine immunoglobulin and anti-rabbit immunoglobulin is reported elsewhere (Townsend et al., 1982). Bovine IgM, IgG_1 and IgG_2 were purified from specific antisera against the three antigens as previously reported (Duffus and Wagner, 1974; Duffus et al., 1978).

RESULTS AND DISCUSSION

The results obtained in the ELISA, using purified immunoglobulins from the specific antisera, were compared to those obtained using whole serum and monospecific antiserum to each immunoglobulin class and subclass.

T. theileri

Specific IgM, G_1 and G_2 activity was detected in the purified immunoglobulin fractions, but when whole serum was used the specific IgG_2 activity against this protozoal antigen was greatly reduced. This was shown in antisera obtained from both calves after a single primary infection, as well as from adult cows.

D. viviparus and IBR

IgM, IgG_1 and IgG_2 fractions from antisera against both pathogens were tested for specific activity. The results were compared to those obtained using whole serum and the monospecific antisera against each immunoglobulin isotype and subisotype. In direct contrast to the T. theileri situation, no reduction in the specific IgG_2 activity occurred using whole sera.

Competitive Inhibition

To examine the possibility of competitive inhibition between different isotypes or subisotypes in more detail, purified immunoglobulins from antisera to T. theileri were mixed in equal concentration in pairs, and then retested in the ELISA using the monospecific antisera. The results of this experiment clearly demonstrated that the specific IgG_1 is responsible for the inhibition of the specific IgG_2. No inhibition is caused by the IgM. These results strongly suggest that competitive binding occurs between specific antibodies for the limited amount of antigen bound to the solid phase. This may well be due to specific immunoglobulins of different subisotypes possessing different avidities.

Although the ELISA is a rapid and sensitive assay for the detection and quantification of class specific immunoglobulins in whole serum, each new system must be separately evaluated using purified immunoglobulin fractions as well as whole serum. As long as this initial precaution is taken, errors caused by competitive binding between different class specific immunoglobulins will be avoided.

REFERENCES

Butler, J.E., McGivern, P.L. and Swanson, P. 1978. Amplification of the enzyme-linked immunosorbent assay (ELISA) in the detection of class-specific antibodies. J. Immunol. Methods 20, 365-383.

Butler, J.E., Winter, A.J. and Wagner, G.G. 1971. Symposium: Bovine immune system. J. Dairy Sci., 54, 1309-1340.

Duffus, W.P.H., Butterworth, A.E., Wagner, G.G., Preston, J.M. and Franks, D. 1978. Antibody-dependent cell-mediated cytotoxicity in cattle: activity against ^{51}Cr-labelled chicken erythrocytes coated with protozoal antigens. Infect. and Immunity 22, 492-501.

Duffus, W.P.H. and Wagner, G.G. 1974. Immunoglobulin response in cattle immunized with Theileria parva stabilate. Parasitology 69, 31-34.

Engvall, E., Jonsson, J. and Perlmann, P. 1971. Enzyme-linked immuno-sorbent assay. II. Quantitative assay of protein antigen, immuno-globulin G, by means of enzyme labelled antigen and antibody coated tubes. Biochem. Biophys. Acta 251, 427-434.

McGuire, T.C., Musoke, A.J. and Kurtti, T. 1979. Functional properties of bovine IgG_1 and IgG_2: Interaction with complement, macrophages, neutrophils and skin. Immunology 38, 249-256.

Townsend, A.J., Duffus, W.P.H. and Lammas, D.A. 1982. The importance of competitive binding in the detection of antigen specific bovine iso-types and subisotypes by the micro-ELISA. (Submitted).

Watson, D.L. 1976. The effect of cytophilic IgG_2 on phagocytosis by ovine polymorphonuclear leucocytes. Immunology, 31, 159-165.

PART IV: APPLICATION OF ELISA TO THE STUDY OF BACTERIA AND MYCOPLASM

NEWER CONCEPTS FOR THE DETECTION OF STAPHYLOCOCCUS ENTEROTOXINS BY ELISA.

Hans Fey

Veterinary Bacteriological Institute University of Bern

ELISA has been introduced into the detection of Staphylococcal enterotoxins by SAUNDERS (1977), then SIMON & TERPLAN (1977) and ourselves together with G.STIFFLER (1977;1978). We deviced a triple ball test yielding a sensitivity of o.1 ng/ml.

Since it is known that a sensitive person falls ill after the ingestion of 1 ug enterotoxin A it is evident that our method is safely below the limit of clinical relevance. Further research should therefore not aim at the increase of the sensitivity of serological methods but at an easy and cheap practicability of the method. An accurate and rapid diagnosis of food poisoning which is most frequently caused by Staphylococci will only become possible when commercial diagnostic kits are available.

Unfortunately there is a serious drawback in our own method. Since it is a competitive technique, the antigen, i.e. the enterotoxin, must be labelled in a fairly pure state. We had no difficulty in producing milligram-amounts of the enterotoxins A,B and C for this purpose, but ran into considerable troubles with the toxins D and E. This will be a limiting factor for potential commercial interest.

Together with WALTER BOMMELI (1980) we used enzyme-labelled protein A successfully in virus serology and in my laboratory the experimental serology is based entirely on this practical tool whenever we are working with antibodies coming from rabbit, man, guinea pig, mouse or swine. It is also used by us for the measurement of human tetanus antitoxin.

However, there is a reservation to be made: It is not recommended for Salmonella serology, where IgM plays an important role (SCHIFFMANN and FEY, in press).

I therefore decided to make use of protein A-phosphatase (SPA-PH) as a universal label in a sandwich enterotoxin ELISA with the following concept:

anti Ent-Enterotoxin-anti Ent-SPA-PH

But it is evident, that SPA-PH, mainly in the absence of enterotoxin, will bind to the Fc-piece of the coating antibody, thus causing severe non-specific uptake of the label.

Therefore I pepsinized the coating antibody which did not work at all, i.e. the uptake of labelled antigen was very bad.

I then became aware of KOPER and NOTERMANS' work (1980) who pepsinized their coating antibody to $F(ab')_2$ and coated it to polystyrene tubes using PBS. When I repeated my experiments with three pH's 9.6, 8 and 7.2 I found that only the latter two allowed a reasonable binding of $F(ab')_2$ to polystyrene. Since then I strongly recommend to try different coating pH's whenever a new system is to be developed.

KOPER and NOTERMANS, who used a sandwich technique, pepsinized their antibody because they realized that in cultures and food extracts, contaminated with pathogenic staphylococci, protein A is present and interferes with serology.

After this experience I worked out a very sensitive method for the measurement of protein A according to the following scheme:

⌇-Tetanustoxoid-human antitoxin-SPA + SPA-PH

SPA competes with SPA-PH for the binding site of the Fc-piece of antitoxin. By using the toxoid/antitoxin system instead of IgG alone as coat the Fc-piece is well exposed and freely accessible.

Being aware of the presence of SPA in considerable amounts in culture supernatants of pathogenic Staphylococci including the respective food extracts and knowing that F(ab')2 does not bind very well to polystyrene I decided to eliminate the protein A by a very simple procedure: I insolubilized porcine IgG with glutaraldehyde. The sediment of ten ml of a 10% suspension was mixed with 10 ml of the culture supernatant and rotated for 30 min. , which was sufficient for the absorption of as much as 250 ug SPA/10 ml (FEY and BURKHARD, 1981).

In order to facilitate the technique by using SPA-PH as a universal label and after all avoiding the labelling of purified enterotoxin I deviced an inhibition ELISA according to the following system:

Anti Ent is incubated with the enterotoxin to be detected. Thereafter ENT insolubilized to a carrier is added. In the presence of enterotoxin the antibody will not bind. In the absence of enterotoxin it will do so. Its presence is demonstrated by SPA-PH.

The carrier for the coating antigen is a tube or a precision polystyrene ball or, eventually, a small nitrocellulose filter pad. The great advantage of the method is the use of a crude culture supernatant as coating agent. It may be necessary to run a first step purification by Amberlite cationic exchange, but that is very easily done. In preliminary trials we could use the supernatants in dilutions of 1/200 or less. Another advantage is the use of crude antiserum as trapping antibody, which however must be free of antibodies against staphylococcal antigens other than enterotoxin. If not it has to be absorbed on a Sepharose column activated with the supernatant proteins from a non-enterotoxigenic Staphylococcus strain. It is essential, however, that protein has been removed from this absorbent as indicated above.

So it would only be necessary to produce fairly purified enterotoxin for the immunization of a rabbit. For this purpose the degree of purity of the immunogen must not be exceedingly high since the resulting antibody can be rendered specific by absorption, a common procedure in Salmonella- and E. coli serology.

This method makes use of the fact that in ELISA only one reagent must be specific, either the coating antigen or the indicator antibody, but not both of them.

It is too early yet to comment about the sensitivity of the method.

Still another possibility for the usage of a single label is the avidin-biotin system. Avidin is relatively inexpensive, commercially available and binds very strongly to biotin. In my laboratory M. SUTER is using it successfully for the detection of equine IgE.

The system works nicely but it is still too premature to speak about its sensitivity.

Quite recently we started with preparing our conjugates with SPDP (Pharmacia) after W. BOMMELI was successful with such a protein A-peroxidase conjugate (personal communication).

Succinimidyl-pyridyldithio-propionate is a heterobifunctional reagent for thiolation and for the production of intermolecular conjugates. We do not hesitate to recommend this very practical procedure which yields highly potent conjugates. EVA ENGVALL (1978) reported on a working dilution of 0.5 ug/ml obtained with her SPA-phosphatase conjugate which she prepared with the two-step glutaraldehyde technique. I possess now conjugates 4 times stronger than that with working dilutions of 1/8000 and more. The same is true for anti enterotoxin IgG-conjugates.

But for the preparation of these antibodies there is still an urgent need for an easy and reproducible method of enterotoxin production. At the present time we depend upon a series of very laborious steps of cationic exchange and gel filtration with heavy losses. I therefore applied the preparative isoelectric focussing in a flat gel and obtained very promising results. The first step is still a cationic exchange on Amberlite which purifies and concentrates the enterotoxin. This product is then submitted to isoelectric focussing.

The gel bed is cut into strips the eluates of which can be examined for enterotoxin using GEDELISA (BRUGGMANN and LUTZ, 1978).

Even with enterotoxin D, which is a very low toxin producer, my coworker CHR. MUELLER reached a very high degree of purification as shown by polyacrylamide electrophoresis.

The next step is the application of chromatofocussing to the same purpose. Using the enterotoxins A, B and C I already demonstrated that this method eventually could be the method of choice.

REFERENCES

Bommeli A., U. Kihm, F. Zindel and H. Fey 1980. Enzyme
    Linked Immuno   Assay and fluorescent antibody
    techniques in the diagnosis of viral diseases using
    staphylococcal protein A instead of anti gamma glo-
    bulins. Vet. Immunol. Immunopath. 1, 179-193.

Bruggmann S. and H. Lutz 1978. Gelelectrophoresis-derived
    enzyme-linked immunosorbent assay (GEDELISA): A new
    technique for the characterisation of antibody speci-
    ficity and the detection of antigens in complex
    mixture. USGEB,Berichte d. 10. Jahresvers., Davos Mai
    Experientia.

Engvall E. 1978. Preparation of enzyme-labelled Staphylo-
    coccal protein A   and its use for detection of
    antibodies. In: Engvall E.   and   A.J. Pesce:
    Quantitative Enzyme Immuno-Assay. Blackwell Sci. Publ.,
    London .

Fey H. and G. Stiffler-Rosenberg 1977. Detection of
    staphylococcal enterotoxin B with a new modification of
    the Enzyme Linked Immuno Sorbent Assay. Experientia 33,
    1678.

Fey H. and G. Burkhard 1981. Sensitive measurement of sta-
    phylococcal protein A and detection of protein A-
    carrying Staphylococcus strains by a competetive ELISA
    method.   J. Immunol. Meth., in press .

Koper J.W., A.M. Hagenaars and S. Notermans 1980. Preven-
    tion of cross- reactions in the Enzyme Linked Immuno
    Assay (ELISA) for the detection of Staphylococcus
    aureus enterotoxin type B in culture filtrates and
    foods. J. Food Safety 2, 35-35 .

Saunders G.C., and M.L. Bartlett 1977. Double-antibody
    solid phase enzyme immunoassay for the detection of
    staphylococcal   enterotoxin A. Appl. Environm. Micro-
    biol. 34, 518-522 .

Schiffmann E. und H. Fey 1981. Entwicklung eines Salmo-
    nella-ELISA, geeignet fhr Massenserologie. Schweiz.
    Arch. Tierheilk. in press.

Simon E. and G. Terplan 1977. Nachweis von Staphylokokken
    Enterotoxin B mittels ELISA-Test. Zbl. Vet.Med.B, 24,
    842-844 .

Stiffler-Rosenberg G. and H. Fey 1978. Simple assay for
    staphylococcal enterotoxins A,B and C: Modification of
    Enzyme Linked Immuno Assay. J. Clin. Microbiol. 8,
    473-479 .

ANTIBODIES, BY ELISA, TO MYCOPLASMAS IN BOVINE SERA

C.J. Howard, R.N. Gourlay, L.H. Thomas, J. Eynon

Agricultural Research Council,
Institute for Research on Animal Diseases,
Compton, near Newbury, Berkshire RG16 0NN, U.K.

ABSTRACT

Antibodies to Mycoplasma dispar and M. bovis were measured by an ELISA in the sera of cattle following vaccination with killed organisms and oil adjuvant. For M. dispar the IgG1 response preceeded the IgG2 response in all cases. However, these responses varied in groups of calves with different ages (average age of groups 16, 59 and 155 days) being greatest in the oldest group and least in the youngest. In contrast, following vaccination with M. bovis little difference was noted in the IgG1 responses in the different age-groups (average ages 16, 55 and 150 days) although the IgG2 response was less in the youngest group. The potential importance of this age effect on the ability to mount an IgG2 antibody response to both mycoplasma species and the ability to respond to M. dispar per se is discussed.

An ELISA has also been used to measure antibody to M. dispar in calves with naturally occurring respiratory disease. Increases in antibody in association with some outbreaks of disease were observed.

INTRODUCTION

A number of species of mycoplasma have been isolated from calves with pneumonia or respiratory disease. Mycoplasma bovis, M. dispar and Ureaplasma sp. are the species most frequently isolated from pneumonic calf lungs in the U.K. and all three have also been proven to be pathogenic for calves (Gourlay and Howard, 1979). Ureaplasma sp. from cattle grow poorly compared to the other two species; furthermore they are serologically complex and based on serological and polypeptide studies appear to comprise three clusters of similar strains. M. bovis and M. dispar are serologically homogeneous.

This communication concerns aspects of the immune response of calves to M. dispar and M. bovis. The purpose of these studies has been to further our understanding of the mechanisms of immunity to mycoplasmas in cattle with an eventual view to controlling infection. An ELISA has been used to examine the antibody response following immunisation and to detect a serological response following natural outbreaks of respiratory disease.

MATERIALS AND METHODS

The system currently used for the ELISA is as follows.

Antigen

Mycoplasmas grown as described previously (Howard et al., 1980) in broth containing foetal calf serum or porcine serum were harvested by centrifugation (10,000 xg, 30 min, $4^{o}C$), washed three times, resuspended in 0.15M NaCl at about 5 mg protein per ml (Lowry) and stored at $-70^{o}C$. This suspension (0.5 ml) was added to 9.5 ml 0.05M carbonate-bicarbonate buffer, pH 10, incubated at $37^{o}C$ for 30 min and stored at $-20^{o}C$. To sensitise trays the suspension in pH 10 buffer was diluted in 0.05M carbonate-bicarbonate buffer pH 9.6 to the previously determined optimum, usually about 1 µg protein per ml (Horowitz and Cassell, 1978).

A method involving treatment of antigens with sodium deoxycholate (Howard, 1981) was used for some tests. Essentially the same results were obtained with antigens treated in either manner except that residual sodium deoxycholate appeared to inhibit antigen binding to plates at higher antigen concentrations.

Anti-globulin sera

Rabbit anti-bovine IgG1, IgG2 and IgA sera were from Miles Labs. and rabbit anti-bovine IgM from Nordic. Horseradish peroxidase (HRP) conjugated with goat-anti-rabbit globulin was obtained from Miles Labs. For the simplified direct ELISA rabbit anti-bovine IgG from Nordic was coupled with HRP (Avrameas and Ternynck, 1971). This reagent detected bovine IgG1 and IgG2, some anti IgG reagents reacted predominantly with only one bovine Ig subclass. Optimum dilutions of anti-globulin sera were determined in the usual manner.

Substrate

Unless stated otherwise the substrate was 5-amino-salicylic acid (5AS) that had been repurified (Ellens et al., 1978). One gram of 5AS was dissolved in 100 ml of stock buffer (2.5 vol. 0.1M $NaH_2 PO_4$, 2.75 vol. 0.1M $Na_2 HPO_4$, 0.05 vol. 0.1M Na_2 EDTA at pH 6.8) together with 900 ml of double distilled, deionised water (DDW) and stored at $-20^{o}C$. For use 10 ml of substrate was mixed with 10 µl of 5% w/v H_2O_2.

Washing

Plates were washed either by hand 6 times with 0.15M phosphate-buffered-saline pH 7.2 (PBS) containing 0.05% Tween 20 (Sigma) or with a plate-washing machine, constructed at Compton, for 3 x 3 sec with 0.005M

Tris-HCl pH 7.3 containing 0.05% Tween 20.

ELISA

All incubations were at room temperature. Antigen suspension, 100 µl per well, in pH 9.6 buffer was added to Linbro EIA microtitration plates. Plates were incubated overnight and washed. 200 µl of 0.1% bovine serum albumin in pH 9.6 buffer was added to each well, plates were then incubated for 30 min and washed. Dilutions of test-sera (100 µl) were made in PBS containing 0.05% Tween. After 90 min incubation followed by washing, 100 µl of rabbit anti-bovine Ig in PBS and Tween was added. Following 90 min incubation and washing, 100 µl HRP conjugated antiglobulin in PBS and Tween was added. After 120 min incubation and washing, 100 µl of substrate was added. After 60 min incubation the OD_{492} nm was measured, using an ELISA plate reader (Titertek, Flow).

To determine the number of units of antibody in a serum, sample test sera were compared with a standard included in all tests. The titre of the standard serum was taken as the reciprocal of the highest dilution that gave an OD twice that obtained with antigen-coated wells that had been treated with all reagents except the test serum (Howard, 1981). The geometric mean titre from five or more determinations was calculated and the number of units of specific IgG1 or IgG2 in the standard serum defined as equal to the titre. The OD values of the dilutions of the test serum were plotted and the number of units of antibody in the test serum determined by comparing their curves with the standard.

Calves

The conventionally reared Ayrshire calves and methods used for immunisation were as previously described (Howard et al., 1980, 1981). Derivation and maintenance of the gnotobiotic Friesian cross calves has been described (Dennis et al., 1976).

Sera from calves in a beef-rearing unit

Sera were collected from five groups of eight calves, selected from groups of about 100, maintained on a beef rearing unit. These animals were bled regularly (about every 30 days) and monitored for respiratory disease over a period of 160 to 220 days, as has been described in detail (Stott et al., 1980). The calves averaged 10 days of age when first bled (time 0 Fig. 6), other details are given in Table 1.

TABLE 1   Details of calves maintained in a beef rearing unit

Calf group No.	No. calves in group	Date[1]	%[2] respiratory disease	%[3] pneumonia
8	114	Jan. 1972	9	1
15	94	June 1973	7	0
17	95	Sept. 1973	33	1
21	100	May 1974	42	2
28	104	Oct. 1975	9	2

(1) Date of first serum sample.   (2) % of calves treated for respiratory disease.   (3) % of deaths ascribed to pneumonia.

Paired sera from calves with respiratory disease

These were taken, at 3 to 4 week intervals, from groups of calves in the acute stage of clinical respiratory disease when first bled.   The animals are described in detail by Thomas et al. (1981).   Some details of numbers of outbreaks and calves are given in Table 2.

RESULTS

Serological response of conventionally reared calves to inoculation of M. dispar

Ayrshire calves were inoculated with formalin-killed M. dispar (1.2 mg protein per dose) combined with incomplete Freund's adjuvant or Marcol 52/Arlacel A (30:70).   Tween 80, 1%, was included in the aqueous phase. Three subcutaneous (s.c.) inoculations of 4 or 5 ml total volume were given at three-weekly intervals.   At the time of the first s.c. injection the three groups of inoculated calves had average ages of 16, 59 and 155 days. The IgG1 and IgG2 antibody responses to M. dispar, given as means for the groups ± the standard error, are shown in Figs. 1 and 2.   No IgA and a very small or no IgM responses were detected in the sera.

The specific IgG1 response was greatest in the oldest and least in the youngest animals.   This effect was particularly pronounced during the first 6 weeks following the primary and secondary injections.   In the youngest group a specific response was barely detectable following a single s.c. inoculation of M. dispar-antigen.   Similar results were obtained for the IgG2 antibody response to M. dispar, no specific IgG2 response was detected

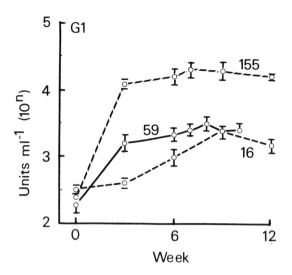

Fig. 1   IgG1 antibody in serum of calves following the subcutaneous
inoculation of formalin-killed M. dispar.   Calves inoculated at weeks
0, 3 and 6 with 1.2 mg antigen-protein with oil adjuvant.   Three
groups of animals injected;━━, 10 calves, average age 16 days;
━━, 5 calves, average age 59 days; ━━, 9 calves, average age 155
days.   Mean IgG1 antibody units plotted ± standard error.

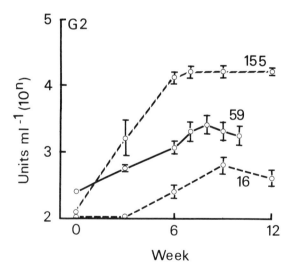

Fig. 2   IgG2 antibody in serum of calves following injection of
M. dispar.   See Fig. 1 for key.

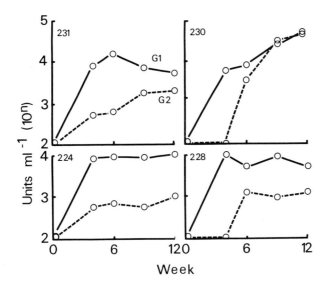

Fig. 3   Antibody response to M. dispar in 4 gnotobiotic calves.
Animals inoculated subcutaneously at 0, 2, 4, 6 and 8 weeks with
killed mycoplasmas with adjuvant and intratracheally at week 9 with
10^9 organisms.   O—O, IgGl; O--O, IgG2;   224, 228, 231, 230,
calf nos.

in the youngest calves following a single s.c. injection.   A comparison of
the IgGl and IgG2 antibody responses within each age group indicated that
IgGl antibody appeared before IgG2 (compare values in Figs. 1 and 2).

Serological response of gnotobiotic calves to M. dispar

Four gnotobiotic calves were inoculated s.c., five times at two-week
intervals, with killed M. dispar (1.2 mg protein) with Freund's incomplete
adjuvant (Fig. 3).   Mycoplasmas were killed by formalin (calves 224 and
231) or cobalt irradiation (calves 228 and 230).   The IgGl response
preceeded the IgG2 response in all four animals.   The number of units of
IgG2 antibody only reached that observed for IgGl in one calf.

Serological response of conventionally reared calves to inoculation of
M. bovis

Three s.c. injections were given of formalin-killed-antigen (1.2 mg
protein) with Freund's incomplete adjuvant, or Marcol-Arlacel, with 1%
Tween in the aqueous phase.   The IgGl responses to M. bovis in the sera of
calves in the three groups, with average ages of 16, 55 and 150 days,

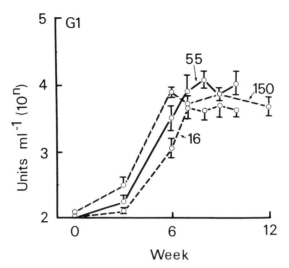

Fig. 4   IgGl antibody in the serum of calves following the
subcutaneous inoculation of formalin killed <u>M. bovis</u>.   Calves
inoculated on weeks 0, 3 and 6 with 1.2 mg antigen-protein with oil
adjuvant.   Three groups of calves injected; ▬ ▬, 5 calves average age
16 days; ▬▬▬, 5 calves average age 55 days; ▬▬▬, 9 calves average
age 150 days.   Mean IgGl antibody units plotted ± standard error.

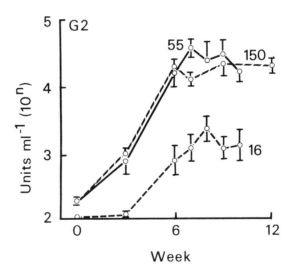

Fig. 5   IgG2 antibody in serum of calves following injection of
M. bovis.   See Fig. 3 for key.

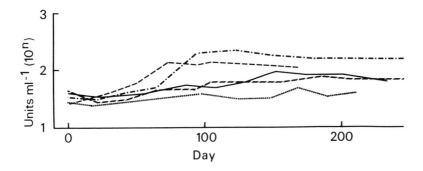

Fig. 6   Antibody to M. dispar in calf sera.   Mean no. units IgG in
five groups of eight calves examined over several months.
━ ━ , group 8; ▬▬ group 15; ▰▰ group 17; ⅰⅰⅰⅰⅰⅰ group 21;
▪ ━ ▪ , group 28.

are shown in Fig. 4.   Only a slight difference was noted between calves of
different ages.   Thus, M. bovis and M. dispar appear to differ in this
respect.   The IgG2 responses are shown in Fig. 5;   similar responses were
observed in the two older groups while in the youngest the IgG2 response
was considerably less.   In the '16 day' group the IgG1 response preceeded
the increase in IgG2 but in the other two groups IgG1 and IgG2 appeared to
be produced at about the same time.

Antibody to M. dispar in sera from calves on a beef rearing unit

Serum collected regularly over a period of 6 to 8 months from groups
of calves held in a beef-rearing unit were examined for IgG antibody to
M. dispar.   HRP coupled anti-bovine IgG was used and the two subclasses of
IgG were not distinguished.   The substrate used was o-phenylenediamine.

The mean responses of five groups of eight calves are depicted in
Fig. 6.   A small increase in the mean number of units of antibody was
observed in two of the groups.

Antibody responses to M. dispar in paired sera from calves with respiratory disease

The number of animals with sera showing four-fold or greater increases
in the number of units of IgG antibody and the number of calves with $>10^3$
units in their sera are shown in Table 2.   Not all outbreaks gave the same
results.   In some, serological evidence was obtained that infection with
M. dispar occurred at the time of the disease outbreak.

TABLE 2   Antibody[1] to <u>M. dispar</u> in sera from calves with
respiratory disease

Outbreak[2]	No. paired sera	No. animals with four-fold increase	No. animals with >10^3 units
A	7	4	6
B	9	2	5
D	6	2	3
E	7	1	2
F	8	0	0
G	8	1	1
H	8	0	2

(1) Units of IgG.   (2) See Thomas et al. (1981 in preparation) for
details.

DISCUSSION

The amounts of IgG1 and IgG2 antibodies have been expressed as
arbitrary units, not as absolute values.   Although the number of Ig
molecules obviously relates to the number of units, other factors such as
antibody affinity affect the values obtained.   Comparisons can therefore be
made between animals but between Ig subclasses reservations are necessary.

Following the <u>s.c.</u> injection of <u>M. dispar</u> IgG1 antibody appeared
before IgG2.   As the age of the calves increased the difference in time of
appearance of IgG1 and IgG2 was less marked.   In the youngest calves the
number of IgG1 units was always greater than the number of IgG2 units.   In
older calves, IgG2 eventually reached the same level as IgG1.   In calves
with an average age of 16 days the number of units of IgG1 antibody to
<u>M. bovis</u> exceeded those of IgG2, whereas in the two older groups IgG2
exceeded IgG1.

The appearance of IgG2 antibody after IgG1, particularly in young
calves, is consistent with other observations on the ontogeny of IgG1 and
IgG2 synthesis in cattle.   Thus, ability to synthesise IgG1 is present by
about day 135 of gestation while ability to synthesise IgG2 appears not to
be well developed until after birth (Schultz, 1973; Tizzard, 1977).

It has been proposed that, in cattle, IgG2 is more effective than IgG1
in promoting neutrophil functions (McGuire et al., 1979; Howard et al.,
1980b; Mossmann et al., 1981) although IgG1 together with complement may be

as effective. An inability to synthesise IgG2 antibody in young calves
following an infection could result in suboptimal neutrophil function in
these animals which is possibly related to increased susceptibility to
certain infectious diseases of neonatal calves.   For the same reason
immunisation of neonatal calves with a variety of antigens might be less
effective than in older animals.

The IgG1 response to M. dispar was markedly less in young calves
compared to older ones whereas, little difference was seen in animals of the
three age groups injected with M. bovis.   Several mechanisms might be
implicated in this observation.   Since calves in the UK are commonly
infected with M. dispar (Gourlay and Howard, 1979) the greater response
seen in older calves may result from priming following colonisation of the
respiratory tract by this mycoplasma.   M. bovis is not endemic and so the
same effect is not observed.   That a specific or non-specific effect of
colostrum is responsible seems unlikely, since gnotobiotic calves not fed
colostrum responded in much the same way as conventionally reared animals.
An alternative explanation is that the ability of calves, and other animals,
to respond immunologically to any given antigen is acquired at different
times in the development of the foetus or neonatal animal (Schultz, 1973;
Tizzard, 1977).   Perhaps the relevant antigens of M. dispar are among those
that are recognised late in immunological ontogeny.

The relatively poor antibody response to M. dispar, in young calves,
could explain another observation.   Characteristically the early experimental lesion observed in the lungs of young gnotobiotic calves, following
the inoculation of M. dispar, is an alveolitis.   In contrast pronounced
perivascular and peribronchial accumulations of lymphocytes occur in the
lungs of gnotobiotic calves inoculated with M. bovis (Gourlay et al., 1976,
1979; Howard et al., 1976).   This lymphocyte accumulation is considered
to be a part of the immune response to respiratory mycoplasmal infections
and a major site of immunoglobulin synthesis (Cassell et al., 1973).
Consequently the inability of young calves to respond immunologically to
M. dispar might be associated with the absence of pulmonary lymphocyte
accumulations.   Furthermore the immunisation of young calves against
M. dispar might be ineffective if an antibody response is lacking.

Serial serum samples taken from the five groups of calves in a beef-
rearing unit revealed no marked antibody increase in association with
outbreaks of respiratory disease; M. dispar is frequently isolated from
calves on the farm in question and the low level of antibody to M. dispar

detected may be typical of animals simply colonised by this mycoplasma without the organism being involved in severe disease.

Of the paired sera taken from calves in groups with clinical respiratory disease 10 of 53 showed a four-fold or greater increase in ELISA antibody to M. dispar. These were derived from 5 of the 7 outbreaks. Thus, M. dispar may be associated with some outbreaks of respiratory disease and it is possible that such seroconversions indicate invasion of the lung tissue and a role in lesion production, rather than simply colonisation of the respiratory tract.

REFERENCES

Avrameas, S. and Ternynck, T. 1971. Peroxidase labelled antibody and Fab conjugates with enhanced intracellular penetration. Immunochemistry, 8, 1175-1179.

Cassell, G.H., Lindsey, J.R. and Baker, H.J. 1974. Immune response of pathogen-free mice inoculated intranasally with Mycoplasma pulmonis. J. Immunol., 112, 124-136.

Dennis, M.J., Davies, D.C. and Hoare, M.N. 1976. A simplified apparatus for the microbiological isolation of calves. Br. Vet. J., 132, 642-646.

Ellens, D.J., de Leeuw, P.W., Straver, P.J. and van Balken, J.A.M. 1978. Comparison of five diagnostic methods for the detection of rotavirus antigens in calf faeces. Med. Microbiol. Immunol., 166, 157-163.

Gourlay, R.N. and Howard, C.J. 1979. Bovine Mycoplasmas. In "The Mycoplasmas vol. II" (Ed. J.G. Tully and R.F. Whitcomb). (Academic Press, N.Y.) pp 49-102.

Gourlay, R.N., Howard, C.J., Thomas, L.H. and Wyld, S.G. 1979. Pathogenicity of some Mycoplasma and Acholeplasma species in the lungs of gnotobiotic calves. Res. Vet. Sci., 27, 233-237.

Gourlay, R.N., Thomas, L.H. and Howard, C.J. 1976. Pneumonia and arthritis in gnotobiotic calves following inoculation with Mycoplasma agalactiae subsp. bovis. Vet. Rec., 98, 506-507.

Howard, C.J. 1981. Mycoplasmacidal action of bovine complement mediated by bovine IgG1, IgG2 or IgM. Vet. Microbiol. In the Press.

Howard, C.J., Gourlay, R.N. and Taylor, G. 1980. Immunity to Mycoplasma bovis infections of the respiratory tract of calves. Res. Vet. Sci., 28, 242-249.

Howard, C.J., Gourlay, R.N. and Taylor, G. 1981. Immunity to mycoplasma infections of the calf respiratory tract. In "The Ruminant Immune System". Adv. Exp. Med. Biol. vol. 137. pp 711-726 (Ed. J.E. Butler) (Plenum, New York).

Howard, C.J., Gourlay, R.N., Thomas, L.H. and Stott, E.J. 1976. Induction of pneumonia in gnotobiotic calves following inoculation of Mycoplasma dispar and ureaplasmas. Res. Vet. Sci., 21, 227-231.

Howard, C.J., Taylor, G. and Brownlie, J. 1980b. Surface receptors for immunoglobulin on bovine polymorphonuclear neutrophils and macrophages. Res. Vet. Sci., 29, 128-130.

Horowitz, S.A. and Cassell, G.H. 1978. Detection of antibodies to Mycoplasma pulmonis by an enzyme-linked immunosorbent assay. Infect. Immun., 22, 161-170.

McGuire, T.C., Musoke, A.J. and Kurtti, T. 1979. Functional properties of bovine IgG1 and IgG2: interaction with complement, macrophages, neutrophils and skin. Immunology, 38, 249-256.

Mossmann, H., Schmitz, B., Possart, P. and Hammer, D.K. 1981. Antibody-dependent, cell mediated cytotoxicity in cattle. In "The Ruminant Immune System". Adv. in Exp. Med. and Biol., 137 pp. 279-292 (Ed. J.E. Butler). (Plenum, New York).

Schultz, R.D. 1973. Developmental aspects of the foetal bovine immune response. Cornell Vet., 63, 507-535.

Stott, E.J., Thomas, L.H., Collins, A.P., Crouch, S., Jebbett, J., Smith, G.S., Luther, P.D. and Caswell, R. 1980. A survey of virus infections of the respiratory tract of cattle and their association with disease. J. Hyg., 85, 257-270.

Thomas, L.H., Gourlay, R.N., Stott, E.J., Howard, C.J. and Bridger, J. 1981. A search for new microorganisms in calf pneumonia. In Preparation.

Tizzard, I.R. 1977. An Introduction to Veterinary Immunology. W.B. Saunders. Philadelphia. pp 155-168.

THE USE OF ELISA TO DETECT ANTIBODIES TO PASTEURELLA HAEMOLYTICA A2
AND MYCOPLASMA OVIPNEUMONIAE IN SHEEP WITH EXPERIMENTAL CHRONIC
PNEUMONIA

W. Donachie and G. E. Jones

Moredun Research Institute, 408 Gilmerton Road, Edinburgh EH17 7JH.

ABSTRACT

Ten untreated sheep and 18 sheep in which chronic pneumonia had
been experimentally reproduced were monitored for serum antibodies to
Pasteurella haemolytica serotype A2 and Mycoplasma ovipneumoniae by
ELISA tests. The pasteurella test utilised a phenol water extract of P.
haemolytica A2 cells as antigen: for the mycoplasma test whole M.
ovipneumoniae cells solubilised in a carbonate:bicarbonate buffer were
used.

A rise in antibody titre in the infected animals was detected at 2
weeks post inoculation (wpi) and a peak in mean titres at 8 wpi for P.
haemolytica and 14 wpi for M. ovipneumoniae. Titres to both organisms
declined slowly thereafter till termination of the experiment at 24.5
wpi.

An indirect haemagglutination (IHA) test for P. haemolytica
serotype A2 antibodies demonstrated a similar pattern of antibody rise
and decline, but at considerably lower titres than provided by the ELISA
test.

It was concluded that the ELISA tests for both P. haemolytica and
M. ovipneumoniae were sensitive and have potential application in the
detection of antibody responses in ovine respiratory disease.

INTRODUCTION

Chronic ovine (atypical) pneumonia is a disease of lambs up to 1
year old (Stamp and Nisbet, 1963). Mycoplasma ovipneumoniae and
Pasteurella haemolytica A biotypes are associated with the disease in
the field (Jones et al, 1979) and inoculation of pneumonic lesion
homogenates containing both organisms induces a proliferative exudative
(PE) pneumonia indistinguishable from the naturally occurring condition
(Jones et al, 1978). Clinical signs of atypical pneumonia are
frequently mild or inapparent, yet its effect on growth and production
may be severe (Jones et al, in preparation). It was thus considered
important to develop methods to assist the detection of atypical
pneumonia and to this end we have investigated the value of ELISA tests
for antibodies to both P. haemolytica and M. ovipneumoniae.

Burrells et al (1979) used an antigen prepared by sodium
salicylate extraction (SSE) of P. haemolytica cells and found their
ELISA much more sensitive than the standard indirect haemagglutination
(IHA) test (Biberstein et al, 1960) for the measurement of antibody to

P. haemolytica.   Subsequently, however, the SSE antigen has been shown
to contain antigens common to all P. haemolytica serotypes resulting in
ELISA cross reactions (Burrells, unpublished observations).   In this
paper we report ELISA results obtained with an antigen prepared by
phenol-water extraction of P. haemolytica biotype A, serotype 2 (A_2).

Several different methods have been used to prepare mycoplasma
antigens for use in ELISA tests, including solubilization in carbonate:
bicarbonate buffer (Horowitz and Cassell, 1978), in sodium dodecyl
sulphate (Bruggman et al, 1977), and in Tween 20 followed by gel
filtration (Nicolet et al, 1981).   Initial trials with M. ovipneumoniae
antigen suspensions treated according to the method of Bruggman et al
(1977) indicated that the antigen produced was sensitive but labile,
even after storage at -20°C (Jones, unpublished observations).   Whole
cell suspensions treated according to the method of Horowitz and Cassell
(1978) were found to be stable if stored at -20°C; their performance
as ELISA antigens is described in this communication.

MATERIALS AND METHODS

Antigens

Mycoplasma: Preparation of washed, whole cell suspensions of
strain 956/2 of M. ovipneumoniae was as previously described (Jones et
al, 1976), except that the medium used was preincubated and shaken at
37°C for 2 days, then filtered through 0.22 μm average pore diameter
(a.p.d.) membrane filters (Millipore UK, Harrow, Middlesex) before use.
The cell suspensions were analysed for protein content by a semi-micro
Kjeldahl method then solubilized in a carbonate: bicarbonate buffer
(CBB) according to the method of Horowitz and Cassell (1978). Aliquots
of the suspension were stored at -20°C until use, when they were
diluted to provide 5 μg protein/ml.

Bacteria: P. haemolytica A_2 cells were grown in nutrient broth
(Oxoid No. 2) for 18 h at 37°C.   Cells were harvested by
centrifugation at 4000 g for 30 minutes then washed twice in distilled
water.   A phenol water extract (PWE) was prepared using the method of
Westphal et al, (1952).   Ten grammes wet weight of cells were
resuspended to 50 ml in distilled water and heated to 68°C.   An equal
volume of 90% phenol at 68°C was added to the suspension and the
mixture kept at 68°C for 10 minutes with vigorous shaking.   The

mixture was quickly cooled to $4^{\circ}C$ on an ice bath then centrifuged at 9000 g for 30 minutes. The aqueous layer was removed, dialysed against running water for 24 hours then concentrated twofold by rotary evaporation before centrifugation at 100,000 g for 2 h. The deposit, resuspended in 5 ml distilled water, was recentrifuged and the resultant pellet taken up in 1 ml distilled water and lyophilised. A concentration of 2 mg/ml in distilled water was used in the ELISA test.

Experimental design

Twenty eight lambs, approximately 10 weeks old, were obtained from a flock in which levels of infection with potentially pathogenic respiratory microorganisms had been found to be very low over 4 years of sampling. Nasal swabs taken from the lambs on day 0 were free of pasteurellae, mycoplasmas and viruses.

Eighteen lambs were inoculated intratracheally on day 0 with 6 ml of a homogenate of pneumonic lung lesions obtained from the abattoir (Jones et al, 1978). This homogenate contained 10^{6} colour changing units (ccu) per 0.2 ml of M. ovipneumoniae and 2×10^{3} colony forming units (cfu) of P. haemolytica A2 with no isolation of other microorganisms. The same animals were inoculated intranasally on day 7 with 1 ml of a culture of P. haemolytica A2 containing 4×10^{6} cfu/ml. The remaining 10 control lambs were untreated throughout. All control lambs and 6 infected lambs were slaughtered at 15.5 wpi; the surviving 8 infected lambs were slaughtered at 24.5 wpi, when they had reached the same mean liveweight as the controls.

Sera

Standard M. ovipneumoniae anti serum:

A vaccine incorporating an aluminium hydroxide adsorbed suspension of strain 956/2 mixed in equal proportions with Bayol and Arlacel (Jones 1978) was administered subcutaneously twice with a 2 week interval to two 3-week old gnotobiotic lambs. The lambs were killed and bled out 7 days after the second vaccination. The sera from both animals were pooled and stored in aliquots at $-20^{\circ}C$ until used at dilutions between 1/2000 and 1/256,000.

Standard P. haemolytica anti-serum:

Sera from sheep shown to have antibody to P. haemolytica A2 in a previous experiment were pooled and stored in aliquots at $-20^{\circ}C$ until used at dilutions between 1/2000 and 1/256,000.

Serology

IHA test: this was carried out as described by Fraser et al (in press).

ELISA tests: the methods used were based on that described by Engvall and Perlman (1972). The tests consisted of 5 steps with 3 washes of 0.05% Tween 20 in phosphate buffered saline pH 7.4 (PBS/Tween) after each step and 200 µl volumes of reagents, at pre-determined optimal dilutions, were used throughout.

For P. haemolytica the steps were: I. Micro ELISA plates (M192A Dynatech Laboratories Ltd., - Billinghurst, Sussex) were coated with PWE antigen diluted 1/200 in carbonate bicarbonate buffer pH 9.6. The plates were incubated at $37^{\circ}C$ for 24 hr then held at $4^{\circ}C$ for 7 days.

II. Standard or test sera were added to all wells except those in column 1 to which diluent was added. Test sera were diluted 1/2000 in PBS/Tween + 0.02% sodium azide before use. The standard serum was made up in 8 two fold dilutions between 1/2000 and 1/256,000. Each sample (test and different dilutions of standard) was tested in duplicate and the plates incubated at room temperature (RT) for 3 h.

III. Pig IgG anti-sheep IgG conjugated with alkaline phosphatase was added to each well and incubated for 3 h at RT.

IV. Substrate (p-nitrophenyl phosphate, Sigma Chemical Co. Poole, Dorset; 1 mg/ml) was added to each well and incubated at RT for 18 h.

V. 3 M NaOH was added to stop the reaction. The results were recorded as optical densities at a wavelength of 405 nm (OD_{405}) using an automatic multichannel spectrophotometer ("Titertek Multiskan",Flow Laboratories, Irvine, Ayrshire).

The steps for M. ovipneumoniae were as follows:

I. The antigen was added to each well and incubated at RT overnight.

II. The standard and test sera were dispensed as for the P. haemolytica ELISA but the plates were incubated for 4 hours at $37^{\circ}C$.

III. Conjugate (as above) was added to all wells and incubated overnight at RT.

IV. Substrate (as above) was added to all wells and incubated for 1 hr at $37^{\circ}C$.

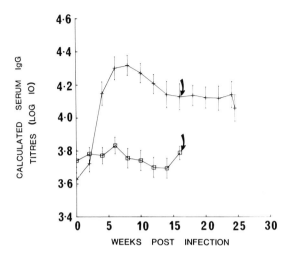

Figure 1.   Mean calculated serum antibody titres ($\log_{10}$) against P haemolytica A2 as detected by ELISA for infected group (+) and control group (□).   Arrow indicates time of first killing at 15.5 wp.i.

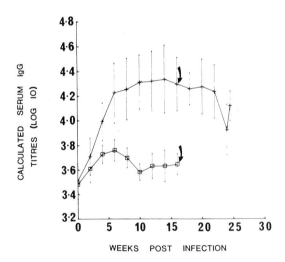

Figure 2.   Mean calculated serum antibody titres ($\log_{10}$) against M. ovipneumoniae as detected by ELISA for infected group (+) and control group (□).   Arrow indicates time of first killing at 15.5 wpi.

V.   As for P. haemolytica ELISA.

Calculation of results

1.   The absorbance figures (A) were converted to $\log_{10}$ values.

2.   The log A values of the standard serum dilutions were plotted against the $\log_{10}$ values of these dilutions to provide a standard graph.

3.   The titre of the standard serum was taken to be that dilution which would give an absorbance value of 0.1 (log 1.0) as negative control sera from SPF and gnotobiotic lambs were never found to exceed this value.

4.   The titres of the test sera are calculated from the formula

$$\text{titre of test serum} = \frac{\text{Reciprocal of dilution of test serum (2000)}}{\text{Reciprocal of dilution of standard serum which would give the same A value as the test serum (read from graph)}} \times \text{titre of standard serum}$$

RESULTS

ELISA.   The calculated mean serum antibody titres against P. haemolytica and M. ovipneumoniae for infected and control animals are shown in Figures 1 and 2 respectively. Mean antibody titres against P. haemolytica in the infected group peaked at 8 wpi (1/27,500) while antibody titres against M. ovipneumoniae peaked at 14 wpi (1/21,480).

   Antibodies against P. haemolytica A2 declined quickly after peaking while those against M. ovipneumoniae persisted at a high level until 24 wpi. The control animals, in both tests, showed no significant rise in mean antibody titre over the duration of the experiment.

IHA - The mean serum antibody titres of the infected group obtained in the IHA test plotted against time are shown in Figure 3. Antibody detected in this test increased quickly to a titre of 1/48 at 4 wpi and declined sharply thereafter. The mean serum antibody titres of the controls remained almost constant (at 1 in 2) throughout the experiment.

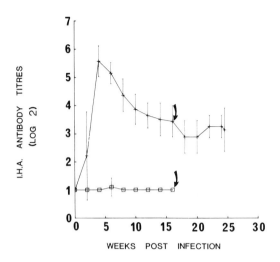

Figure 3.   Mean serum antibody titre (log$_2$) against P. haemolytica as detected by IHA for infected group (+) and control group (□).   Arrow indicates time of first killing at 15.5 wpi.

Necropsy - The principal pathological and microbiological findings are shown in Table 1. PE pneumonia was detected in all infected animals but not in any control animal. Lungs from all infected animals and 3 controls yielded M. ovipneumoniae; P. haemolytica was recovered from the lungs of 2 infected animals killed at 15.5 wpi.

Table 1.   Principal pathological and microbiological findings in infected and control groups at necropsy.

Group	No. in group	No. with PE pneumonia	No. positive for	
			M. ovipneumoniae	P. haemolytica
Infected	14	14	14	2
Control	9	0	3	0

DISCUSSION

Sheep in which pneumonia had been experimentally reproduced with suspensions containing P. haemolytica and M. ovipneumoniae showed rises in antibody titre to these two organisms by ELISA tests. Group mean titres to the bacterium rose more quickly than those to the mycoplasma, peaking at 8 weeks for the former and 14 weeks for the latter. Reasons for this difference are uncertain but may involve a greater invasiveness or antigenicity of the bacterium compared with the mycoplasma. One possibility, that the response to P. haemolytica was anamnestic and that to M. ovipneumoniae was primary, is a less likely explanation since low levels of antibody to both organisms appeared to be present in pre-inoculation sera, suggesting prior exposure of the animals to the two agents. Whatever the cause, the ELISA test for P. haemolytica would seem to be more useful diagnostically in the early phases of PE pneumonia. The relatively rapid decline in titres to P. haemolytica compared with M. ovipneumoniae probably reflects the early elimination of the bacterium and the lengthy persistence of the mycoplasma in lesions of PE pneumonia (Gilmour et al, in press), suggesting that the ELISA test for M. ovipneumoniae antibodies may be more useful diagnostically in the subacute phase of the disease.

None of the 9 control sheep showed significant rises in antibody titre to pasteurella or mycoplasma above the levels present at the start of the experiment, despite the isolation of M. ovipneumoniae from the lungs of 3 sheep at slaughter. This finding corroborates earlier observations (Jones, unpublished observations) that simple pulmonary colonisation with M. ovipneumoniae is insufficient to induce seroconversion, and that lung consolidation is necessary before significant rises in antibody are detected.

Phenol-water extracts of serotypes of P. haemolytica have been shown to contain the serotype specific antigen for that serotype (Donachie, unpublished observations). This extract contains lipopolysaccharide (Wilkinson, 1977) and as P. haemolytica serotypes may share antigenic determinants in this component this may decrease the specificity of the ELISA test and contribute to the "background" level of antibody detected. Difficulty in binding polysaccharide antigens to polystyrene has been noted previously (Barret et al, 1980). This problem was overcome in these studies by incorporation of a prolonged binding step (Dahlberg et al, 1980) of 24 h incubation at $37^{o}C$ followed by 7 days at $4^{o}C$.

The IHA test was less sensitive than the ELISA, but demonstrated maximum titres at an earlier stage, suggesting that a different antibody was assayed. The IHA test measures only antibodies to those antigens which have affinity for erythrocyte membrane sites while all antigens binding to the well are available for antibody-antigen reactions in the ELISA test.

The ELISA test for M. ovipneumoniae antibodies used whole cell antigen solubilized in CBB and proved extremely sensitive in these studies. However, this antigen has been found to give positive results with hyperimmune sera to a variety of mycoplasma species (Jones, unpublished observations) and it may prove necessary to develop a more specific antigen for future use.

In conclusion it would seem that the ELISA has potential for serodiagnosis of pneumonia, as the combination of high serum antibody titres to both P. haemolytica and M. ovipneumoniae which are easily detected by the assay, are correlated with consolidated lesions. However a more specific antigen for both assays would give greater confidence in the test and make it a more powerful diagnostic tool.

REFERENCES

Barret, J.D., Amman, A.J., Stenmark, S. and Wara, D.W. (1980).
Immunoglobulin G and M antibodies to pneumococcal polysaccharide
detected by enzyme-linked immunosorbent assay. Inf. & Immun. 27,
411-417.

Biberstein, E.L., Gills, M. and Knight, H. (1960).   Serological types
of Pasteurella haemolytica. Cornell Vet. 50, 223-300.

Bruggman, S., Keller, H., Bertschunger, H.U. and Engberg, G. (1977).
Quantitative detection of antibodies to Mycoplasma suipneumoniae in
pigs' sera by an enzyme-linked immunosorbent assay. Vet. Record,
101, 109-111.

Burrells, C., Wells, P.W and Dawson, A.McL. (1979).   The quantitative
estimation of antibody to Pasteurella haemolytica in sheep using a
micro enzyme-linked immunosorbent assay (ELISA).   Vet. Microbiol. 3,
291-301

Dahlberg, T. and Branefors, P. (1980).   Enzyme-linked immunosorbent
assay for titration of Haemophilus influenzae capsular and O
antigen antibodies.   J. clin. Micro. 12, 185-192.

Fraser, J., Laird, S. and Gilmour, N.J.L. (1982).   A new serotype
(Biotype T) of Pasteurella haemolytica.   Res. vet. Sci. (in
press).

Gilmour, J.S., Jones, G.E., Keir, W.A. and Rae, A.G.   Long-term
pathological and microbiological progress in sheep of experimental
disease resembling atypical pneumonia.   J. comp. Path. (in
press).

Horowitz, S.A. and Cassell, G.A. (1978).   Detection of antibodies to
Mycoplasma pulmonis by an enzyme linked immunosorbent assay.   Inf.
& Immun. 22, 161-170.

Jones, G.E., Foggie, A., Mould, D.L. and Livitt, S. (1976).   The
comparison and characterisation of glycolytic mycoplasmas isolated
from the respiratory tract of sheep. J. med. Microbiol. 9, 39-51.

Jones, G.E. (1978).   Studies on mycoplasmas of the respiratory tract of
sheep. PhD. Thesis University of Edinburgh.

Jones, G.E., Gilmour, J.S. and Rae, A.G. (1978).   Endobronchial
inoculation of sheep with pneumonic lung-tissue suspensions and
with the bacteria and mycoplasmas isolated from them.   J. comp.
Path. 88, 85-96.

Jones, G.E., Buxton, D. and Harker, D.B. (1979).   Respiratory
infections in housed sheep, with particular reference to
mycoplasmas. Vet. Microbiol. 4, 47-49.

Jones, G.E., Field, A.C., Gilmour, J.S., Rae, A.G., Nettleton, P.F. and
McLauchlan, M. (1982).   Effects of experimental chronic pneumonia
on bodyweight, feed intake and carcass composition of lambs.   Vet.
Record (in press).

Nicolet, J. and Paroz, P. (1980).   Tween 20 soluble proteins of
Mycoplasma hyopneumoniae as antigen for an enzyme-linked
immunosorbent assay. Res. vet. Sci. 29, 305-309.

Stamp, J.T. and Nisbet, D.I. (1963).   Pneumonia of sheep. J. comp.
Path. 73, 319-328.

Westphal, O., Luderitz, O. and Bister, F. (1952).   Uber die Extraction
von Bacterien mit Phenol/Wasser. Z. Naturforschung, 76, 148-155.

Wilkinson, S.G. (1977). Composition and structure of bacterial lipopolysaccharide.   In "Surface Carbohydrates of the Prokaryotic
Cell". (Ed. I.W. Sutherland, Academic Press London) 97-175.

PART V: APPLICATION OF ELISA TO THE STUDY OF VIRUSES

DEVELOPMENT AND APPLICATION OF ELISA FOR VETERINARY DIAGNOSIS
AND RESEARCH ON ENTERIC AND OTHER VIRUSES

D.J. Reynolds

Institute for Research on Animal Diseases,
Compton, Newbury, U.K.

ABSTRACT

Direct, indirect and sandwich ELISA techniques, with their many modifications for individual antigens are used to detect and quantitate viruses for veterinary diagnosis. The indirect and blocking assays provide sensitive methods for serological screening. Rapid results combine with economy and safety of reagents to facilitate the handling of large numbers of samples. Epidemiological studies are now possible on enteric viruses which are non-cultivable or propagated only with difficulty; such investigations were previously not possible or were too laborious to perform. Sources of discrepancy between ELISA and other diagnostic tests exist, such as immune complexes, inactivated or non-infectious virus antigens and serotypic variation. Comparative studies to determine the specificity and sensitivity of each virus immunoassay are necessary and if careful standardization is adopted, the ELISA technique is likely to be widely accepted in veterinary research and diagnosis.

INTRODUCTION

An effective enzyme-linked immunosorbent assay (ELISA) was described nearly a decade ago (Engvall and Perlman, 1972). The development of ELISA techniques for detection and quantitation of viral antigens and antibodies followed, relying on preparation of enzyme conjugates with high enzymatic and immunological activity. A comprehensive booklet including the various types of assays and their application was published in 1979 (Voller et al., 1979). For animal viruses, ELISA has been widely applied and can present many advantages for rapid diagnosis and research purposes. Comparison with other established methods of virus identification provides essential information on sensitivity, specificity and future potential applications of individual assays.

ANTIGEN DETECTION

Methods

The detection by immunoassay of virus-specific antigens permits rapid diagnosis of infections. Technical variations of 3 basic heterogeneous non-competitive ELISA methods have been described, namely direct, indirect

and sandwich assays (Yolken et al., 1977; Ellens and De Leeuw, 1977;
Crowther and Abu-ElZein, 1979a).   In the direct and indirect assay for
foot-and-mouth disease virus (FMDV), purified FMDV was adsorbed onto a
plastic microplate and detected by either enzyme-labelled FMDV-antibody
(direct) or FMDV-antibody followed by an enzyme-labelled anti-species
conjugate (indirect).   Between 5-30 ng/ml of purified FMDV can be measured,
compared with 1 μg/ml by complement fixation (Crowther and Abu-ElZein,
1979a).   The sandwich ELISA is capable of detecting antigen with 2 or more
binding sites.   Plates are coated with a capture antibody prior to
addition of test antigen and then treated with an appropriate direct or
indirect detection system.   Homogeneous ELISA utilizes steric hindrance at
the enzyme active site, when labelled antibody/antigen complexes form, so
avoiding necessity for separation of unbound material (Rubenstein, 1978).
Essential requirements of this technique are a pure, standard antigen with
high specific-activity enzyme label.   Assays for monitoring therapeutic
levels of potentially toxic drugs and antibiotics have been developed
(EMIT, Syva Co., USA); as yet these methods have been applied to haptens
rather than viral antigens and work with only selected enzymes.

Enteric viruses

Sandwich ELISA methods have been particularly favoured for virus in
faeces and secretions, where the proportion of virus-specific protein
antigen is relatively low (Herrman et al., 1979).   Diagnosis of enteric
virus infection often relies on identification of faecal virus.   ELISA and
RIA were as sensitive as electron microscopy (EM) for human rotavirus
(Yolken et al., 1977) and in an initial comparison between ELISA and EM,
Ellens and De Leeuw (1977) detected 10^5 bovine rotavirus particles per gram
of infected calf faeces.   Virus shedding from experimentally-infected
calves showed good correspondence between ELISA and EM for rotavirus
(Bachmann, 1979); ELISA and haemadsorption-elution-haemagglutination assay
for bovine coronavirus (Ellens et al., 1978c) and between ELISA and EM for
CV777, a non-cultivable porcine enteric coronavirus (Callebaut and Debouck,
1981).   Distinction between rotaviruses from different animal species by
incorporation of a blocking-step in the sandwich ELISA was described by
Yolken et al. (1978).   Subsequently, the importance of subgroup and
serotype specificity has been recognized (Kapikian et al., 1981).   All
sandwich ELISAs are dependent on the antisera used to develop capture and
detector systems, thus using heterologous antisera (for example bovine

rotavirus antiserum for human rotavirus detection) measures components which differ from the homologous system.

Other viruses

Double-sandwich ELISA for FMDV has been used for typing virus from epithelial samples and with appropriate antisera and dilutions, cross-reactions due to subunit and non-structural proteins (which present problems in CF) could be avoided (Crowther and Abu-ElZein, 1979b). This approach has been applied to other viruses, including African swine fever (Wardley et al., 1979) detecting 50-500 HA 50/well and feline leukaemia virus for which a commercial kit is available (Leukassay-F, C-Vet, UK) for use in Europe and USA. Equine infectious anaemia major group antigen (p29) could be detected above 2.5-5 ng/0.1 ml, which was sufficiently sensitive for end-point detection in routine virus infectivity assays (Shen et al., 1979).

Comparison with other tests

Five diagnostic methods for rotavirus detection in field samples were compared by Ellens et al., 1978. 49/98 were ELISA-positive and 39 by indirect immunofluorescence (IIF) or EM, 42 by CF and 30 by immunoelectro-phoresis. Bachmann (1979) using a similar ELISA in comparison with immune-EM found 18/136 rotavirus-positive faeces were ELISA-negative. Comparisons of this sort reveal the potential sensitivity of ELISA (versus CF and electrophoresis), together with important discrepancies.

(1) ELISA and EM

Immune complexes may be present during convalescence, late in the virus infection process. Antibody produced may mask antigenic sites so that detection by ELISA is blocked, although characteristic single or grouped particles, coated with immunoglobulin, can still be visualized by EM (Almeida, 1979). Faecal samples examined at 7 and 8 days after experimental infection with bovine coronavirus (Fig. 1) were ELISA negative, coronavirus-antibody complexes were visualized by EM and antigen-containing cells were found in the gut of calf A at post-mortem examination the next day (Reynolds, D.J., unpublished).

Major variations between virus subgroups or serotypes, which present identical EM appearance, could be overlooked by ELISA (Bridger, 1980). As

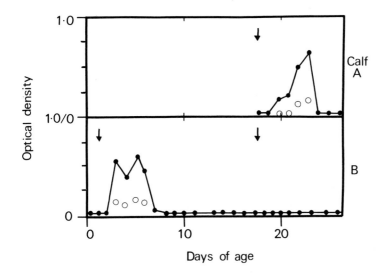

Fig. 1   Faecal samples examined daily by Bovine coronavirus sandwich
ELISA.   (Infection indicated ↓ , test well ● , test well + specific
blocking antiserum, incorporated before enzyme-labelled antiserum ○ .)

in any immunological assay critical evaluation of antiserum specificity
demands that all potential antibody/virus reactions occurring in tests
should ultimately be understood.

Viral subunits may or may not be recognized by EM but can retain
antigenicity for ELISA.

(2)   ELISA and virus isolation or IIF

During transit to diagnostic centres, pH and temperature changes may
result in loss of infectivity without altering antigenicity.

Cytotoxicity and bacterial contamination can cause serious problems
for direct virus isolation but not for immunoassay methods.

Non-cultivable viruses and agents such as adeno- and coronaviruses,
being difficult to cultivate in vitro from field samples, can be identified
by their specific antigens rather than growth characteristics or morphology

Low level shedding of readily cultivable agents may fall below ELISA
detection limits.   After amplification in cell culture a recognisable
cytopathic effect may be demonstrated from an inoculum of low initial
titre.

FeLV isolation (VI) and immunofluorescence (IF) correlated well, as did ELISA-negative samples and VI or IF tests (Jarrett et al., 1981). However, at least 30% of ELISA-positive diagnoses were negative by VI or IF (Table 1). This discordance when investigated, was not apparently

TABLE 1 A comparison of virus isolation (VI), immunofluorescence (IF) and leukassay F ELISA (LF) for the diagnosis of feline leukaemia virus. (Jarrett, J.O., Golder, M.C. and Weijer, K., 1981)

	Comparison	No. of discordants/ No. of tests	Discordance %
Overall	VI : IF	6/412	1.5
	VI : LF	23/412	5.6
	IF : LF	23/412	5.6
Positive	LF : VI	23/72	31.9
	LF : IF	22/72	30.6
	VI : LF	0/49	0
	VI : IF	2/49	4.1
	IF : VI	4/51	7.8
	IF : LF	1/51	1.9

due to differences in sensitivity of the tests in use, virus inactivation prior to isolation attempts or transient viraemia. It was suggested that FeLV could be present in these cats in a latent carrier state, producing only circulating antigen, not whole infectious virus. Alternatively endogenous FeLV-related genes may be present in the DNA of all cat cells and expression of cross-reactive endogenous antigen, without appearance of infectious virus occurred as a result of transient natural FeLV. The prognosis for discordant ELISA-positive, virus-negative cats was uncertain but they did not seem to constitute a risk for virus spread. Thus, FeLV ELISA has presented problems in interpretation, whilst possibly revealing new aspects of the infection itself.

Applications of ELISA for virus detection

The advantage of a specific, sensitive and rapid screening test has been particularly exploited in epidemiological surveys for infection by enteric viruses (De Leeuw et al., 1980). Regular screening of faecal virus excretion by ELISA has highlighted the frequency of infection in clinically normal animals (Reynolds, D.J., unpublished observations). Development of immunoassays for uncultivable agents such as Norwalk virus

have made studies possible of prevalence prior to virus characterization
in vitro (Greenberg, 1978).   The high handling capacity and rapid results,
without necessity for expensive capital equipment, make ELISA attractive
for routine detection of enteric viruses in faeces.   However new,
previously unidentified agents, would not be detected if this test was used
alone and a combination with other approaches may be required in some
circumstances.

ANTIBODY DETECTION
     For epidemiological surveys of new or emergent infections, rapid
specific results are often required.   Immunoassays can be adapted to
detect and quantitate total or class-specific immunoglobulin levels directed
against whole virus or individual subcomponents.   The ELISA titre measured
results from a primary combination of both precipitating and non-precipita-
ting antibody and antigen, which has varied significance in terms of
biological activity, such as virus neutralization or complement fixation.

Methods and applications of ELISA serology

Indirect ELISA
     Where viral antigens can be obtained by in vitro culture, adsorption
to a microplate provides an ideal solid phase for non-competitive ELISA
(Voller et al., 1976).   The alternative, growth and fixation of infected
cell monolayers in microtrays (Saunders, 1977) has been less widely applied.
Having obtained antigen-coated wells, test-serum dilutions followed by
enzyme-labelled anti-species reagents are added.   After incubation with
the enzyme substrate, increases in optical density are proportional to test
antibody binding.   Modifications of this regime have been discussed by
several authors (Bullock and Walls, 1977; Bidwell et al., 1977) who stress
the necessity for standardization of procedures and reagents before
acceptable diagnostic serology can be performed by ELISA.
     Serology of infectious bovine rhinotracheitis (IBR) has been
conveniently adapted to a micro-ELISA (Payment et al., 1979; Herring
et al., 1980).   In the first description, antigen adsorbed on to plates
was from infected cell-cultures disrupted by freeze-thawing and purified
by density gradient centrifugation, whilst released virus used in the
second method was suitable without purification.   When ELISA was compared

with VN, all VN-positive sera were ELISA positive; however antibody to
non-neutralizing components might result in higher ELISA values or a
proportion of sera which were VN-negative and ELISA-positive.
Additionally, where an IgM neutralizing response was present, indirect
ELISA using enzyme-labelled antibody to bovine IgG could produce
discrepancies in titre between VN and ELISA.

Soluble antigen prepared from African swine fever (ASF) infected cells
was used to develop an ELISA which would detect 5 ng amounts of ASF-antibody
(Hamdy et al., 1979) and produced good differentiation of normal and
convalescent pig sera (Wardley et al., 1979).   An indirect immunofluorescence test for feline infectious peritonitis (FIP) antibody, using
porcine transmissible gastroenteritis virus was extended for use as an
ELISA (Osterhaus et al., 1979).   Inevitably the responses were to cross-
reacting group antigens but this assay has enabled work on the seroepidemiology of FIP to be conducted.   Descriptions of assays for other veterinary
viruses have included those where herd screening for evidence of infection
may be particularly required, rather than individual diagnoses.   Aujeszky's
disease, enzootic bovine leukosis and Maedi/Visna, amongst others can
now be tackled using ELISA methodology (Briaire et al., 1979; Ressang
et al., 1978; Houwers and Gielkins, 1979).   For use in disease
recognition and control programmes good standardization is again emphasized
by individual authors before ELISA should be adopted.

Class-specific immunoglobulins

Solid phase non-competitive antibody ELISA may be extended to measure
responses to individual virus antigens (Macnaughton et al., 1981) and
class-specificity of the immunoglobulin (Corthier and Franz, 1981).   Thus,
subdivision of component parts of an immune response to virus infection may
be achieved by immunoassay.   Diagnosis of recent infection can be
established by an IgM response, subsequent to clinical symptoms with or
without virus excretion.   IgM determination for rubella, cytomegalovirus,
measles and herpes virus infections of man have provided rapid diagnostic
tests, some of which are commercially available (e.g. Enzygnost, Hoechst).
After mucosal infection, protective local immunity may be mediated
predominantly by certain immunoglobulin classes.   Corthier and Franz
(1981) demonstrated anti-rotavirus IgA in porcine milk by ELISA, avoiding
the laborious immunoglobulin separation techniques required previously

(Bohl et al., 1975). These studies of potentially protective antibodies, by ELISA, require careful assessment as non-neutralizing (so probably non-protective) antibodies can be measured effectively. FeLV-neutralizing antibody appeared to correlate well with protection against reinfection and passive protection by maternal antibody. ELISA-serology revealed cats which were antibody positive but not protected from infection. Thus VN-antibody was of greater value than ELISA in prognosis of FeLV (Jarrett, 1981).

Staphylococcal protein-A in ELISA serology

Staphylococcal protein-A (SpA) interacts with the crystallizable fragment of IgG molecules from many species, so that a single enzyme-labelled SpA can be used in place of a range of anti-species conjugates. Important precautions were required to avoid non-specific reactions, including serum-free medium for antigen production. There were promising results for a range of porcine, equine, bovine, feline and human viruses (Bommeli et al., 1980; Potgieter et al., 1980).

ELISA-blocking tests

Where the sandwich-antigen ELISA was modified to include a test-serum before incubation with the enzyme-labelled reagent, "blocking" or reduction in enzyme-substrate reaction was proportional to test antibody levels (Ellens et al., 1978a; Bartz et al., 1980). Antigen, including faecal virus, did not require purification and binding antibody of any specificity could be measured. Ellens (1978a) determined rotavirus antibody in bovine serum and colostrum, finding that VN levels correlated well with ELISA-blocking. Bovine coronavirus serology has been possible at Compton using a similar approach. Figure 2 shows the development of ELISA-blocking antibody in a calf following oral inoculation and 2 parenteral hyper-immunizations. End-points were calculated as the last serum dilution to produce an optical density less than 50% of the positive control value. The availability of blocking assays allowed initiation of epidemiological studies of CV777 infection which could not otherwise have been studied until in vitro culture was achieved (Callebaut and Debouck, 1981).

FURTHER DEVELOPMENTS FOR ELISA

Initially, improvements to existing ELISA tests for antigen or antibody should be encouraged, so that their diagnostic and prognostic value can be

120

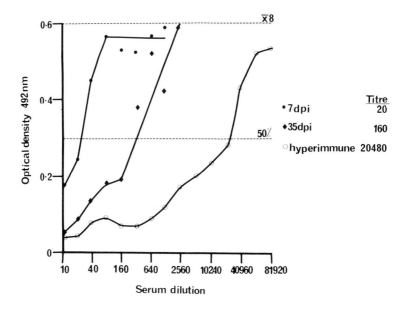

Fig. 2 Development of antibody to bovine coronavirus in a calf in
an ELISA-blocking test.

fully assessed. Monoclonal antibodies directed against individual
antigenic determinants, with differing activities may make future
refinements possible. Screening of supernatant fluids from potential
antibody-producing hybridomas can be rapidly performed by enzyme or
radioimmunoassay. The sensitivity of assays may be improved by adoption
of new techniques for conjugation or modifications, such as the use of
anti-enzyme conjugates which amplify ELISA further. The comparison of
virus strains, particularly where isolation or purification are difficult,
can be facilitated as has been shown for human rotavirus (Zissis and
Lambert, 1980). The in vivo significance of ELISA data requires
additional investigation and in vaccine production, quantitative immunoassay
may improve our understanding of the viral components required for effective
immunization.

REFERENCES

Almeida, J.D. 1979. Morphology and antigenicity of rotavirus. Les
colloques de l'INSERM - Viral Enteritis, 90, 379-392.
Bachmann, P.A. 1979. Rotavirusnachweis in Faezes : Erfahrungen mit dem
Enzyme Linked Immunosorbent Assay (ELISA). Zbl. Vet. Med. B,
26, 835-842.

Bartz, C.R., Conklin, R., Steele, J.H. and Glass, S.E.   1980.   Rotavirus
    antibody in chickens as measured by Enzyme-Linked Immunsorbent Blocking
    Assay.   Am. J. Vet. Res., 41, 969-971.

Bidwell, D.E., Bartlett, A. and Voller, A.   1977.   Enzyme Immunoassays
    for viral diseases.   J. Inf. Diseases, 136 Suppl., 274-278.

Bohl, E.H., Gupta, P., Olquin, M.V.F. and Saif, L.J.   1972.   Antibody
    responses in serum, colostrum and milk of swine after infection or
    vaccination with transmissible gastroenteritis virus.   Infect.
    Immunity, 6, 289-301.

Bommeli, W., Kihm, U., Zindel, F. and Fey, H.   1980.   Enzyme linked
    immunoassay and fluorescent antibody techniques in the diagnosis of
    viral diseases using Staphylococcal Protein-A instead of anti-gamma
    globulins.   Vet. immunol. and immunopathol., 1, 179-193.

Briaire, J., Meloen, R.H. and Barteling, S.J.   1979.   An Enzyme Linked
    Immunosorbent Assay (ELISA) for the detection of antibody against
    Aujeszky's Disease Virus in pig sera.   Zbl. Vet. Med. B., 26, 76-81.

Bridger, J.C.   1980.   Detection by electron microscopy of caliciviruses,
    astroviruses and rotavirus-like particles in the faeces of piglets
    with diarrhoea.   Vet. Rec., 107, 532-533.

Bullock, S.L. and Walls, K.W.   1977.   Evaluation of some of the parameters
    of the Enzyme-Linked Immunospecific Assay.   J. Inf. Diseases,
    136 Suppl., 279-285.

Callebaut, P.E. and Debouck, P.   1981.   Some characteristics of a new
    porcine coronavirus and detection of antigen and antibody by ELISA.
    Proc. Vth Int. Congress of Virology.   Strasbourg, France, 1981, 420.

Corthier, G. and Franz, J.   1981.   Detection of antirotavirus
    immunoglobulins A, G and M in swine colostrum, milk and feces by
    Enzyme-Linked Immunosorbent Assay.   Infect. Immunity, 31, 833-836.

Crowther, J.R. and Abu-ElZein, E.M.E.   1979a.   Detection and
    quantification of Foot and Mouth disease virus by enzyme-linked
    immunosorbent assay techniques.   J. gen. Virol., 42, 597-602.

Crowther, J.R. and Abu-ElZein, E.M.E.   1979b.   Application of enzyme-
    linked immunosorbent assay to the detection and identification of Foot
    and Mouth disease viruses.   J. Hyg. Camb., 83, 513-519.

De Leeuw, P.W., Ellens, D.J., Straver, P.J., van Balken, J.A.M.,
    Maerman, A. and Baanvinger, T.   1980.   Rotavirus infections in
    calves in dairy herds.   Res. vet. Sci., 29, 135-141.

Ellens, D.J. and De Leeuw, P.W.   1977.   Enzyme-linked immunosorbent assay
    for diagnosis of rotavirus infection in calves.   J. Clin. Micro.,
    6, 530-532.

Ellens, D.J., De Leeuw, P.W. and Straver, P.J.   1978a.   The detection of
    rotavirus specific antibody in colostrum and milk by ELISA.
    Ann. Rech. Vét., 9, 337-342.

Ellens, D.J., De Leeuw, P.W., Straver, P.J. and van Balken, J.A.M.   1978b.
    Comparison of five diagnostic methods for the detection of rotavirus
    antigens in calf faeces.   Med. Microbiol. Immunol., 166, 157-163.

Ellens, D.J., van Balken, J.A.M. and De Leeuw, P.W.   1978c.   Diagnosis
    of bovine coronavirus infections with haemadsorption-elution-
    haemagglutination assay (HEHA) and Enzyme-linked immunosorbent assay
    (ELISA).   Proc. 2nd Int. Sym. on Neonatal Diarrhoea.   Oct. 3-5th
    1978.   Univ. of Saskatchewan, Canada.   321-330.

Engvall, E. and Perlmann, P.   1972.   Enzyme-linked immunosorbent assay
    (ELISA).   III. Quantitation of specific antibodies by enzyme-labelled
    anti-immunoglobulin in antigen-coated tubes.   J. Immunol., 109,
    129-135.

Greenberg, H.B., Wyatt, R.G., Valdesuso, J., Kalica, A.R., London, W.T., Chanock, R.M. and Kapikian, A.Z. 1978. Solid phase microtiter radioimmunoassay for the Norwalk strain of acute non bacterial, epidemic gastroenteritis virus and its antibodies. J. Med. Virol., 2, 97-108.

Hamdy, F.M. and Dardiri, A.H. 1979. Enzyme-Linked immunosorbent assay for the diagnosis of African swine fever. Vet. Rec., 105, 445-446.

Herring, A.J., Nettleton, P.F and Burrells, C. 1980. A micro-enzyme-linked immunosorbent assay for the detection of antibodies to infectious bovine rhinotracheitis virus. Vet. Rec., 107, 155-156.

Herrmann, J.E., Hendry, R.M. and Collins, M.F. 1979. Factors involved in Enzyme-linked immunoassay of viruses and evaluation of the method of identification of enteroviruses. J. clin. Micro., 10, 210-217.

Houwers, D.J. and Gielkins, A.L. 1979. An ELISA for the detection of Maedi/Visna antibody. Vet. Rec., 104, 611.

Jarrett, J.O. 1981a. Serology of feline leukaemia virus infections. Vet. Rec., 108, 465.

Jarrett, J.O., Golder, M.C. and Weijer, K. 1981. A comparison of three methods of Feline Leukaemia diagnosis. Personal communication.

Kapikian, A.Z., Cline, W., Greenberg, H., Wyatt, R., Kalica, A., Banks, C., James, H., Flores, J. and Chanock, R. 1981. Studies of rotaviruses by IAHA: distinctness of IAHA and neutralization antigens. Proc. Vth Int. Congress of Virology, Strasbourg, France. 194.

Macnaughton, M.R., Hasony, H.J., Madge, H. and Reed, S.E. 1981. Antibody to virus components in volunteers experimentally infected with human coronavirus 229E group viruses. Infect. Immunity, 31, 845-849.

Osterhaus, A.D.M.E., Kroon, A. and Wirahadiredja, R. 1979. ELISA for the serology of FIP virus. Vet. Quarterly, 1, 59-62.

Payment, P., Assaf, R., Trudel, M. and Marois, P. 1979. Enzyme-linked Immunosorbent assay for serology of infectious bovine rhinotracheitis virus infections. J. Clin. Microbiol., 10, 633-636.

Potgieter, L.N.D., Rouse, B.T. and Webb-Martin, T.A. 1980. Enzyme-Linked immunosorbent assay, using Staphylococcal protein-A for detecting virus antibodies. Am. J. vet. Res., 41, 978-980.

Ressang, A., Gielkins, A.L.J., Quak, S., Mastenbroek, N., Tuppert, C. and Castro, A. de. 1978. Studies on bovine leukosis virus. VI. Enzyme linked immunosorbent assay for the detection of antibodies to bovine leukosis virus. Ann. rech. vét., 9, 663-666.

Rubenstein, K.E. 1978. Homogeneous enzyme immunoassay today. Scand. J. Immunol., 8, Suppl. 7, 57-62.

Saunders, G.C. 1977. Development and evaluation of an enzyme-labelled antibody test for the rapid detection of hog cholera antibodies. Am. J. vet. Res., 38, 21-25.

Shen, D.T., Crawford, T.B. and Gorham, J.R. 1979. Enzyme-linked immunosorbent assay (ELISA) for detection of equine infectious anaemia antigen. J. equine med. surgery, 3, 303-307.

Voller, A.D., Bidwell, D.E. and Bartlett, A. 1976. Microplate enzyme immunoassay for the immunodiagnosis of virus infections. In N.R. Rose and H. Friedman (eds), Manual of Clinical Immunology, American Society for Microbiology, Washington, 506-512.

Wardley, R.C., Abu-ElZein, E.M.E., Crowther, J.R. and Wilkinson, P.J. 1979. A solid phase enzyme-linked immunoassay for the detection of African swine fever virus antigen and antibody. J. Hyg. Camb., 83, 363-369.

Yolken, R.H., Kim, H.W., Clem, T., Wyatt, R.G., Kalica, A.R., Chanock, R.M. and Kapikian, A.Z.   1977.   Enzyme-linked immunosorbent assay (ELISA) for detection of human reovirus-like agent of infantile gastro-enteritis.   Lancet, II, 263-267.

Yolken, R.H., Barbour, B., Wyatt, R.G., Kalica, A.R., Kapikian, A.Z. and Chanock, R.M.   1978.   Enzyme-linked immunosorbent assay for identification of rotaviruses from different animal species. Science, 201, 259-261.

Zissis, G. and Lambert, J.P.   1980.   Enzyme-linked immunosorbent assays adapted for serotyping of human rotavirus strains.   J. Clin. Micro., 11, 1-5.

DETECTION OF CANINE PARVOVIRUS IN FECAL SAMPLES BY ELISA.
APPLICATION TO ROUTINE SCREENINGS AND A COMPARISON WITH
HEMAGGLUTINATION.

P. Have

State Veterinary Institute for Virus Research,
Lindholm, DK-4771 Kalvehave, Denmark.

SUMMARY.

The conditions of an enzyme-linked immunosorbent assay of canine parvovirus are outlined. The assay is slightly more sensitive than hemagglutination and could be applied to feline panleucopenia virus and mink enteritis virus without altering conditions.
Analysis of fecal samples from dogs with gastroenteritis compared favourably with hemagglutination tests. No samples positive in hemagglutination were found negative by Enzyme immunoassay, whereas a number of samples negative in hemagglutination were positive by the latter test.
A final evaluation of the specificity of the enzyme-linked immunosorbent assay cannot be made by comparison with hemagglutination alone but should include additional evidence for the presence or absence of canine parvovirus in fecal samples.

INTRODUCTION.

The worldwide introduction of canine parvovirus (CPV) into the dog population some 3-4 years ago has created a rather unusual disease-situation, resulting from rapid dissemination of this relatively pathogenic virus into a totally susceptible population. Soon after its introduction similarities with feline panleucopenia were recognized and the relatedness of CPV with feline panleucopenia virus (FPV) and mink enteritis virus (MEV) noted (Appel and others 1979).

The laboratory diagnosis of CPV-infection principally relies on measurement of the strong humoral antibody response that accompany infection and/or detection of CPV excreted with feces, which, in clinically affected dogs, may reach very high levels (Carmichael and others 1980).

Canine parvovirus hemagglutinates red blood cells from a number of species (Carmichael and others 1980), the most sensitive being those of porcine and rhesus macaque origin. Hemagglutination-inhibition is easy to perform and sufficiently sensitive to provide serological evidence of natural exposure to CPV, however a high level of CPV-antibodies persists for years and thus is not in itself indicative of recent infection.

Excretion of CPV with feces shows a highly variable picture as assessed by hemagglutination. Some cases excrete a high level of CPV for several days whereas others present low and transient levels of CPV in feces (unpublished observation). Ill-defined hemagglutinins may be encountered in fecal samples from dogs, most often at relatively low levels (Carmichael and others 1980, Klingeborn and Moreno-López 1980). Accordingly, the presence of CPV-hemagglutinin should always be confirmed by its ability to be inhibited by a suitable high-titered reference serum.

Hemagglutination is at present almost universally adopted as the only practical method for large scale screening of fecal samples for CPV. Considering the theoretical and practical potentials of enzyme immunoassays it was found interesting to investigate, whether such methods might provide additional, and perhaps improved, ways of analysing samples for CPV.

MATERIALS AND METHODS.
Sera.

A positive reference-antiserum to CPV, produced in SPF-dogs, was kindly supplied by Dr. L. E. Carmichael, Cornell University, N. Y. This serum is used to check the specificity of HA-activity in feces.

A pool of dog sera having a hemagglutination-inhibition (HI) titre to CPV of 5120 was made from samples submitted for diagnostic purposes. The globulin fraction of this pool was precipitated with ammonium sulphate and dialysed against phosphate-buffered saline (PBS).

Antiserum to CPV was produced in rabbits immunized with CPV obtained from fecal material and purified by rate-zonal centrifugation in a sucrose gradient. Rabbit antiserum to MEV, purified by rate-zonal and isopycnic banding in sucrose and cesium chloride gradients respectively, was kindly provided by Dr. J. C. Lei, this institute.

HA and HI tests.

These were performed essentially as described by Klingeborn and Moreno-López (1980), except that fecal suspensions after clarification were added bovine serum albumin (BSA) to 1%
final concentration for use in both HA-test and ELISA.

ELISA

Roundbottomed microplates (NUNC, Roskilde, Denmark, cat.
no. 62162) were used throughout.

Plates were coated overnight at $4^{O}C$ with 0.1 ml/well of
the globulin fraction of pooled dog sera, diluted 1:5000 in
50 mM carbonate-buffer, pH 9.6. After three 5 min washes in
PBS-0.05% Tween 20 0.1 ml of fecal suspension was added to 4
wells per sample and allowed to react at $37^{O}C$ for 1 hour. A
blank control and a positive control was set up with each plate. After washing as above 0.1 ml of a 1:1000 dilution of rabbit anti-CPV or rabbit anti-MEV serum in PBS-0.5% BSA was added to each well and left at $37^{O}C$ for 1 hour. Following washing
as above 0.1 ml of peroxidase-conjugated swine anti-rabbit Ig
(DAKO, Copenhagen, cat. no. P 217) diluted 1:200 in PBS-0.5%
BSA was added. The conjugate was pretreated with 25 microli-
ters of dog serum per ml of conjugate to minimize cross-reactivity with canine immunoglobulins. After 1 hour at room temperature plates were washed with PBS-Tween and citrate-phosphate buffer, pH 5, followed by the addition of 0.1 ml of substrate (5 mM o-phenylenediamine (SIGMA), 3.5 mM H_2O_2 in citrate-phosphate buffer). The enzyme reaction was allowed to proceed for 15 min and stopped by the addition of 0.1 ml 1 M
sulphuric acid. Absorbance values at 492 nm were recorded in a
Beckman 151 spectrocolorimeter using water as reference.

RESULTS.

In initial experiments it immediately became clear, that
the rabbit antiserum to CPV was unsuitable as a reagent in this
type of enzyme immunoassay, due to a strong reactivity with the
globulin fraction of dog serum. Absorption of the rabbit antiserum with glutaraldehyde-insolubilized whole dog serum eliminated the reactivity completely. However, indirect evidence

suggested that the specificity of this serum was still not satisfactory, presumably due to incomplete purification of the
immunizing material. The data reported in the following are
therefore obtained exclusively with rabbit antiserum to MEV.

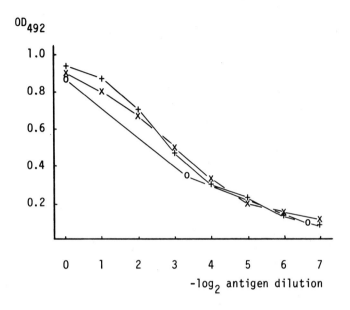

Fig. 1. Titration in CPV-ELISA of FPV (commercial vaccine
for use in dogs) + - +, MEV (field isolate) o - o, CPV
(field isolate, diluted to have a HA-titre of 10) x - x.

Figure 1 gives representative titrations of FPV, MEV and
CPV. Background values were in general around 0.1. The FPV used
was an inactivated, non-adjuvanted commercial vaccine for use
in dogs. The MEV was from a field case of mink enteritis (kindly supplied by Dr. J. C. Lei, this institute). In terms of absolute sensitivity hemagglutination by CPV does not differ significantly from CPV-ELISA, as the lower useful limit of the
latter test (2 x background) corresponds to a HA-titre of approx. 0.5 (fig. 1). When testing goose parvovirus (GPV) and
porcine parvovirus (PPV) in a similar manner no reaction above
background was noted in any dilution tested.

Analysis of 404 fecal samples submitted from clinical cases of vomiting and diarrhea is summarized in fig. 2. The samp-

les were tested undiluted (i.e. as 10% suspensions) and ELISA OD values recorded. It follows from the figure that a large fraction (72%) of the samples form a homogenous group with OD values less than 0.4, hence specific detection of CPV is precluded in this interval.

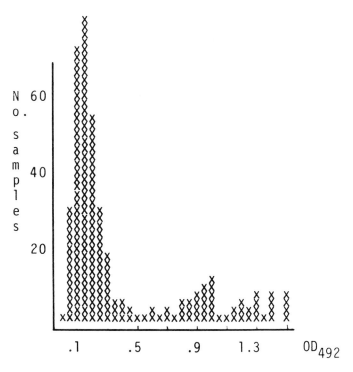

Fig. 2. Analysis with CPV-ELISA of 404 fecal samples from dogs with clinical gastroenteritis.

In fig. 3 the samples from fig. 2 having an OD higher than 0.4 are plotted against the corresponding HA-titres together with a few samples with HA-titres of 640 or higher but OD values less than 0.4. The latter samples could not be confirmed as CPV positive by HI. It should be remembered that the plot is not strictly correlative since ELISA OD values originate from testing only one dilution and thus do not represent a titration. No attempt was made to confirm HA-titres less than

640. Of the 99 samples having OD 0.4 or higher 58 have confirmed HA-titres of 640 or higher. The remaining 41 samples have HA-titres of 320 or lower, however,only very few show no HA-response at all. This is opposed to the samples with OD less than 0.4 where the majority present no HA-activity (not shown).

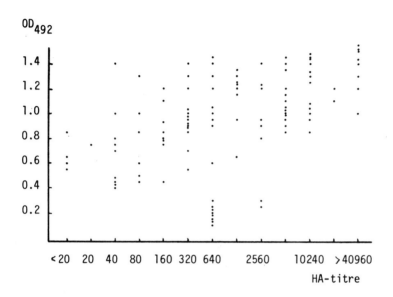

Fig. 3. Association between ELISA OD-values and HA-titre in those fecal samples having OD-value higher than 0.4 or HA-titre at least 640. Same samples as in fig. 2.

Further insight into the relation between hemagglutination an ELISA can be gained from fig. 4 which summarizes the results of daily sampling of feces from a dog with confirmed CPV-infection (serum HI-titre day 1 = 40, day 6 = 2560) and a dog with non-CPV gastroenteritis (serum HI-titre day 1 and 7 less than 20). During the first four days a uniformly high HA-activity as well as ELISA OD values are seen in samples from the CPV-infected dog. After the fourth day HA-activity drops rapidly to a undetectable level whereas the corresponding OD values decline more slowly and still remain appreciably high on day six when no HA-activity is evident. The other dog having a non-CPV disease, which on clinical grounds was suspect of CPV-infection, remained negative in both tests throughout.

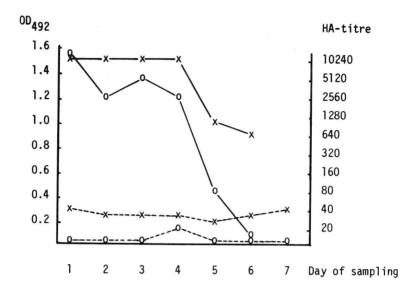

Fig. 4. ELISA and HA examination of fecal samples obtained daily from a dog with confirmed CPV-gastroenteritis ——— and from a dog with non-CPV gastroenteritis (hemorrhagic) -----. (x) ELISA OD values, (o) HA-titres.

DISCUSSION.

The present study tentatively establishes conditions for an enzyme immunoassay of CPV, applicable to large scale screening of fecal samples for the diagnosis of CPV-infection.

The selection of appropriate immunizing material for preparation of rabbit antisera seems to be critical and in this respect virus of fecal origin may be less than ideal, as seen from the results obtained with rabbit anti-CPV serum. Based on the close antigenic relationship between CPV and FPV/MEV, rabbit antiserum to MEV was subsequently used for further studies. As expected, this set-up of reagents allowed detection of not only CPV but also FPV and MEV. Its use with the two latter viruses has not been investigated in detail.

Enzyme immunoassay of CPV appears to provide only slightly higher absolute sensitivity than hemagglutination. On the other hand, the sensitivity of HA is very much dependent on careful selection of red blood cells of individual pigs. The occurrence of non-specific hemagglutinins in feces further limits the usefulness of HA-testing and it has been repeatedly observed, as also illustrated in fig. 4, that CPV hemagglutinin activity may be low, and sometimes incomplete, in face of a strong response in ELISA clearly specific to CPV. From this and from the data in fig. 3 it can be concluded that fecal samples found to contain CPV by hemagglutination will also be detected by ELISA. A number of samples can be expected to produce low or no HA-activity and still retain significant reactivity in ELISA. Whether all the samples in fig. 3 having HA-titre 320 or less belong to this category cannot be stated with certainty.

A final evaluation of the specificity of the enzyme immunoassay of CPV is not possible from data of hemagglutination alone, but will require additional evidence such as infectivity testing, electron microscopic examination and indirect evidence i.e. confirmed antibody response.

REFERENCES.

Appel. M.J.G., F.W.Scott & L.E.Carmichael (1979). Isolation and immunisation studies of a canine parvolike virus from dogs with haemorrhagic enteritis. Vet.Rec. 105, 156-159.

Carmichael, L.E., J.C.Joubert & R.V.H.Pollock (1980). Hemagglutination by canine parvovirus: Serologic studies and diagnostic applications. Am. J. Vet. Res. 41, (5), 784-791.

Klingeborn, B. & J.Moreno-López (1980). Diagnostic experience from an epidemic of canine parvoviral enteritis. Zbl. Vet. Med. B 27, 483-488.

COMPARISON OF AN IMMUNOFLUORESCENT TEST AND AN ELISA FOR THE RAPID
DIAGNOSIS OF INFECTIOUS BOVINE RHINOTRACHEITIS IN EXPERIMENTALLY
INFECTED ANIMALS.

P.F. Nettleton, J.A. Herring, J.M. Sharp, A.J. Herring and
A. McL. Dawson

Moredun Research Institute, Edinburgh

ABSTRACT

Five, 3 to 8 week old calves were infected intranasally with one or
other of two strains of infectious bovine rhinotracheitis virus, and the
amount of virus in nasal secretions was monitored daily over the next 8
days using standard virus isolation procedures and rapid immunofluorescence (IF) and ELISA methods.

Despite a difference in the pathogenicity of the 2 strains which was
reflected in the amounts of live virus excreted, all five calves showed
consistent patterns of virus excretion as detected by the 3 methods.
Infectious virus was isolated from all calves over the first 7 days and
all but one calf on the 8th day with peak excretion levels occurring
between days 2 and 6. One animal was positive by the IF test on day 1 but
otherwise the 2 rapid methods detected virus only between 2 and 7 days
post infection. During this time 83% of samples in the IF test and 77% of
samples in the ELISA test were shown to contain virus. It was concluded
that the ELISA test was as sensitive as the IF test in establishing a
rapid diagnosis of IBR infection and could be adapted for use under field
conditions.

INTRODUCTION

Bovine herpesvirus 1 (BHV1) infection in cattle has been associated

with respiratory, ocular, reproductive, central nervous system, enteric,

neonatal and dermal disease (Gibbs and Rweyemamu, 1977). A particularly

severe form of infectious bovine rhinotracheitis (IBR) due to BHV1

infection emerged in north-east Scotland during the winter of 1977-78

(Wiseman and others, 1978) and spread quickly so that the disease is now a

major economic problem in beef fattening units and dairy herds in many

parts of Britain (Wiseman and others, 1979). Severe IBR is characterised

by respiratory tract and ocular disease (Wiseman and others, 1980; Allan

and others, 1980) and although a tentative diagnosis can be made on

clinical and epidemiological grounds laboratory confirmation is advisable

since other similar syndromes occur (Obi and others, 1981). It is also

likely that as the disease becomes established in the national herd it

will become more difficult to differentiate from other respiratory

infections. Traditional laboratory procedures of virus isolation and
typing require expensive tissue culture facilities and are relatively slow
usually providing only a retrospective confirmation of infection.

Now that a live vaccine is available (Tracherine, Smith Kline Animal
Health) which is effective in preventing the spread of IBR to adjacent
groups of cattle (Imray, 1980) a rapid confirmatory test would be of value
to veterinary practitioners faced with a respiratory disease outbreak
possibly caused by IBR virus.

Rapid methods of diagnosing IBR infection using immunofluorescent
(IF) tests have been described. Smears made from cells derived from nasal
scrapings allowed a diagnosis to be reached (Chennekatu and others, 1966)
but smears of nasal swabs on microscope slides have also been used
successfully (Terpstra, 1979). With the recent development of enzyme-
linked immunosorbent assay (ELISA) systems rapid diagnosis of virus
infections such as hepatitis B (Wolters and others, 1976) and rotavirus
(Ellens and De leeuw, 1977) has become feasible. In view of the need for
a rapid diagnostic test for IBR infections an IF test and an ELISA test
have been evaluated using experimentally infected calves from which the
level of virus in nasal secretions was also monitored by isolation in
tissue culture.

MATERIALS AND METHODS

Virus.   2 strains of IBR virus (designated 460/2 and 523/3) were used.
These had been isolated from dexamethasone treated calves used to study
the re-excretion of virus from vaccinated and challenged animals
(Nettleton and Sharp, 1980). Both strains were passed 3 times at limiting
dilution in secondary bovine embryo kidney (BEK) cells and stocks were
prepared in a semicontinuous cell line of embryonic bovine trachea (EBTR)
cells.

Cell cultures and virus growth.   BEK cells were grown as previously
described (Snodgrass and others, 1976), EBTR cells were grown until
confluent in Eagles '59' medium supplemented with 10% adult bovine serum
and containing penicillin, streptomycin, polymixin-B and mycostatin at 100
i.u., 100 μg., 50 i.u., and 50 units per ml. respectively. After removal
of growth medium, washing in Hank's B.S.S. and virus adsorption at 37°C
for 1 hour, both types of cell monolayers were maintained in serum-free
'199' medium supplemented with 0.5% bovine serum albumin (BSA), 0.1%

lactalbumin hydrolysate (LAH) and 0.1% yeast extract, and containing penicillin, streptomycin and polymixin-B in the same concentrations as used in the growth medium. At 72 hours post-infection cultures were frozen and thawed once, clarified at 2000 g for 15 minutes and the supernates stored at -70°C.

All cell cultures were screened for the presence of contaminating bovine virus diarrhoea virus using an indirect immunofluorescence test (Nettleton, Herring and Corrigall, 1980).

Experimental animals. Five, 3 to 8 week old Jersey bull calves free from antibodies to IBR virus were housed singly or in pairs in loose boxes. Two calves, aged 6 and 8 weeks, received 6.7 $\log_{10}$TC1D$_{50}$ of virus strain 523/3 and three calves, aged 3, 4 and 8 weeks, received 6.9 $\log_{10}$TC1D$_{50}$ of virus strain 460/2. Virus was given as a 5 ml intranasal dose divided equally between each nostril.

The calves were examined clinically before infection and daily for the next 8 days. Following examination 2 nasal swabs (Exogen Ltd) were collected and each swab was used to make a smear on 2 microscope slides before one was placed into 4 ml. Hank's BSS containing 1% BSA 300 i.u./ml penicillin, 300μg/ml streptomycin, and 50 i.u./ml Polymixin B (VTM) for virus isolation and the other was placed into 2 ml. ELISA washing and diluting (W/D) buffer for ELISA assay.

Virus isolation. Swabs in VTM were sonicated for 30 seconds in an ultrasonic water bath (Engisonic Ltd., model B32) and 0.2 ml of $\log_{10}$ dilutions of medium was inoculated on to duplicate tubes of EBTR cells. After 1 hour the inoculum was washed off with Hanks BSS containing antibiotics and 1 ml of maintenance medium was added to each tube. The cultures were examined for up to 6 days to detect virus cytopathic effect and the concentration of virus in the starting material was calculated according to the method of Spearman and Karber (Lennette and Schmidt, 1969).

Preparation of hyperimmune serum. Clarified harvests of EBTR cells infected with a field isolate of IBR virus (strain 8301) were centrifuged at 40,000 g for 1 hour and the pelletted virus resuspended in 1/20th of the original volume in phosphate buffered saline (PBS) pH 7.2. Virus was then centrifuged at 95,000 g for 1 hour in a Beckman SW40Ti rotor down a 10% to 25% ficoll step gradient. The virus banding on top of the 25% ficoll was harvested, diluted five times in 1MNaCl, 0.1M Tris, 0.01M EDTA (TNE) buffer and pelletted at 95,000 g for 40 minutes. Virus pellets were redissolved in 0.5 ml PBS and emulsified with an equal volume of adjuvant.

A single rabbit received two 0.3 ml subcutaneous injections of virus in complete Freund's adjuvant, followed at 3 weekly intervals, by the same dose of virus in incomplete Freund's and purified virus without adjuvant given intravenously. 10 days later the rabbit was exsanguinated and the serum, which had a reciprocal neutralising antibody titre of 1024 in a microtitre test employing 40 $T.C.I.D._{50}$/well of the IBR Oxford strain, was stored at -20°C.

Indirect immunofluorescent test (IFT)

In order to reduce non-specific fluorescence, the hyperimmune rabbit serum was absorbed with an uninfected EBTR cell lysate followed by an equal volume of nasal secretion, collected by tampon, from IBR-antibody free, clinically healthy calves. This absorbed serum was further diluted with PBS to give a final working dilution of 1:1000.

The acetone fixed nasal smears were successively incubated at 37°C for 30 minutes with the absorbed serum, and fluorescein labelled sheep anti-rabbit immunoglobulin (Wellcome reagents) with 3 washes of PBS in between. After further washing and counterstaining with 0.005% Evan's blue the smears were mounted in buffered glycerol, pH 8.2 and examined with a Leitz Ortholux microscope using an incident u-v light source. Known positive and negative nasal smears were included in each test.

ELISA Test

IgG was prepared from the same hyperimmune rabbit serum using a protein-A sepharose column (Goding, 1976) and half of this specific anti-IBR virus IgG was conjugated with alkaline phosphatase, Sigma type VII (Sigma Chemical Company, Poole, Dorset) by the method of Engvall and Perlmann (1972) and stored in 150 μl aliquots at -20°C.

The reagents for the test were the same as those already described (Burrells, Wells and Dawson, 1979) except that the buffer used for diluting the conjugate and for washing the plates consisted of 1 litre of PBS containing 20.45 g of NaCl, 0.05% Tween 80 and 0.01M EDTA (W/D buffer). Tests were carried out in polystyrene microtitre plates (type M129A, Dynatech Laboratories Ltd) using 100 μl volumes of all reagents. The wells on half the plate were sensitised overnight at 4°C with a 1/50 dilution of anti-IBR IgG (containing 5-11 mgm protein/ml) made in carbonate coating buffer, all other wells receiving only coating buffer. Plates were washed 3 times with W/D buffer, virus suspensions were added to duplicate sensitised wells and a single unsensitised well, and the plates incubated for 2 hours, after which the virus suspensions were aspirated and the washing procedure was repeated. Alkaline phosphatase-conjugated rabbit anti-IBR IgG (conjugate) diluted in W/D buffer was then added to all wells and the plates were again incubated for 2 hours at room temperature before being washed as before. Enzyme substrate was then added to all wells and after a further 2 hours at room temperature the level of absorbance at OD_{405} in each well was measured using a Titertek Multiskan multichannel spectrophotometer (Flow Laboratories). Eight wells exposed only to coating buffer, conjugate and enzyme substrate were used as a blank and a virus suspension with a known absorbance value was included in each test. All nasal secretions were tested at least twice and the mean absorbance of all the test wells calculated. All virus suspensions added to unsensitised wells gave absorbance values $<$ 0.01 OD_{405}. Pre-infection samples added to sensitised wells had absorbance values in the range 0.00 - 0.05 OD_{405}. The minimum absorbance value consistently detectable by eye was 0.08 and samples with mean values $>$0.08 were considered positive.

RESULTS

Clinical examination of the calves revealed a difference in pathogenicity between the 2 virus strains used. Strain 523/3 produced pyrexia ($>$ 40°C) in both calves for 3 and 4 days respectively, between the third and sixth day post-infection and serous nasal discharge was apparent at this time. Ulceration of the nasal mucosae developed on day 6 and persisted until the end of the experiment by which time the nasal discharge was mucopurulent. Calves receiving strain 460/2 did not develop pyrexia and the only clinical sign of infection was ulceration of the

nasal mucosae from day 6 onwards accompanied by slight mucopurulent
discharge.

This difference in pathogenicity was reflected by the levels of live
virus excreted by calves receiving the 2 strains. Figures 1 and 2
summarise the virus excretion patterns, as measured by virus isolation,
IFT and ELISA, from calves receiving 523/3 and 460/2 virus respectively.

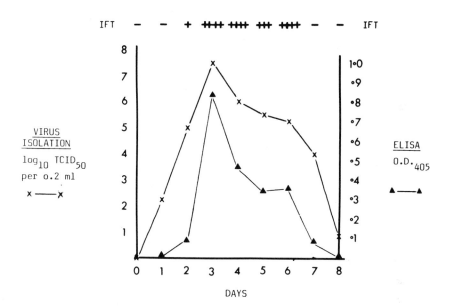

Fig. 1.   Virus excreted by calves
          receiving strain 523/3. Virus
          isolation and ELISA values are
          the mean results from 2 calves.
          IFT results are shown as No. of
          positive slides/day.

The more pathogenic 523/3 strain resulted in the mean excretion of 5.0 –
7.5 $\log_{10}TClD_{50}$/0.2 ml VTM between 2 and 6 days post-infection whereas
over the same period only 4.0 – 5.0 $\log_{10} TClD_{50}$0.2 ml was excreted by
calves receiving strain 460/2. ELISA values from calves receiving strain
523/3 were consequently higher over the period of peak virus excretion but

138

it was interesting that ELISA values on days 2 and 7 were higher from calves receiving strain 460/2 suggesting that greater amounts of non-infectious antigen were produced by this strain. Evidence to support this was provided by the IFT which also detected virus earlier and later from calves receiving the less pathogenic strain.

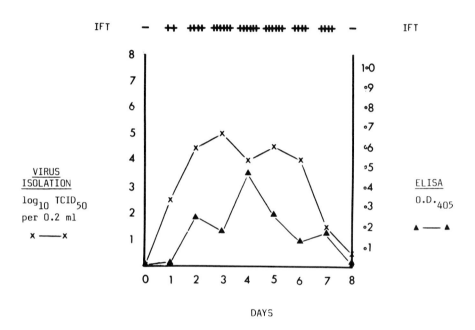

Fig. 2.   Virus excreted by calves receiving strain 460/2.   Virus isolation and ELISA values are the mean results from 3 calves. IFT results are shown as No. of positive slides/day

In spite of the quantitative differences between the virus excretion pattern provoked by the 2 strains some important findings emerge about the comparative efficiency of the three methods of virus detection when the results from all 5 calves are considered together.   The number of calves excreting virus on each day as detected by the 3 methods, is shown in Table 1

Table 1. Number of calves from which
virus was detected by each
of the three methods

DAY	VIRUS ISOLATION	IFT	ELISA
1	5	1	0
2	5	4	3
3	5	5	4
4	5	5	5
5	5	5	5
6	5	4	3
7	5	2	3
8	4	0	0
TOTAL	39	26	23

Clearly, virus isolation was the most efficient method of detecting virus,
with only 1 calf on the 8th day not excreting virus. There was little
difference between the number of samples shown to be positive by the rapid
diagnostic tests although the IFT was slightly better, detecting 67% of
samples shown to contain infectious virus as against the 59% detected by
ELISA.

DISCUSSION

Isolation of virus from nasal swabs in tissue culture was the most
sensitive method of confirming IBR virus infection. Peak infectious virus
excretion occurred on day 3 post infection, fell off slowly over the next
3-4 days and was at a low level by day 8, so that 1 of 5 calves was
negative on this day. Other workers have shown that virus may be isolated
from calves for up to 11 days (Gibbs and Rweyemamu, 1977).

Of the rapid diagnostic tests the IFT detected all animals as positive between day 3 and day 5. One animal was detected on day 1, and between days 2 and 7 83% of all samples were positive by this method. These results are in close agreement with those of Terpstra (1979) who, using a direct IFT, also showed that fluorescence was detectable from the second till the seventh day after infection and was most distinct between 3 and 5 days. The ELISA test detected virus only between days 2 and 7 during which time 77% of all samples were positive; as with the IFT virus was most readily detectable from all animals between day 3 and day 5. Previous reports of the detection of herpes virus in clinical samples by ELISA are limited, and this may be because herpes simplex virus and cytomegalovirus have been shown to be more difficult to detect than some other human viruses notably respiratory syncytial virus and coxsackievirus (McIntosh et al, 1980).

In considering the application of either rapid test for use in the diagnosis of field infections of IBR the following points should be considered. Both methods are inferior to virus isolation in cell cultures but have the advantages that they do not require expensive tissue culture facilities and provide a rapid answer. The IFT can be undertaken only in a laboratory with a fluorescent microscope and good staining facilities, and interpretation of the fluorescence is subjective. While the ELISA requires a greater preparation and consumption of reagents it can be performed with very limited facilities and provide an unequivocal result.

The most important point, however, is that both rapid tests are only of value between day 2 and 7 post infection. In the clinical disease this period coincides with pyrexia and serous nasal discharge. Since veterinary attention may be sought only for animals with a mucopurulent discharge, it is essential that, for a rapid diagnosis of IBR, several animals in the group should be examined and samples collected from at least three with pyrexia. Only then will a negative result from a rapid diagnostic test rule out the possibility of an IBR infection.

REFERENCES

Allan, E.M., Pirie, H.M., Msolla, P.M., Selman, I.E. and Wiseman, A. 1980.
The pathological features of severe cases of infectious bovine
rhinotracheitis. Vet. Rec. 107, 441–445.
Burrells, C., Wells, P.W. and Dawson, A. McL. 1978/1979. The quantitative
estimation of antibody to Pasteurella haemolytica in sheep sera using
a micro-enzyme-linked immunosorbent assay (ELISA). Vet. Micro., 3,
291–301.
Chennekatu, P.P., Gratzek, J.B., Ramsey, F.K. 1966. Isolation and
characterisation of a strain of infectious bovine rhinotracheitis
virus associated with enteritis in cattle: pathogenesis studies by
fluorescent antibody testing. Am. J. Vet. Res. 27, 1583–1590.
Ellens, D.J. and De Leeuw, P.W. 1977. Enzyme-linked immunosorbent assay
for diagnosis of rotavirus infections in calves. J. Clin. Micro,
6, 530–532.
Engvall, E. and Perlmann, P. 1972. Enzyme-linked immunosorbent assay,
ELISA. III. Quantitation of specific antibodies by enzyme labelled
anti-immunoglobulin in antigen coated tubes. J. Immunol. 109, 129–
135.
Gibbs, E.P.J. and Rweyemamu, M.M. 1977. Bovine herpesviruses. Part I.
Bovine herpesvirus I. Vet. Bull., 47, 317–343.
Goding, J.W. 1976. Conjugation of antibodies with fluorochromes:
modifications to the standard methods. J. Immunol. Methods. 13, 215–
226.
Imray, W.S. 1980. Use of a modified live infectious bovine rhinotracheitis
vaccine in the field. Vet. Rec. 107, 511–512.
Lenette, E.H. and Schmidt, N.J. 1969. Diagnostic procedures for viral and
rickettsial infections. 4th Edition. (American Public Health
Association Inc).
McIntosh, K., Wilfert, C., Chernesky, M., Plotkin, S. and Mattheis, M.J.
1980. Summary of a workshop on new and useful techniques in rapid
viral diagnosis. J. Inf. Dis., 142, 793–802.
Nettleton, P.F., Herring, J.A. and Corrigall, W. 1980. Isolation of bovine
virus diarrhoea virus from a Scottish red deer. Vet. Rec. 107, 425–
426.
Nettleton, P.F. and Sharp, J.M. 1980. Infectious bovine rhinotracheitis
virus excretion after vaccination. Vet. Rec., 107, 379.
Obi, T.U., Wiseman, A., Selman, I.E., Allan, E.M. and Nettleton, P.F. 1981.
An infectious bovine rhinotracheitis-like respiratory syndrome in
young calves. Vet. Rec. 108, 400–401.
Snodgrass, D.R., Herring, J.A. and Gray, E.W. 1976. Experimental rotavirus
infection in lambs. J. comp. Path. 86, 637–642.
Terpstra, C. 1979. Diagnosis of infectious bovine rhinotracheitis by
direct immunofluorescence. Vet. Quart. 1, 138–144.
Wiseman, A., Msolla, P.M., Selman, I.E., Allan, E.M., Cornwell, H.J.C.,
Pirie, H.M. and Imray, W.S. 1978. An acute severe outbreak of
infectious bovine rhinotracheitis: clinical, epidemiological,
microbiological and pathological aspects. Vet. Rec. 103, 391–397.
Wiseman, A., Msolla, P.M., Selman, I.E., Allan, E.M. and Pirie, H.M. 1980.
Clinical and epidemiological features of 15 incidents of severe
infectious bovine rhinotracheitis. Vet. Rec. 107, 436–441.
Wiseman, A., Selman, I.E., Msolla, P.M., Pirie, H.M. and Allan, E. 1979.
The financial burden of infectious bovine rhinotracheitis. Vet. Rec.
105, 469.
Wolters, G., Kuijpers, L., Kacaki, J. and Schuurs, A. 1976. Solid-phase
enzyme-immunoassay for detection of hepatitis B surface antigen.
J. Clin. Path, 29, 873–879.

THE RELATIVE EFFICIENCY OF TWO ELISA TECHNIQUES

FOR THE TITRATION OF FMD ANTIGEN

E Ouldridge, P Barnett and M M Rweyemamu

Wellcome Foundation Limited,
Wellcome Foot and Mouth Disease Laboratory,
Ash Road,
Pirbright, Woking,
Surrey, England.

ABSTRACT

The ability of indirect enzyme linked immunosorbent assays (ELISA), indirect sandwich ELISA, reverse passive haemagglutination (RPH), solid phase agglutination with coupled erythrocytes (SPACE) and complement fixation tests (CF) to detect FMDV antigen were compared.

Indirect sandwich ELISA and RPH were found to be most sensitive detecting as little as 0.02 µg/ml 140S antigen. CF, SPACE and indirect ELISA were less sensitive, detecting a minimum of 0.2 to 0.4 µg/ml 140S antigen. RPH, SPACE and indirect sandwich ELISA were most discriminating for homologous 140S; differentiating between 140S particles and trypsin treated 140S and not appreciably detecting 12S or heterotypic 140S antigen. Indirect ELISA and CF were found to be relatively nonspecific. They did not differentiate between 140S and trypsin treated 140S. Both these latter rests showed strong heterotypic reaction especially when using sera taken after revaccination.

For the measurement of 140S particles, in tissue culture antigens either RPH or indirect sandwich ELISA systems would be suitable. SPACE and indirect sandwich ELISA might be suitable for detecting 140S in samples of complex composition (e.g., vaccines).

INTRODUCTION

The immunoassay commonly used by FMD investigators to quantify the immunogen has been the complement fixation test (CFT) (Brown and Newman, 1963; Bradish et al., 1964). Other tests such as the radial diffusion test (Cowan and Wagner, 1970), single radial haemolysis (Rweyemamu et al., 1980), and the antibody combining test. (Terpstra et al ., 1976), have had a limited application in vaccine antigen titrations. The major drawback of the CFT has been its relative nonspecificity. It detects both the immunogenic antigens - the 140S and 75S particles (Rowlands et al., 1975, Rweyemamu et al., 1979), and the non immunogenic capsid protein subunits - 12S particles (Brown, 1972). Furthermore it does not distinguish between the intact capsid and the trypsin cleaved capsid which for most virus strains is of diminished immunogenicity (Wild and Brown; Bachrach et al., 1975). Because of these criticisms of CFT, assessments of 140S mass detected by sucrose density sedimentation (Barteling and Meloen, 1974) have increasingly been used for the measurement of FMD immunogen. However, this assay does not distinguish between mixtures of virus types or between the intact capsid and trypsin cleaved capsids.

With the recent advent of new immunoassay systems such as Radio-immunoassays (Hunter, 1973), Enzyme-linked immunosorbent assays (ELISA) (Voller et al., 1978), Red blood cell agglutination assays (Coombs, 1981) and Fluoroimmunoassays (Katsh et al., 1974), it seems possible to develop inproved immunoassays for measurements of the FMD immunogen. In this paper the indirect ELISA, the indirect sandwich ELISA (Abu El-Zein and Crowther 1979, a; b). Reverse passive haemagglutination (RPH) (Coombs, 1981) and solid phase agglutination with coupled erythrocytes (SPACE) (Bradburne et al., 1979) have been adapted for use with FMD and their specificity and sensitivity compared with CFT and the potential sensitivity of 140S mass determinations.

The details of each of these immunoassays are described elsewhere (Ouldridge et al., 1982). The antigen preparations used were sucrose density gradient purified preparations of homologous (strain: O_1BFS 1860) 140S, 12S and trypsin-cleaved 140S and heterotypic 140S (strain: SAT 2 Tan 5/68). Sensitivity was defined as the minimum concentration of homologous 140S detected and specificity was defined as the ability of the test to distinguish between homologous 140S and the other preparations.

THE INDIRECT ELISA AND THE INDIRECT SANDWICH ELISA

Both the indirect and the indirect sandwich ELISA techniques (Abu El-Zein and Crowther, 1979 a and b) were investigated. Figure 1 outlines the procedures adopted. For the indirect ELISA, serial dilutions of antigen were adsorbed to wells of PVC microtitre plates, reacted with guinea pig anti-virion serum and then rabbit anti guinea pig IgG antibody conjugated to horse radish peroxidase. The final reaction was detected using o-phenylenediamine as the substrate. For the indirect sandwich ELISA, rabbit anti-FMDV serum was adsorbed to wells of PVC microplates, reacted with dilutions of antigen and thereafter, the same procedure as the indirect ELISA was followed. Typical results obtained in both test systems are summarised in Figs 2 and 3, and the greater specificity of the indirect sandwich ELISA is apparent since it readily distinguished intact virion from trypsin-cleaved virion and 12S subunits and heterotypic virion. End points for each titration were

144

FIGURE 1

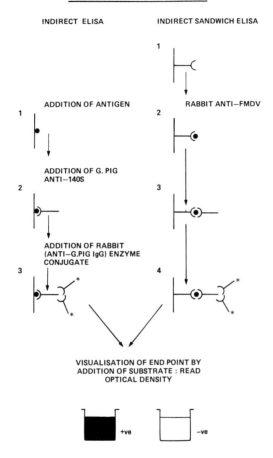

SCHEMATIC PROCEDURE FOR ELISA

INDIRECT ELISA INDIRECT SANDWICH ELISA

RABBIT ANTI—FMDV

ADDITION OF ANTIGEN

ADDITION OF G. PIG
ANTI—140S

ADDITION OF RABBIT
(ANTI—G.PIG IgG) ENZYME
CONJUGATE

VISUALISATION OF END POINT BY
ADDITION OF SUBSTRATE : READ
OPTICAL DENSITY

+ve   −ve

FIGURE 2:   A plot of the optical densities obtained in an indirect ELISA
using serum from, primovaccinates and varying concentrations
of homologous 140S (140) homologous trypsin-treated 140S
(140TT) virion subunits (12S) and heterotypic 140S.

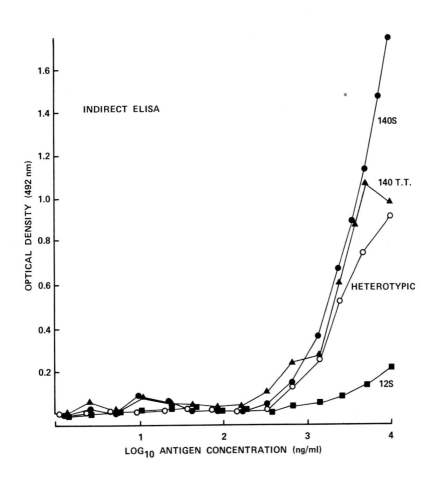

FIGURE 3: A plot of the optical densities obtained in an indirect sandwich ELISA using homologous serum from primovaccinates and varying concentrations of homologous 140S (140), homologous trypsin-treated 140S (140TT), virion subunits (12S) and heterotypic 140S.

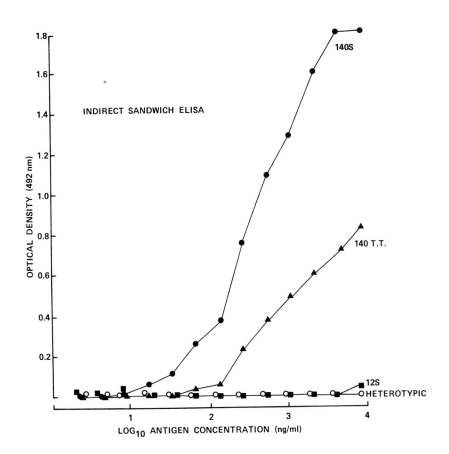

taken as the minimum detectable positive reaction. Using this criterion, the indirect sandwich ELISA was about ten times more sensitive than the indirect ELISA.

COMPARISON OF THE SENSITIVITY AND SPECIFICITY OF ELISA SYSTEMS WITH OTHER IMMUNOASSAYS

The indirect ELISA and the indirect sandwich ELISA were compared with RPH, SPACE and C.F.

Both RPH and SPACE tests involve the coating of sheep or goat erythrocytes with anti-FMDV IgG, using chromic chloride (Fig 4). For the RPH test, coated erythrocytes were incubated at $37^{\circ}C$ for 30 minutes and haemagglutination was determined. For ease of detection of the 50% end point, plates were left in the refrigerator for 2-3 hours to allow non-agglutinated erythrocytes to settle beofre final reading of the HA titres. The principle difference in the procedure for SPACE was that anti-FMDV IgG was initially adsorbed to microtitre plate wells, then reacted with serial dilutions of antigen before the addition of erythrocytes. Haemagglutination was determined similarly.

Complement fixation tests were performed as a checkerboard (Forman, 1974) using 3 units of complement and fixation at $37^{\circ}C$ for one hour. The 50% dilution end point for each antigen was determined using the optimum dilution of serum.

The same homologous virion preparation was used to determine the limits of detection for each test. Table 1 shows that the indirect sandwich ELISA and RPH were most sensitive, detecting as little as 0.02 to 0.05 µg 140S/ml. This compares well with the sucrose density method used in our laboratory for 140S assessment which has a detection limit at about 0.05 µg 140S/ml (Terry G.M. personal communication).

The relative specificity of the tests was compared by calculating ratios of the minimum concentration of intact virion to the minimum concentration of trypsin cleaved virion, virion subunit or heterotypic virion detected in each test. Table 1 also shows that while RPH, SPACE and the indirect sandwich ELISA were very discriminating, the indirect ELISA was even less discriminating than complement fixation.

The indirect sandwich ELISA, RPH and SPACE all distinguished between intact virion and trypsin cleaved virions while barely detecting virion subunits or heterotypic virion.

148

FIGURE 4

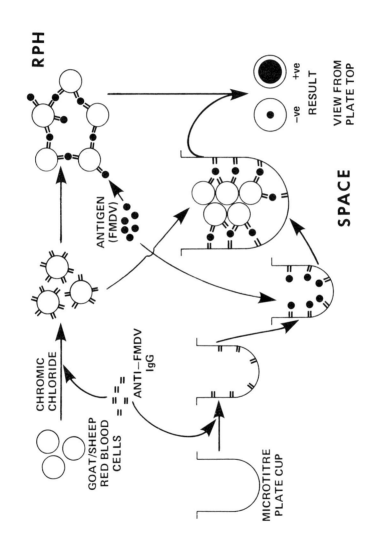

SCHEMATIC PROCEDURE FOR RPH AND SPACE TESTS

RPH

GOAT/SHEEP RED BLOOD CELLS

CHROMIC CHLORIDE

ANTIGEN (FMDV)

ANTI–FMDV IgG

MICROTITRE PLATE CUP

SPACE

–ve   +ve
RESULT
VIEW FROM PLATE TOP

TABLE 1: A comparison of the sensitivity and specificity of CF, RPH, SPACE, indirect ELISA and indirect sandwich ELISA.

Test	Serum	Sensitivity (Minimum detectable 140S μg/ml)	Specificity *		
			Trypsin treated 140S	12S	Heterotypic 140S (SAT 2 TAN 5/68)
Complement fixation	primovaccinate	0.39	2	43	>64
	revaccinate	0.28	1	4	8
R.P.H.	primovaccinate	0.05	8	256	>256
S.P.A.C.E.	primovaccinate	0.20	16	>128	>128
Indirect sandwich ELISA	primovaccinate	0.02	8	>512	>512
	revaccinate	0.02	4	128	128
Indirect ELISA	primovaccinate	0.251	1	13	1
	revaccinate	0.158	1	32	1

*Ratio of homologous 140S antigen concentration to concentration of the following antigens at their respective end points for each test.

THE EFFECT OF SERUM ON TEST SPECIFICITY

The effect of serum quality on the specificity of complement and the two ELISA's was examined. Table 1 shows that while serum from primovaccinates could distinguish between homologous and heterotypic virion in complement fixation, serum from revaccinates did not so readily do so. Serum from revaccinates was also marginally less discriminating in the indirect sandwich ELISA. The indirect ELISA showed such poor specificity anyway, that a comparison between sera from primovaccinates and revaccinates was not possible.

DISCUSSION

The object of this work was to develop or adapt immunoassays for the specific and sensitive measurement of the FMDV immunogen. Of the tests examined RPH and the indirect sandwich ELISA were found to be the most sensitive and most specific. These tests would therefore seem to be the most suited for routine titration of vaccine antigens. In view of its simplicity, the RPH test may be the method that is most readily adaptable for routine work by laboratories that are not equipped for ELISA. However, the indirect sandwich ELISA has a greater potential for quantification particularly where it is essential to detect minor virion degradation i.e. VP1 proteolysis.

REFERENCES

Abu El-Zein, E.M.E. and Crowther, J.R. 1979a. Detection and Quantification of foot and mouth disease virus by enzyme labelled immunosorbent assay techniques. J. Gen. Virol. 42, 567-602.

Abu El-Zein, E.M.E. and Crowther, J.R. 1979b. Application of the enzyme linked immunosorbent assay to the detection and identification of foot and mouth disease viruses. J. Hyg. Camb. 83, 513.

Bachrach, H.L., Moore, D.M., McKercher, P.D. and Polatnick, J. 1975. Immune and antibody responses to an isolated capsid protein of foot and mouth disease virus. J. Immunol. 115, 1636-1641.

Barteling, S.J. and Meloen, R.H. 1974. A simple method for quantification of 140S particles of FMD virus. Arch ges. virusforsch. 45, 362-364.

Bradish, C.J., Jowett, R. and Kirkham, J.B. 1964. The fixation of complement by virus-antibody complexes: equivalence and inhibition in the reactions of the viruses of tomato bushy stunt and foot and mouth disease with rabbit and guinea pig antisera. J. Gen. Microbiol, 35, 27-51.

Bradborne, A.F., Almeida, J.D., Gardener, P.S., Moosai, R.B., Nash, A.A. and Coombs, R.R.A. 1979. A solid-phase system (SPACE) for the detection and quantification of Rotavirus in faeces. J. Gen. Virol. 44, 615-623.

Brown, F. 1972. Structure-function relationships in foot and mouth disease virus. In Immunity in Viral and Rickettsial Diseases. Editors A. Kohn and M.A. Klingberg, Plenum Publishing Corpn.

Brown, F and Newman, J.F.E. 1973. In vivo measurement of the potency of inactivated foot and mouth disease vaccines. J. Hyg. Camb. 61, 345-351.

Coombs, R.R.A. 1981. Assays using red blood cells as markers in "Immuno-Assays for the 80s" (edited by A. Voller, A. Bartlett and D. Bidwell) (MTP Press Limited, Lancaster, England) pp. 17-34.

Cowan, K.M. and Wagner, G.G. 1970. Immunochemical studies of foot and mouth disease VIII. Detection and quantification of antibodies by radial immunodiffusion. J. Immunol. 105, 557-566.

Forman, A.J. 1974. A study of foot and mouth disease virus strains by complement fixation II a comparison of tube and microplate tests for the differentiation of strains. J. Hyg. Camb. 72, 407.

Hunter, W.M. 1973. Handbook of Experimental Immunology. 1, (ed. D.M. Weir) (Blackwell, Oxford).

Katsh, S., Leaver, F.W., Reynolds, J.S, and Katsh, G.F. 1974. A simple rapid fluorimetric assay for antigens. J. Immunol. Methods. 5, 179-187.

Ouldridge, E., Barnett, P. and Rweyemamu, M.M. 1982. A comparative assessment of five immunoassays for the specific detection and quantification of the FMDV immunising antigen. (In Press).

Rowlands, D.J., Sangar, D.V. and Brown, F. 1975. A comparative chemical serological study of the full and empty particles of foot and mouth disease virus. J. Gen. Virol. 26, 227-238.

Rweyemamu, M.M., Terry, G. and Pay, T.W.F. 1979. Stability and immunogenicity of empty particles of foot and mouth disease. Arch. Virol. 59, 69-79.

Rweyemamu, M.M., Parry, N.R. and Sargent, J. 1980. The application of a single radial haemolysis technique to foot and mouth disease virus-antibody study. Arch. Virol. 64, 47-55.

Terpstra, C., Frenkel, S., Straver, P.J., Barteling, S.J. and van Bekkum, J.G. 1976. Comparison of laboratory techniques for the evaluation of the antigenic potency of foot and mouth disease virus culture and vaccines. Vet. Microbiol. 1, 71-83.

Voller, A., Bidwell, D.E. and Bartlett, A. 1976. The application of microplate enzyme-linked immunosorbent assays to some infectious diseases. First International Symposium on Immunoenzymatic Techniques INSERM Symposium No 2. pp 167-173, (ed Feldman et al) (North-Holland pub. Co. Amsterdam).

Wild, T.F. and Brown, F. 1967. Nature of the inactivating action of trypsin on foot and mouth disease virus. J. gen. Virol. 1, 247-250

THE USE OF AN INDIRECT SANDWICH ELISA ASSAY
FOR THE DIFFERENTIATION OF FMD VIRUS STRAINS

E J Ouldridge, P Barnett, P Hingley, M Head and M M Rweyemamu

Wellcome Foundation Limited,
Wellcome Foot and Mouth Disease Laboratory,
Ash Road,
Pirbright, Woking,
Surrey, England

ABSTRACT

An indirect sandwich ELISA technique is described which can be used for the differentiation of FMD virus strains. A technique using a fixed concentration of virus with varying dilutions of serum was investigated. Sigmoid curves were obtained for the homologous and heterologous reactions. A mathematical model was devised to fit curves using all the data. This model estimates the characteristics of each curve which may be interpreted as measures of the number of reacting antigenic sites, the antigen heterogeneity and the average affinity of the antigen-antibody reaction.

This test was applied to a study of relationships between type O FMDV strains of recent epidemiological significance. The exact biological significance of relationships determined by ELISA is at present unknown. However, when these results were compared with r values from micro-neutralisation tests only one example in seven demonstrated a discrepancy in the inter-strain relationship.

INTRODUCTION

One of the principal characteristics of FMDV is its serological diversity. There are seven distinct serotypes which demonstrate no cross protection and over 60 subtypes which demonstrate only partial cross protection (Pereira, 1977). Intratypic serological differentiation of virus strains, therefore, constitutes a major activity of FMD laboratories engaged in epidemiological studies and those involved in vaccine selection. In our laboratories the reference test system for this purpose is the two dimensional microneutralisation test (Rweyemamu et al, 1978). This test selectively measures differences in the major immunogenic site of FMDV. Complement fixation, the other assay system widely used for strain differentiation (Forman, 1974) lacks specificity (Rweyemamu et al., 1980). In recent studies of the suitability of ELISA (enzyme linked immunosorbent assays) for the detection of FMDV antigen, it was observed that the indirect sandwich ELISA technique preferentially measured the major immunogenic site (Ouldridge, Barnett and Rweyemamu, 1981). Here we investigate its potential for FMDV strain differentiation.

METHODS

The procedure for the indirect sandwich ELISA was essentially that described by Abu El-Zein and Crowther (1979). Firstly an optimum dose of rabbit anti FMDV IgG was adsorbed to wells of PVC microplates. This was then reacted with dilutions of purified virion, followed by dilutions of guinea pig FMDV antiserum and anti-guinea pig IgG-horse radish peroxidase conjugate. The presence of horse radish peroxidase was detected using o-phenylenediamine as the substrate. The optical density of the reaction was determined using a Titertek Multiskan spectrophotometer.

The virus strains used in this study were obtained from the world reference laboratory for FMD, at the AVRI, Pirbright, except for strain O K83/79 which was obtained from the Wellcome Institute for FMD, Nairobi, Kenya. They were typed by WRL as belonging to serotype O and comprised 3 categories:-

    i)   Reference subtype O_1 virus: O_1 Lausanne 65

    ii) Vaccine strains: O_1BFS 1860 and O K83/79

    iii) Isolates from recent outbreaks: O Jersey 1/81, O Austria 1/81, O Malaysia 1/80, O Thailand 1/80 and O Thailand 3/80.

All tests used purified 140S preparations of these antigens (Brown and Cartwright, 1964).

Anti O_1BFS 1860 sera were used to evaluate the relationships between the 8 virus strains. The rabbit serum was raised against live virus and the guinea pig against purified AEI inactivated 140S antigen (Rweyemamu et al., 1978).

THE VARIABILITY OF THE TEST

In the first series of experiments, considerable day-to-day and plate to-plate variation was observed in the intensity of colour development of the enzyme reaction. Figure 1 shows titrations of the guinea pig O_1BFS 1860 serum against a constant homologous antigen dose performed on four separate occasions. Although the curves were all sigmoid and each curve clearly followed the same pattern, i.e. plateau values could be expected to occur at similar serum dilutions, the actual optical density of the plateau values was variable. This suggested an experiment-to-experiment variability of the maximum capacity for colour development. This capacity was standardised by expressing the results as the percentage of a potential reaction determined in each experiment. For these experiment

154

we standardised the 100% reaction as the optical density of the reaction at
a 0.12μg/well concentration of the homologous antigen with the antiserum
diluted 1/100.   Expressing all results as a percentage of this reference
reaction, standardised reaction curves could be drawn which demonstrated
little experiment-to-experiment variability (Figure 2).   Consequently,
all homologous and heterologous reactions have been expressed as
percentages of the reference reaction (designated here as PR).   The
experiments presented in this paper used a reference reaction determined
for each experiment.   However, the variability of the test was further
reduced if the reference reaction was performed on each plate and the
results on each plate calculated with this individual reference
reaction.

GENERATION OF SATURATION PROFILES FOR HOMOLOGOUS AND HETEROLOGOUS REACTIONS
     In an experiment to compare homologous and heterologous preparations,
3 type O viruses, BFS 1860, Jersey 1/81 and Lausanne 65 were tested
against the O_1BFS 1860 antiserum using a constant dose of antigen.   The
responses obtained were sigmoid for both the homologous and heterologous
preparations.   It was readily apparent from this study that whereas the
saturation curve for O_1Lausanne 65 virus was almost coincidental with that
of the homologous virus (O_1BFS 1860), that for O Jersey 1/81 was
considerably depressed.   This suggested that there were some antigenic
sites on O_1BFS 1860 virus which were not shared with O Jersey 1/81.
     The sigmoid nature of these relationships suggested that it was
appropriate to find a suitable mathematical treatment for the
determination of the characteristics of each response.   By representing
the monospecific antibody-antigen reaction as:-

     Ab + Ag $\rightleftarrows$ AbAg

The association constant K can be defined as

     $$K = \frac{[AbAg]}{[Ab][Ag]}$$

where $[Ab]$, $[Ag]$ and $[AbAg]$ are the concentrations of antibody,
antigen and antigen-antibody complex at equilibrium.

FIGURE 1: The variability of ELISA optical density values.

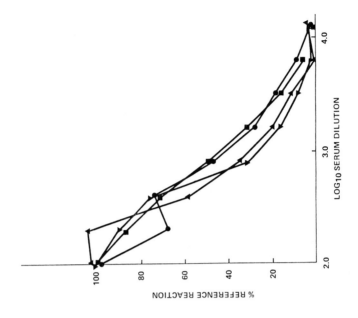

FIGURE 2: Standardisation of ELISA values.

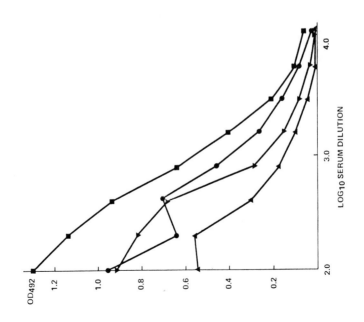

Manipulation of this expression gives:

$$\frac{[Ab\ Ag]}{[Ag] + [AbAg]} = \frac{K[Ab]}{1 + K[Ab]}$$

The indirect sandwich ELISA measures PR. The value of PR for any given antibody concentration is defined as

$$PR = \frac{[AbAg]}{[Ag] + [AbAg]} \cdot PR_{max}$$

where PR_{max} is the value of PR at saturation.

By substitution from the previous equation

$$PR = \frac{PR_{max} \cdot K[Ab]}{1 + K[Ab]}$$

In order to account for the heterogeneous nature of the antibody and antigen populations (Eisen and Siskind, 1964) the above expression was modified thus:-

$$PR = \frac{(\bar{K}[Ab])^{\underline{a}}}{1 + (\bar{K}[Ab])^{\underline{a}}} \cdot PR_{max}$$

where $\bar{K}$ is a mean association constant and $\underline{a}$ is a measure of the antigen heterogeneity. PR_{max} is proportional to the number of antigenic sites available.

Using this equation and a suitable computer package programme (BMDP 3R), saturation curves can be fitted to estimate values of PR_{max}, $\bar{K}$ and $\underline{a}$.

USE OF SATURATION VALUES FOR SEROLOGICAL COMPARISON OF VIRUS STRAINS

From the above it appeared that homologous and heterologous strains generate varying saturation profiles, with different maximum saturation values. This study was extended to assess profiles generated by 8 different type O FMDV strains and whether these were influenced by the dose of antigen employed in the test. The profiles generated at antigen doses of 0.12μg/well and 0.06μg/well are depicted in Figures 3 and 4.

FIGURE 3: Computer fitted homologous (O_1BFS 1860) and heterologous PR curves for 0.12µg antigen dose.

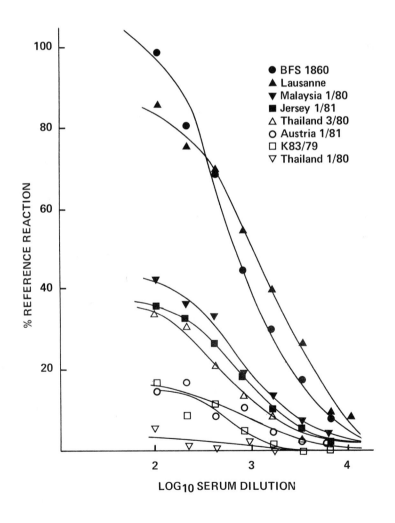

FIGURE 4: Computer fitted homologous (O_1BFS 1860) and heterologous PR curves for 0.06µg antigen dose.

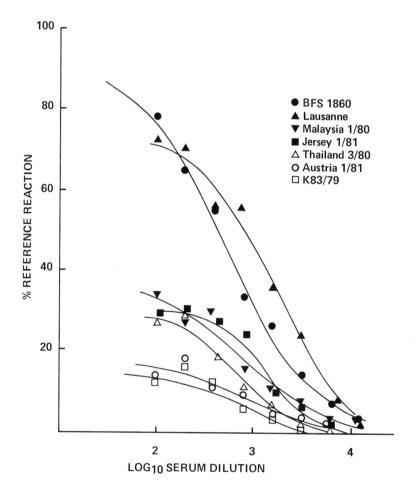

TABLE 1: Showing a comparison of relationships measured by indirect sandiwch ELISA and neutralisation.

Ratio $\frac{PR_{max}(het)}{PR_{max}(BFS)}$	BFS 1860	Lausanne 65	Jersey 1/81	Austria 1/81	Malaysia 1/80	Thailand 1/80	Thailand 3/80	K83/79
0.12µg dose	1.00	0.80	0.32	0.18	0.42	–	0.32	0.16
0.06µg dose	1.00	0.78	0.33	0.15	0.41	0.22	0.36	0.13
r value from 2DMN**	1.00	0.50	0.79	0.22*	≥1.00	0.23*	N.D.	0.19*

*   Values of r significantly different from 1.00 at p = 0.05.

N.D. Not done

**   Two dimensional microneutralisation

r = $\frac{\text{titre of serum to heterologous virus}}{\text{titre of serum to homologous virus}}$

159

The values of $\bar{K}$ and a obtained from the calculated saturation curves did not vary significantly from strain to strain. However, significant variations were observed in the values of PR_{max}. Therefore this seemed to be the most useful variable for the comparison of serological relationships. The ratios of heterologous to homologous (O_1BFS 1860) PR_{max} were constant for the two antigen doses studied (Table 1) and therefore presumably independent of antigen dose. Consequently, the PR_{max} ratios were compared with r value relationships (ratio serum titre heterologous:homologous virus strains) determined in two dimensional microneutralisation tests, and these r values were similar to the PR_{max} ratios.

By examination of the saturation profiles, the viruses tested seem to be readily separated into four groups. BFS 1860 and Lausanne 65 both reacted strongly, Malaysia 1/80, Jersey 1/81 and Thailand 3/80 showed good reactions. Austria 1/81 and K83/79 reacted moderately and Thailand 1/80 showed a barely detectable reaction.

REFERENCES

Abu Elzein, E.M.E. and Crowther, J.R. 1979. Application of the enzyme linked immunosorbent assay for the detection and identification of foot and mouth disease viruses. J. Hyg. (Camb.) 83, 513.

Brown, F. and Cartwright, B. 1964. Purification of radioactive foot and mouth disease virus. Vet Bull 34, 882.

Eisen, H.N. and Siskind, G.W. 1964. Variations in affinities of antibodies during the immune response. Biochemistry 3, 996.

Forman, A.J. 1974. A study of foot and mouth disease virus strains by complement fixation. I. A model for the fixation of complement by antigen/antibody mixtures. J. Hyg. (Camb.) 72, 397.

Ouldridge, E., Barnett, P. and Rweyemamu, M.M. 1981. A comparative assessment of five immunoassay for the specific detection and quantification of the FMDV immunising antigen. Proceedings of ELISA: its role in Veterinary research and diagnosis. Guildford, September.

Pereira, H.G. 1977. Subtyping of foot and mouth disease virus. Dev. Biol. Stand. 35, 167-174.

Rweyemamu, M.M., Booth, J.C., Head, M. and Pay, T.W.F. 1978. Micro-neutralisation tests for serological typing and subtyping of foot and mouth disease virus strains. J. Hyg. (Camb.) 81, 107-123.

Rweyemamu, M.M., Ouldridge, E.J., Hingley, P.J. and Head, M. 1980. Further studies on the effect of antiserum quality on strain specificity in foot and mouth disease virus strain differentiation. F.A.O. Vienna.

ELISA FOR DETECTION OF BOVINE CORONAVIRUS
IN FAECES AND INTESTINAL CONTENTS

A. Meyling

State Veterinary Serum Laboratory
Bülowsvej 27, 1870 Copenhagen V., Denmark

ABSTRACT

A double-sandwich enzyme-linkes immunosorbent assay (ELISA) to detect bovine coronavirus in faeces and intestinal contents of calves has been developed. A potent antiserum for the Nebraska bovine coronavirus was produced by immunizing rabbits with a brain suspension from baby rabbits infected with the Nebraska bovine coronavirus adapted to baby mice. Immunoglobulins from this antiserum were used as catching antibody and for preparation of a horse-radish peroxidase conjugate.

The ELISA-technique was found to be 8 to 16 times more sensitive than hemagglutination for detecting virus in infective tissue culture medium. In experimentally infected calves, coronavirus could be detected by ELISA before, during, and after the diarrheic period.

ELISA detected coronavirus in intestinal contents of 24 (96%) of 25 calves that had been found positive by FA. The FA-negative samples had corrected OD-values < o.1. When a corrected OD-value < o.1 was used for discriminating between positive and negative samples of faeces from diarrheic calves, 53 (12%) of 432 were found positive in the coronavirus ELISA.

INTRODUCTION

Viruses that cause or are found to be associated with diarrhea in the newborn animal are usually difficult to grow in tissue culture. Therefore enzyme-linked immunosorbent assays (ELISA) have become of widespread application for diagnosis of these agents. For rotaviruses several techniques have been published and some have formed the basis for development of commercial kits (Grauballe et al., 1981).

Bovine coronavirus causing neonatal diarrhea in calves, either alone or in combination with other agents, are difficult to isolate, and so far only few strains have been adapted to tissue culture. Electron microscopy of intestinal contents or faeces is a rather unreliable way of diagnosing the infection, because the characteristic fringes of the particles may be lost, or because evaluation may be confused by similar fringe-like structures from the intestinal epithelium.

Immunofluorescent staining of gut sections is another way
of diagnosing the infection on autopsy material (Mebus et al.,
1973). In the living animal, ELISA (Ellens et al., 1978), a
hemadsorption-elution-hemagglutination assay HEHA) (van Balken
et al., 1978/1979), or counter-current electrophoresis may be
used (Dea et al., 1979).

In the present report an ELISA technique for the detection
of bovine coronavirus in faeces and intestinal contents is described, and the results are compared with those obtained by
fluorescent antibody staining of colon sections and by HEHA on
faeces samples.

MATERIAL AND METHODS

Experimental animals and samples

Two calves that had been 'caught' at parturition and immediately brought to an isolated room were fed milk replacer and
infected by oral inoculation with faeces from a gnotobiotic calf
infected with the Danish isolate of bovine coronavirus (Bridger
et al., 1978). Faeces samples were taken daily from the rectum.

Faeces samples from 432 calves with diarrhea, submitted to
the laboratory for bacteriological and virological examination,
were examined by ELISA for corona- and rotaviruses. Samples
were stored at $-2o^{\circ}C$ until examined within a week.

Colons from 111 calves from field cases of neonatal calf
diarrhea were processed for immunofluorescense and 10% suspensions of mixed intestinal contents were tested by ELISA.

Virus and antisera

The tissue-culture adapted Nebraska calf diarrhea coronavirus was passed in primary embryonic calf kidney (BEK) cultures and then adapted to baby mice. The clarified medium from
BEK cultures were inoculated intracerebrally into one-day-old
baby mice. In the first passage 2 of 1o mice died on day 3 p.i.
and the remaining 8 mice became ill on day 4-5. They were killed when showing symptoms, and from their brains a clarified
1o% suspension was made and injected into new litters. After 5
passages, baby rabbits were injected i.c. with the mouse-brain
suspension. The rabbits were killed after 48 hours and a clar-

ified suspension of their brains was mixed with an equal amount of Freunds incomplete adjuvant and used as antigen.

Rabbits that had been found free from antibodies to bovine rotavirus and coronavirus by indirect immunofluorscence (IFA) were bled 3 times before immunization to provide preimmune serum. The rabbits were given intradermal injections of o.2 ml antigen at intervals of 3 weeks over 3 months.

Immunoglobulins (Ig) from the rabbit antiserum for bovine coronavirus and from the preimmune sera were isolated on DEAE -sephadex A 5o$^{(R)}$ as described elsewhere (Harboe and Ingild, 1973).

Conjugation with horse-radish peroxidase (Sigma, RZ value 3.o) was performed by the pericdate method (Willson and Nakane, 1978). The conjugate had a protein concentration of 2.1 mg/ml and was used in a 1:2oo dilution.

ELISA procedure

The procedure has been described in detail elsewhere (Grauballe et al., 1981). Flat-bottom, irradiated, polystyrene microtest plates (A/S Nunc$^{(R)}$) were used.

The wells in the microtest plates were coated with the Ig fraction of the rabbit antiserum for bovine coronavirus diluted in o.o5M carbonate buffer, pH 9.6. An amount of 1oo µl was added to each well. In each test plate, rows of wells coated with anti-coronavirus Ig alternated with rows coated with the same amount of preimmune Ig. The plates were incubated for 24 h at room temperature. The fluid contents were then thrown out and the plates washed 4 times in PBS with o.5M NaCl and o.o5% Tween 2o, pH 7.2.

Specimens, i.e., 1o% suspensions of faeces or intestinal contents were diluted in washing fluid to which had been added 5 g/l of bovine serum albumin. An amount of 1oo µl of each specimen was added to two wells coated with anti-coronavirus Ig and two wells coated with preimmune Ig. The plates were incubated for 3 hours at room temperature and washed 3 times, whereupon 1oo µl of conjugate dilution was added to each well. After 3o min. incubation the plates were washed again and 1oo µl

of the substrate solution (20μl 30% H_2O_2 in a solution of 40 mg
1.2 phenylene-diamine hydrochloride in citrate-phosphate buffer
(34.7 mM citric acid, 66.7 mM Na_2HPO_4, pH 5.0) was added. The
reaction was stopped after 15 min. by adding 100μl of 2N H_2SO_4
per well. The results were read in the Titertek Multiscan(R)
photometer at 492nm.

To test the specificity of the ELISA reaction a blocking
test was performed. A 1:10 dilution of an immune serum against
the Danish isolate of bovine coronavirus from a gnotobiotic
calf was added to the test wells after these had reacted with
positive specimens and then been incubated for one hour. Other
wells reacted with the same specimens were treated with a 1:10
dilution of bovine fetal serum. If the OD_{492} values of the
wells treated with immune serum were reduced by more than 50%,
blocking had occurred. The serum used in the blocking reactions had an H.I. titer of 1:128 and an IFA titer of 1:2560.

The rotavirus ELISA used on this material was performed as
described above. Ig of bovine-rotavirus rabbit antiserum prepared against immunoprecipitates, and a conjugate prepared from
the same antiserum were used as catching antibody. Preparation
of the antiserum has been described elsewhere (Grauballe et al.,
1977).

Fluorescent antibody technique (FA)

A fluorescein-conjugate produced from a goat antiserum for
Nebraska bovine coronavirus, together with a fluorescein conjugate of preimmune serum, was used for staining of acetone-fix-
ed cryostat sections of colon and of coronavirus-infected BEK
cells in 24-well cluster plates (Nunc(R)).

Hemadsorption-elution-hemagglutination assay (HEHA) was
performed as described by van Balken et al. (1978/1979).

Hemagglutination

An 0.5% suspension of freshly collected mouse erythrocytes
in PBS, pH 7.2, with 0.2% bovine serum albumin, was added in 50
μl amounts to dilutions of virus in round-bottom microtiter
plates. Complete agglutination endpoint was read after 3 hours
at room temperature.

Nebraska bovine coronavirus in tissue culture

To compare the sensitivity of the ELISA with that of hem-agglutination and infectivity tests, clarified medium of BEK--cells grown in 5o ml bottles and infected with the Nebraska bovine coronavirus was tested by ELIDA and hemagglutination, and for infectivity in BEK cells in 24-well cluster plates (Nunc[R]). Medium was harvested daily after flasks had each been inoculated with 1 ml virus containing $1o^3$ $TCID_{5o}$.

RESULTS

The catching antibody

A 1% solution of the anti-coronavirus Ig had an H.I. titer of 1:512 and an indirect immunofluorescence titer of 1:512o. The optimal concentration of catching antibody was determined by testing different dilutions of a coronavirus-containing fae-ces sample from an experimentally infected calf. The OD_{492} values of different antigen dilutions formed a plateau from 5 to 1o µg Ig/ml. Consequently 5 µg Ig/ml was used in the test.

ELISA-reactivity of the Nebraska coronavirus in BEK-cells

To compare the sensitivity of the ELISA with hemagglutin-ation and infectivity, clarified tissue culture fluids from in-fected BEK-cultures were tested on different days p.i.. Taking a difference of o.1 in OD_{492} values between test wells and con-trol wells as endpoint, ELISA titers were 8 to 16 times higher than hemagglutination titers, and one ELISA unit was equivalent to $3.9 \times 1o^1$ to $1.2 \times 1o^2$ $TCID_{5o}$ of the bovine coronavirus in BEK-cultures.

Experimentally infected calves

Two conventional, colostrum-deprived calves were experim-entally infected with the Danish isolate of bovine coronavirus. One calf developed diarrhea on day 3 p.i. but had faeces of normal consistency again on day 4. The OD_{492} values of the faeces samples were increased on days 2 to 6 p.i. Rotavirus ELISA gave negative results until day 15 p.i..

Another calf inoculated with the same virus had watery

Fig. 1

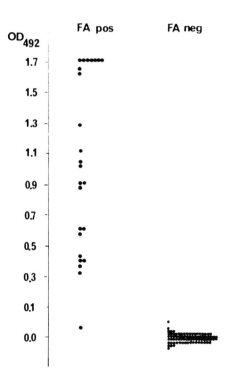

Fig. 1   Corrected ELISA OD_{492} values for 111 samples
of intestinal contents from calves examined for bovine
coronavirus by FA on cryostat sections of colon.   25
samples were FA-positive, 86 FA-negative.

diarrhea from day 2 to day 4 p.i. when the faeces became muco-
id. Faeces samples from this calf showed strong ELISA reactivity from day 2 to day 8 p.i. The sampling from this calf continued until day 3o. On day 18 a second episode of diarrhea
occurred. On this occasion the ELISA gave positive reactions
for both rota- and coronavirus. The calf had been infected
accidentally with rotavirus.

Naturally infected animals

Intestinal contents from 111 calves that had been examined by FA staining of colon sections were also examined by ELISA.
Twenty-five cases were positive by FA and 86 were negative.
The OD-values of the test wells minus the OD-values of the control wells are plotted in Fig. 1. It appears that none of 86
suspensions from FA-negative colons had corrected OD-values
above o.1, and that this value therefore may be used to discriminate between a positive and a negative ELISA reaction. Of
25 FA-positive samples 24 had corrected OD-values above o.3,
and one had an OD-value of o.o4 (^{P}/N-value 1.4). The average
^{P}/N-values (the OD-value of the test well divided by the OD-
-value of the control well) for samples with corrected OD-values higher than o.3 was >12 (4.3 to >22), whereas for FA-negative samples it was 1 (o.8 to 1.7).

Fifty-three samples (12%) were found positive by the coronavirus ELISA and 157 (36%) by the rotavirus ELISA, when 432
samples were examined and the above-mentioned criterion used
(Table 1). Twenty-eight (6.4%) samples were positive in both
tests. The average ^{P}/N-value was 14.5 (2.8 to >3o) for positive samples and 1.o (o.6 to 1.7) for negative samples.

To compare the ELISA with the HEHA, 1o4 samples were tested. Coronavirus agglutinins were detected by HEHA in 9 of 17
faeces samples which were positive by the ELISA, while 85 samples were negative in both tests and 3 samples positive in the
HEHA but negative in the ELISA.

DISCUSSION

The ELISA-technique for detection of bovine coronavirus

reported on in this paper seems to be sensitive and specific.
It was 8 to 16 times more sensitive than hemagglutination for
testing of tissue culture medium infected with the Nebraska bovine coronavirus.

In experimentally infected animals positive ELISA reactions
could be found before, during, and after the diarrheic phase.
One of the calves became accidentally infected with rotavirus.
The rotavirus excretion that followed was associated with a renewed excretion of coronavirus, as demonstrated by ELISA. It
is not known whether the renewed excretion of coronavirus was
due to reinfection or to a reactivation of the original infection. In a comparison between immunofluorescence and ELISA,
coronavirus was detected by ELISA in 24 (96%) of 25 cases that
had been evaluated as positive by FA. On examination of faeces
samples from the field, ELISA was found to be more sensitive
than the rather laborious HEHA test, a finding which is in
agreement with previously reported results (Ellens et al., 1981).
The corrected OD-values for specimens of intestinal contents
from, respectively, FA-positive and -negative cases were clearly separated in that all of 86 FA-negative cases had OD-values
lower than o.1. When this value was used for discriminating
between positive and negative reactions on faeces samples, 56
(12%) of 432 diarrheic samples were found to contain coronavirus, and these positive samples had ^{P}/N-values higher than
2.8, whereas the highest ^{P}/N-value for negative samples was 1.7.

For all samples evaluated as positive the specificity of
the test was ascertained by blocking with an anti-coronavirus
serum from a gnotobiotic calf. That no false positive reactions
were revealed by this test is hardly surprising, since a preimmune serum was used in the control wells, and a serological
control thereby included in the measurement of the reactivity
of each specimen.

REFERENCES

Bridger, Janice, C., Woode, G.N. and Meyling, A. 1978. Isola-
    tion of coronavirus from neonatal calf diarrhea in Great
    Britain and Denmark. Vet. Microbiol. 3, 1o1-113.
Dea, S., Roy, R.S. and Begin, M.E. 1979. Counterimmunoelectro-
    osmophoresis for detection of neonatal calf diarrhea coro-

navirus: Methodology and comparison with electron microscopy. J. Clin. Microbiol. 1o, 24o-244.

Ellens, D.J., van Balken, J.A.M. and de Leeuw, P.W. 1978. Diagnosis of bovine coronavirus infections with hemadsorption-elution-hemagglutination assay (HEHA) and with enzyme-linked immunosorbent assay (ELISA). Proc. Second International Symposium on Neonatal Diarrhea, 321-329.

Grauballe, P.C., Genner, J., Meyling, A. and Hornsleth, A. 1977.
Rapid diagnosis of rotavirus infections: Comparison of
electron microscopy and immunoelectro-osmophoresis for detection of rotavirus in human infantile gastroenteritis.
J. gen. Virol. 35, 2o3-218.

Grauballe, P.C., Vestergaard, B.F., Meyling, A. and Genner J.
1981. Optimized enzyme-linked immunosorbent assay for detection of human and bovine rotavirus in stools: Comparison with electron-microscopy - immunoelectro-osmophoresis
and fluorescent antibody techniques. J. med. Virol. 7,
29-4o.

Harbo, N. and Ingild, A. 1973. Immunization of immunoglobulins,
estimation of antibody titre. Sand. J. Immunol. 2 (suppl.
1), 161-164.

Mebus, C.A., Stair, E.L., Rhodes, M.B. and Twiehaus, M.J. 1973.
Pathology of neonatal calf diarrhea induced by a coronavirus like agent. Vet. Pathol. 1o, 46-64.

van Balken, J.A.M., de Leeuw, P.W., Ellens, D.J. and Straver,
P.J., 1978/1979. Detection of coronavirus in calf faeces
with a hemadsorption-elution-haemagglutination assay (HEHA).
Vet. Microbiol. 3, 2o5-211.

Willson, M.B. and Nakane, P.K. 1978. Immunofluorescence and
related staining techniques, eds. W. Knapp, K. Holubar and
G. Wick (Elsevier/North Holland Biomedical Press, Amsterdam), p. 215.

TABLE 1   Results of corona- and rotavirus ELISA tests
on 432 faeces samples from diarrheic calves

Corona-virus	Rota-virus	Number of samples			
+	o	25	5.7%	Coronavirus total	53 12%
+	+	28	6.4%		
o	+	129	3o.o%	Rotavirus total	157 36%
o	o	25o	58.o%		

ELISA FOR THE DETECTION OF VIRUS AND ANTIBODIES
IN PIGS WITH EPIDEMIC DIARRHEA

P. Debouck, M. Pensaert and P. Callebaut

Laboratory of Virology
Faculty of Veterinary Medicine
State University of Gent
Casinoplein 24, B-9000 Gent, Belgium

ABSTRACT

An ELISA was developed for the specific detection of the coronavirus-like agent (CVLA) in feces of pigs affected with porcine epidemic diarrhea (PED) type II. An ELISA blocking assay was used for the detection of antibodies to this agent. Feces of pigs with PED type I, either following a natural or experimental infection, also reacted in the ELISA for the detection of CVLA. Convalescent sera from these pigs reacted in the ELISA blocking assay for the detection of CVLA antibodies, whereas pre-infection sera scored negative. It was, therefore, concluded that both type I and type II of PED are caused by the same virus or by an antigenically closely related virus.

INTRODUCTION

Porcine epidemic diarrhea (PED) has been described in two forms with a different clinical picture. In PED type I, only older pigs are affected (Anon, 1972). Until now, the causative agent was unknown although a viral etiology was suspected, and diagnosis of PED type I was only possible by recognizing this particular clinical picture.

In PED type II, clinical signs are very similar to those seen in outbreaks of transmissible gastroenteritis (TGE) although mortality in piglets is lower than in TGE (Wood, 1977). A coronavirus-like agent (CVLA) unrelated to known porcine coronaviruses, has been isolated from piglets affected with PED type II (Chasey and Cartwright, 1978; Pensaert and Debouck, 1978). Diagnosis of type II field outbreaks is possible by immunofluorescent staining of small intestinal sections of sick piglets (Debouck et al., 1980). A reliable method for the specific detection of CVLA in feces or a serologic test to demonstrate a seroconversion was not available until now, hampering the diagnosis in field cases where no sick piglets were available.

To solve this problem, we developed an ELISA for the detection of CVLA and an ELISA blocking assay for the detection of antibodies against CVLA. Both ELISA for antigen and antibody detection also made it possible to investigate feces and paired serum samples obtained from pigs affected with PED type I.

MATERIALS AND METHODS

Details on the reagents, protocol, sensitivity and specificity of both ELISA methods will be fully described elsewhere (Callebaut et al, submitted for publication), but are summarized underneath.

ELISA for antigen detection:

The ELISA for the detection of CVLA antigen is performed by a sandwich technique. The antibodies used for coating the microtiterplates and for the production of a horseradish peroxidase conjugate against CVLA, originate from a serum of a caesarean-derived colostrum-deprived (CDCD) pig which was hyperimmunized with the CV777 strain of the CVLA (Debouck and Pensaert, 1980). Each fecal sample is tested twice. Before adding the conjugate, one well is incubated with a negative swine serum and the other well with a specific anti-CVLA serum. A fecal sample is regarded as positive when the absorbance in the first well is higher than or equal to the cut-off value and at the same time the reaction is blocked ⩾50% by the positive serum in the second well. The cut-off value (1 ELISA unit) was taken as the mean absorbance of known negative fecal samples to which 3 times the standard deviation was added.

ELISA for antibody detection:

The ELISA for the detection of antibodies against CVLA is a blocking assay which is very similar to the ELISA for antigen detection. The reference antigen is a CVLA virus stock obtained by perfusion of the intestines of an experimentally infected CDCD pig (Debouck and Pensaert, 1980) diluted to contain 16 ELISA units. Unknown sera are tested for their capacity to block the reaction of the antigen with the specific conjugate.

The amount of specific antibodies is determined by testing two-fold dilutions of the serum, starting with a dilution of 1/5. The endpoint is the dilution by which the reaction is blocked ⩾50%. Titers are recorded as the reversal of this dilution.

Collection of specimens from pigs affected with PED type II

Fecal specimens were collected from 8 CDCD piglets experimentally infected with CV777, and from 23 pigs and sows naturally affected with PED type II.

Sera were collected at various time intervals (table I) from 4 CDCD pigs experimentally infected with CV777 and from 25 sows from 3 different farms, affected with PED type II.

Collection of specimens from pigs affected with PED type I

Feces were collected from 22 diarrheic sows out of 17 different farms where a typical PED type I outbreak was observed. With a bacteria free filtrate of one of these fecal samples, it was possible to reproduce the disease by oral inoculation of a sow and of a pig at slaughterweight. The incubation period was 2 days. Another pig of the same age became contact infected 3 days later (Pensaert, unpublished). Feces were collected from those 3 animals during the acute phase of diarrhea.

Paired serum samples were obtained from two sows from a PED type I field infection and from the 3 experimentally inoculated pigs.

RESULTS

CVLA antigens could consistently be detected by ELISA in feces of the piglets experimentally inoculated with the CV777 isolate, up to the second day of diarrhea. Feces collected during the third to the fifth day of diarrhea scored inconsistently positive.

Feces collected from diarrheic pigs and sows naturally affected with PED type II and obtained during the first days of the outbreak scored all positive in the ELISA. Feces collected from 5 pigs that had recovered for more than one week scored negative.

Antibodies to CVLA could be detected by ELISA in post-infection sera of pigs experimentally infected with CV777 or naturally affected with PED type II, but not in sera collected at the time of inoculation or in the acute phase of diarrhea respectively (table 1).

TABLE 1   Demonstration of CVLA antibodies by ELISA blocking assay, in sera of pigs experimentally infected with CV777 (up) or naturally affected (below) with PED type II.

Time of serum collection	No +/No tested	Range of titer
Preinoculation	0/4	−
15 d.p.i.[x]	0/4	−
43 d.p.i.	4/4	40 − 80
135 d.p.i.	3/3	20 − 80
Onset of diarrhea	0/8	−
30 days later	8/25	5 − 160
45 days later	10/12	5 − 160
60 days later	8/8	10 − 80
180 days later	22/22	10 − 160

[x] d.p.i. : days post inoculation

Twenty of the 22 fecal samples collected from sows with PED type I and fecal specimens obtained from the 3 experimentally infected animals also reacted positively in the ELISA for detection of CVLA antigen.

The results of the ELISA blocking assay for the detection of CVLA antibodies in the paired serum samples collected from experimentally and naturally infected pigs with PED type I, are presented in table II.

174

TABLE II   Titer of CVLA antibodies as determined by
            ELISA blocking assay in sera of pigs experi-
            mentally (up) or naturally infected (below)
            with PED type I.

	First serum	Second serum
Sow	< 5[a]	10 (24)[c]
Pig	< 5	10 (48)
Contact infected pig	< 5	10 (48)
Sow A	< 5[b]	20 (35)
Sow B	< 5	20 (35)

a   collected before inoculation
b   collected at onset of diarrhea
c   delay between collection of first and second serum
    in days

CONCLUSIONS

The ELISA for the detection of CVLA antigen can be used
for the diagnosis of PED in young as well as in older pigs,
provided that fecal samples are collected during the acute
phase of diarrhea. The negative results obtained with some
fecal specimens collected during the third to the fifth day of
diarrhea may be due to the formation of aggregates between CVLA
antigen and locally produced specific antibodies. However,
electron microscopic examination of these specimens did not
reveal such aggregates nor single coronavirus-like particles.

Diagnosis of PED can also be made by the demonstration of
a specific antibody seroconversion to CVLA when paired sera are
examined. From Table I it can be deduced that the second serum
should be collected rather late (6 weeks after onset of
diarrhea) to assure that the pig has detectable antibody titers. There are possible explanations for the unusual long lag
time for antibody production to be detected by this ELISA
blocking assay. This ELISA may be not sensitive enough, or we
deal with an infectious agent with poor antigenic capacities.

Feces and sera collected from experimentally or naturally
infected pigs with PED type I scored positive in an ELISA

using reagents obtained from pigs experimentally infected with
the CV777 isolate originating from a typical PED type II outbreak. These data substantiate the hypothesis that both type I
and type II of PED are caused by the same or an antigenically
closely related virus. Whether the difference in clinical
signs between type I and type II outbreaks is due to occurrence
of related antigenic types of the virus, to differences in
virulence between antigenically identical virus isolates or to
farm-dependent circumstances is a subject of further investigations.

REFERENCES

Anon. 1972. Vet. Rec., 90, (Suppl) 95, 49.
Chasey, D. and Cartwright, S.F. 1978. Virus-like particles
    associated with porcine epidemic diarrhea. Res. Vet.
    Sci., 25, 255-256.
Debouck, P. and Pensaert, M. 1980. Experimental infection of
    pigs with a new porcine enteric coronavirus, CV777. Am.
    J. Vet. Res., 41, 219-223.
Debouck, P., Callebaut, P. and Pensaert, M. 1980. The diagno-
    sis of coronavirus-like agent (CVLA) diarrhea in suckling
    pigs. Laboratory diagnosis in neonatal calf and pig
    diarroea. Current topics in veterinary medicine and ani-
    mal science. Ed. P.W. de Leeuw and P.A.M. Guinée.
    Martinus Nijhoff Publishers, 13, 59-61.
Pensaert, M.B. and Debouck, P. 1978. A new coronavirus-like
    particle associated with diarrhea in swine. Arch. Virol.,
    58, 243-247.
Wood, E.N. 1977. An apparently new syndrome of porcine epide-
    mic diarrhea. Vet. Rec., 100, 243-244.

Acknowledgement: These studies were supported by the Institute
    for the Encouragement of Research in Industry and Agricul-
    ture (IWONL), Brussels, Belgium.

APPLICATION OF ENZYME IMMUNOASSAYS IN RINDERPEST RESEARCH

J. Anderson and L.W. Rowe

Animal Virus Research Institute, Pirbright, Woking,
Surrey, GU24 ONF, England.

ABSTRACT
    The indirect ELISA has been used for the detection of
IgG, IgA and IgM antibodies to rinderpest virus in
experimentally infected cattle and the results compared to
those obtained by the virus neutralisation test, in order
to study the ontogeny of the immune response.
    The IgG assay has been applied to large scale
epidemiological surveys of field and abattoir sera and the
problems of non-specific reactions and the establishment of a
meaningful reference negative serum are discussed.
    The ELISA is also being used for the detection of
specific viral cytopathic effect in the micro-virus
neutralisation test, allowing visual rather than microscopic
reading of the test.

INTRODUCTION

    Rinderpest is primarily a disease of cattle, although it
may infect sheep, goats and pigs, and has been controlled in
recent years by the use of an attenuated vaccine. Due to a
resurgence of the disease in some African and Middle Eastern
countries it is important to maintain surveillance of the
immune status of the animals at risk. The main methods for
the detection of antibody to rinderpest virus have been the
virus neutralisation test (VNT) and the haemagglutination
inhibition test (HI), both of which are time consuming,
laborious and require a good supply of tissue culture
materials and clean sterile glassware. The indirect enzyme-
linked immunosorbent assay (ELISA) has been applied
successfully to the detection and quantification of antibodies
to many viral diseases of veterinary importance. Such tests
have proved to be reproducible, sensitive and capable of

assaying large numbers of samples. It was therefore decided
to apply the ELISA to the detection of antibodies to
rinderpest virus.

INDIRECT ELISA

A solid-phase microplate indirect ELISA was developed
using rigid flat bottomed polystyrene ELISA plates (Dynatech,
England). Full details of the test procedure are described by
Anderson et al (in press). The standard indirect ELISA as
described by Voller et al (1979) was used for detecting anti-
rinderpest IgG antibodies (see Table 1).

a) Ag + Ab + Rabbit anti-bovine IgG conjugate + substrate
         ↑ 1/2 ↑   ↑
         W   W   W

b) Ag + Ab + Rabbit anti-bovine IgA serum + Protein A conjugate + substrate
         ↑ 1/2 ↑   ↑   ↑
         W   W   W   W

c) Ag + Ab + Rabbit anti-bovine IgM serum + Protein A conjugate + substrate
         ↑ 1/100 ↑   ↑   ↑
         W   W   W   W

Tables 1a, b and c. Protocols for the detection of
a) IgG, b) IgA and c) IgM by ELISA.

In order to avoid preparing anti-bovine IgA and IgM conjugates
for the detection of these specific sub-classes, an extra step
was used in the test. Immunoglobulin sub-class antisera were
added at an optimal dilution established by previous
titration. These were then detected by the addition of S.
aureus Protein 'A', conjugated to horse-radish peroxidase

(HRPO). The substrate used was orthophenylene diamine and the optical density (OD) readings at 492 nm were measured using a multichannel spectrophotometer (Titertek Multiskan, Flow Laboratories, U.K.).

(a) Establishment of optimal antigen dilution

The antigen was prepared from infected secondary bovine kidney (BK) tissue culture supernatant by clarification at 1800 g followed by centrifugation at 100,000 g for 60 minutes at 4C. The resulting pellet containing virus was resuspended by sonication in 1/100 of the original volume of phosphate buffered saline (PBS).

The optimal test antigen dilution was established by titrating an antigen dilution series against a constant dilution of positive VNT serum using standard conditions. The results are shown in Fig.1 where a maximum OD reading was obtained from 1/2 to around 1/64 antigen dilution, after which the OD reading decreased with the change in antigen concentration. The uninfected tissue culture antigen control gave only low reactions at high concentrations and these were eliminated above a dilution of 1/8. Consequently, a dilution of 1/50 was used in subsequent tests. All fresh antigen preparations were titrated in this way before use.

(b) Establishment of optimal test serum dilutions

In order to select a single dilution of test serum for use in the assays, it was essential to titrate a number of sera over a full two-fold dilution series.

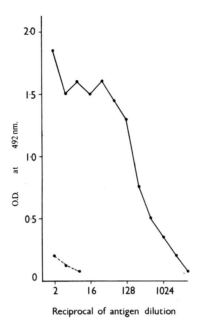

Fig. 1. Establishment of the optimum antigen dilution
for use in the test. Rinderpest antigen pellet (————),
negative control antigen (— — — —).

This was done to determine whether there was an inhibitory

effect at high serum concentrations and also to determine the

levels of non-specific activity present in negative sera.

Known susceptible and known convalescent cattle sera

previously examined by VNT were tested under standard

conditions described for IgG, IgA and IgM assays (Tables 1a, b

and c). Typical results for IgA and IgM are shown in Figs 2

and 3. The results for IgG were essentially the same as for

IgA. Negative sera, even at a dilution of 1/2 in the IgG and

IgA titrations showed very low ODs when compared to the

positive sera. There was no inhibitory effect at high serum

concentrations. On the basis of these results, dilutions of

1/2 were used for the detection of IgA and IgG, thus allowing
accurate dilution of the sera directly in the plates.

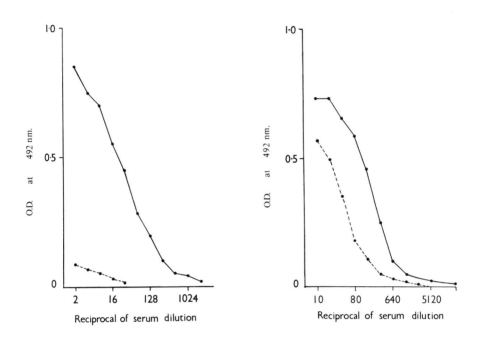

Fig. 2. Establishment of optimal test serum dilution for
the IgA assay. Positive serum (———), negative serum (— — —).

Fig. 3. Establishment of optimal test serum dilution for
the IgM assay. Positive serum (———), negative serum (— — —).

Results for IgM were different, in that significantly
high levels of colour were produced by negative sera at
dilutions down to 1/100. Consequently test sera were diluted
1/100 for IgM assays, as this produced the highest
differential between positive and negative whilst retaining
the sensitivity for low levels of IgM.

ONTOGENY OF THE IMMUNE RESPONSE

Before applying the ELISA to field surveys, it was decided to examine the chronological development of IgM, IgG and IgA and to compare this response with the development of neutralising antibody as detected by the VNT. The latter test was performed using virus-serum mixtures incubated at 4C. for approximately 16 hours, residual infectivity being detected using secondary BK cells (Plowright and Ferris, 1961). Four cattle were inoculated with an attenuated strain of rinderpest virus and blood for serum was collected daily. The animals were challenged at 10 week post-infection with a virulent strain of rinderpest virus.

Figure 4 shows the ELISA results for the individual cattle after infection with rinderpest virus and compares the antibody responses with the development of neutralising antibody.

In order to establish a common base line the background levels of non-specific activity have been subtracted from the total OD reading. The neutralising antibody preceded the first ELISA detectable antibody (IgM) by 1-2 days. It then rose steadily from day 6 to day 10 and maintained a high level throughout the experiment. The IgM response rose sharply between days 8 to 12 and returned to 0 day levels by day 68. The IgG response was detected 2-3 days later than IgM, and was maintained at a high level until challenge. The IgA levels followed a similar pattern to that of IgG. Both these levels fluctuated slightly after challenge but there was no overall increase. The IgM levels did not rise significantly above the background level after challenge.

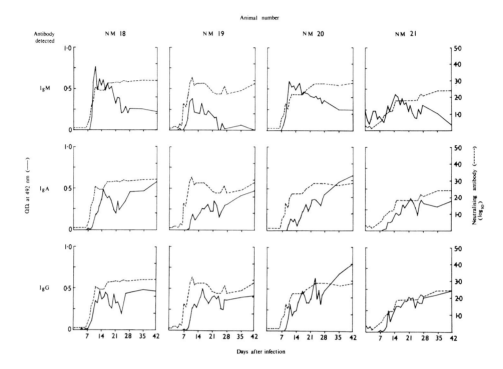

Fig. 4. A comparison of ELISA results (———) and VNT results (— — —) from four experimentally infected cattle.

None of the animals showed any clinical signs of the disease; nor was there any virus detected in the blood and nasal swabs in the two week period after challenge.

The detection of neutralising antibody 1-2 days earlier than the detection of IgM antibodies by ELISA may be due to the high dilution of serum (1/100) used in detecting IgM by ELISA, compared to that used in the VNT (1/4). Another reason for this difference in sensitivity may be that the early neutralising antibody may have a low affinity for the ELISA antigen and longer incubation times may be needed for the detection of such antibodies.

Although the number of animals examined was small, there was a marked variation in the levels of non-specific activity from animal to animal and it may be noted that low levels of IgM and neutralising antibody were detected in the pre-inoculation serum of animal NM21.

From this work, it was decided that the IgG assay would be the method of choice for field surveys as this resulted in low background levels, correlated well with the VNT, and the sera could be accurately and conveniently diluted directly on to the plates.

ELISA FOR FIELD SURVEYS

In order to discriminate between positive and negative readings in the ELISA and to establish a reference negative serum, it was necessary to examine the background levels of activity present in negative sera. Negative sera from three geographical areas were examined to establish whether there was a difference in the population mean or the standard deviation about the mean in sera from different regions which would necessitate the establishment of a reference negative serum for each area studied. One hundred sera were obtained from Britain and Turkey (disease-free countries) and Bangladesh (non-disease free country but VNT negative sera) using the standard ELISA; the population mean ($\bar{x}$) standard deviation (SD) and distribution of the OD readings were determined and are shown in Fig.5. There was little

184

difference between the population mean and the standard
deviation from each region and one reference negative serum
would suffice for all three regions.

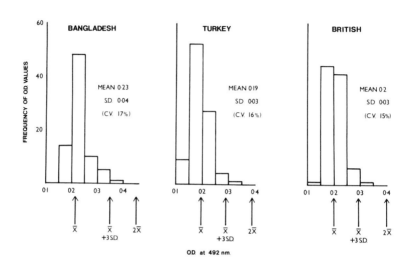

Fig. 5. A comparison of the distribution of OD values
obtained by ELISA from three negative populations.

Consequently a pool of the Bangladesh sera giving the
population mean OD was made, and this was used as the
reference negative in all further tests. The OD readings of
the negative populations do not have a normal distribution but
are skewed to the right. Consequently a cut-off point of $\bar{x}$ + 3
SD would result in false positive results. It was therefore
decided that any serum giving an OD higher than $2\bar{x}$ would be
designated as positive.

Bangladesh field sera (307) were obtained from a region
which has not undergone a rinderpest vaccination campaign.
These were examined by VNT and ELISA and overall there was

good agreement between the two tests, where only 2% were
negative VNT/positive ELISA and 1% positive VNT/negative
ELISA.

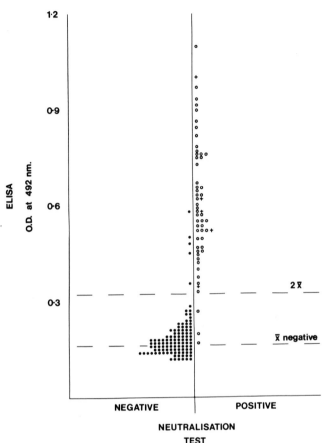

Fig. 6. A comparison of ELISA and VNT results from
Bangladesh cattle sera (166). Negative VNT (●), trace VNT (+)
positive VNT (o).

The results of 166 sera examined within one test are shown
in the scattergram Fig.6 - (VNT antibody titres of 0.3 -0.45
SN50 were expressed as a trace positive, and antibody titres
over 0.45 SN50 were expressed as positive.).

Nigerian abattoir sera (116) were obtained from a
region which had been regularly vaccinated against rinderpest.

186

The results for VNT and ELISA are shown in Fig.7. Overall
there were 4% VNT negative/ELISA positive and 4% VNT
positive/ELISA negative

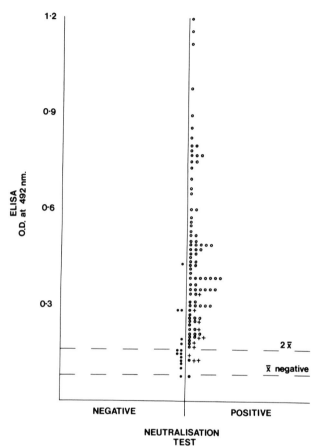

Fig. 7. A comparison of ELISA and VNT results from Nigerian
cattle sera (116), negative VNT (●), trace VNT (+), positive
VNT (o).

All of the ELISA negative/VNT positive sera were
examined by ELISA for the presence of IgM antibodies and were
found to have high levels. These animals could therefore have
been at an early stage in the development of their immune
response to either rinderpest infection or vaccination but
this would appear unlikely as we have shown that there is only

a two-day interval between the detection of IgM and IgG.
It is possible that it could be a non-specific neutralising
antibody as shown by one of the experimental animals (see
previous section). The distribution of OD readings in Fig.8
show two distinct populations in the Bangladesh sera whereas
the Nigerian sera show a continuous spectrum of OD readings.

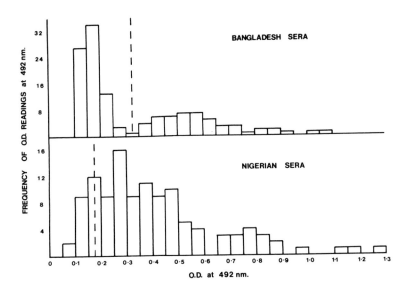

Fig. 8. A comparison of the distribution of OD reading
obtained by ELISA from Bangladesh and Nigerian cattle sera.
(----- represents 2x reference negative value.)

The lack of a distinct negative and positive
population in the Nigerian samples could be due to a gradation
in response to rinderpest vaccine producing a complete
spectrum of antibody levels, thus explaining the increased
numbers of sera giving only trace levels of neutralising
antibody. It could also be due to higher levels of non-

specific activity being present in abattoir sera compared to field sera resulting in an overlap between high non-specific readings and low positive readings. A pooled British abattoir serum gave an OD reading of 65% higher than the mean for 100 British field sera. However, more work must be carried out to elucidate this problem..

Generally, there was a good agreement between the ELISA and the VNT results and the use of ELISA in field surveys would give a true indication of the immune status of the animal population.

NEUTRALISATION - ELISA

The micro virus neutralisation test (VNT) has been developed for the detection of antibodies to rinderpest virus (Rowe and Anderson, in preparation). As rinderpest virus infection does not result in detachment of infected cells the test cannot be read by vital staining of the remaining viable cells, and must be read microscopically. This is time consuming and requires a skilled worker to discriminate between virus specific cytopathic effect (CPE) and non specific cytotoxicity. It was decided to apply an indirect immunoperoxidase technique to detect virus infected cells in the plates on completion of the VNT.

The VNT was performed as described by Rowe and Anderson (in preparation), then the plates were fixed for 1 hour using 10% formaldehyde solution in PBS. Rabbit anti-rinderpest virus serum was then added, at a dilution established by previous titration, and specific binding of antibody was detected by the addition of S. aureus PA conjugated to HRPO.

The substrate (OPD) was added and the reaction stopped by the addition of IM sulphuric acid.

The optimal time for fixation of plates was 5-6 days after infection. Once fixed, the enzyme assay could be performed at the convenience of the experimenter, plates being stored in the interim at 4C. Very low background ODs were observed with uninfected cells and thus results could easily be read by eye (see Fig.9).

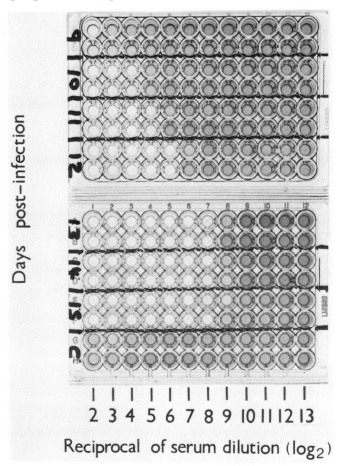

Fig. 9. A typical example of a micro virus neutralisation test visualised by the use of ELISA. Duplicate serum samples from a steer experimentally infected with rinderpest virus are diluted across the plate from left to right. The numbers 9, 10, 11, 12, 13, 14 and 15 denote days post infection. A negative control serum (C) is also included.

There was a good agreement between microscopic and ELISA reading of the test, the ELISA consistently giving serum titres 0.3-0.5 log10 SN50 higher than microscopic reading.

The VNT was performed using constant virus against dilutions of serum, and the criterion for positive antibody by microscopic reading was the complete neutralisation of the virus input, i.e. the absence of any CPE. The amount of colour development using the ELISA technique was dependent on the number of virus infected cells present in the well; therefore a reduction in virus input resulted in a reduction in colour, making the ELISA reading more sensitive for the detection of low levels of antibody.

The advantages of the neutralisation - ELISA over the microscopic reading of plates are that it is easily read by eye, can be read by unskilled technicians and could be used for the viruses which do not produce a marked cytopathic effect on cells, or have a slow growth rate which would make development of a standard virus-neutralisation test difficult.

The advantages of the neutralisation - ELISA over the standard indirect ELISA are that it only detects neutralising antibody and it could be used for examining exotic animal sera where non-specific levels in negative sera are not known or where anti-species sera are not available.

This technique is currently being brought into routine use in this laboratory and we are examining its suitability for other viruses.

REFERENCES.

Plowright, W. and Ferris, R.D. 1961. Archiv fur die gesamte Virusforschung, 11, 516.

Voller,A., Bidwell, D.E. and Bartlett, A. 1979.
    In "The enzyme linked immunosorbent assay (ELISA).
    A guide with abstracts of microplate applications".
    Dynatech Europe, Borough House, Rue du Pre, Guernsey,
    U.K.

DEVELOPMENT OF A SEROLOGIC ELISA FOR EQUINE INFECTIOUS ANEMIA

AND APPLICATION OF A SIMILAR ASSAY IN MAEDI/VISNA CONTROL IN THE FIELD

Arno L.J. Gielkens and Dirk J. Houwers

Central Veterinary Institute, Department of Virology,

8221 RA Lelystad, The Netherlands

ABSTRACT

An enzyme-linked immunosorbent assay (ELISA) was developed for the detection of antibodies against equine infectious anemia virus (EIAV). Of 472 sera from a sero-negative horse population that were examined, 467 showed a positive/negative (P/N) ratio lower than 2 and only 5 between 2 and 4. Thus a P/N ratio of 5 was chosen as lower limit for positive test samples. The sensitivity of the assay was compared with that of a standard immunodiffusion (ID) test using sera from naturally and experimentally infected horses. ELISA detected a higher number of positive samples and was more sensitive in detecting an early immune response. Preliminary results obtained with a double antibody sandwich (DAS) blocking assay are also discussed.

An indirect ELISA for the detection of antibodies against maedi/visna virus (MVV) has been applied in the framework of field experiments on the control of maedi/visna. As part of these experiments a number of flocks is tested for MVV-antibodies every six months and the reactors and their progeny are culled. The results indicate that reactor-free flocks can be achieved in this manner within reasonable time, depending on the initial percentage of reactors and the consequent culling of all progeny. ELISA proved to be of great value in these experiments and will be applied in a recently launched official control and accreditation scheme in the Netherlands.

INTRODUCTION

After the introduction of the enzyme-linked immunosorbent assay (ELISA) (Van Weemen and Schuurs, 1971; Engvall and Perlmann,1971) and the application of this method for virological diagnosis (Voller and Bidwell, 1975), many virological laboratories have started the development of enzyme-immunoassays for the detection of viral antigens and antibodies. Today, there is consensus that in many fields ELISA provides a rapid, sensitive and specific alternative to standard diagnostic methods. An additional advantage of ELISA is its suitability for screening large numbers of samples.

In our institute several ELISA-tests for the detection of viral antigens and antibodies were developed and some have been employed routinely for some years now. Double antibody sandwich (DAS) assays are used for the detection of bovine rotavirus and coronavirus in faecal extracts (Ellens et al. 1978a, 1978b) and for group-specific antigen of avian leukosis virus in many different substrates (De Boer et al., in preparation). Indirect assays were developed for the detection of antibodies against Aujeszky's disease virus (Briaire et al., 1979), bovine leukosis virus (Gielkens et al., 1981; Ressang et al., 1978, 1981) and maedi/visna virus (Houwers and Gielkens, 1979).

The agar-gel immunodiffusion test (ID) is generally accepted as a practical and suitable method for the serological diagnosis of equine infectious anemia (EIA) in Europe and the United States. In this test a crude concentrate of cultured virus, containing the group-specific antigen p24 as major viral component, is used as antigen. The method is specific and rather sensitive, but requires expertise to interpret the results.

Persistent infection with maedi/visna virus (MVV) usually induces specific antibodies which can be demonstrated by agar-gel precipitation and complement fixation. Experience in the past showed that these tests may present difficulties with respect to reproducibility of results in and between laboratories. These observations stimulated our search for a sensitive and reproducible serological method, which led to the development of an indirect ELISA (Houwers and Gielkens, 1979). A detailed report on this ELISA is given by Houwers et al. (1982).

In this report an ELISA for EIAV-antibodies is presented. In addition, preliminary results of field experiments on the control of maedi/visna in sheep are discussed, in which the above mentioned MVV antibody-ELISA plays a crucial role.

MATERIALS AND METHODS

Viruses and cells

EIAV was grown in an embryonic mule skin cell line chronically infected with the virus (kindly provided by Dr. W.A. Malmquist, National Animal Disease Center, Ames, Iowa). The virus containing culture fluid was collected from cells grown in maintenance medium supplemented with one per cent foetal calf serum (FCS) with a Bellco autoharvester at 4 h intervals.

Preparation of EIAV-antigen

For virus purification, one litre of culture fluid was clarified
by centrifugation at 8,500 x g for 20 min and the virus was then collected
by centrifugation at 8,500 x g for 16 h at 4°C. The supernatant was carefully removed and the pellet resuspended in PBS. This suspension was clarified at 700 x g for 5 min, layered on a cushion of 20% (w/v) of sucrose
in 10 mM Tris-hydrochloride pH 7.4 and centrifuged at 42,000 x g for 2 h
at 4°C in a Spinco type 40 rotor. Finally, the virus pellet was resuspended in one ml of PBS and stored at -20°C.

Indirect ELISA

The indirect ELISA-tests for the detection of antibodies against EIAV
and MVV were performed essentially as described for bovine leukosis virus
(Gielkens et al., 1981).

(i) Antigen coating.

The wells of polystyrene microtitre plates (Cooke M-129A) were coated
with an optimal concentration of EIAV-antigen in 10 mM sodium carbonate
buffer pH 9.5. After incubation for 6 h at 37°C, plates were stored at
4°C or at -20°C. Prior to use the plates were washed with deionized water
containing 0.05% of Tween-80 (wash fluid).

(ii) Incubation with serum.

Sera were diluted 1:20 in PBS-Tween (0.01 M phosphate buffer pH 7.3, 500
mM NaCl, 1 mM EDTA and 0.05% Tween-80) supplemented with 10% FCS and 0.05%
of N-Acetyl-L-Cysteine. After incubation for 1 h at 37°C in a water bath
the plates were rinsed ten times.

(iii) Incubation with conjugate.

HRPO (grade I, Boehringer, Mannheim, West Germany) labelled anti-species
IgG-conjugates were prepared according to the modified periodate method
described by Wilson and Nakane (1978). Plates were incubated for 1 h at
37°C and rinsed ten times.

(iv) Incubation with enzyme substrate.

A purified preparation of 5-aminosalicylic acid (5-AS) was prepared as
described previously (Ellens and Gielkens, 1980). Substrate was dissolved
at a concentration of 1 mg/ml in 10 mM phosphate buffer pH 6.8, containing 0.1 mM of Na_2EDTA. The final pH of this solution was 6.0. Just before
use 100 µl of a 0.5% solution of hydrogen peroxide in deionized water
was added per 10 ml of substrate solution.

The absorbance at 474 nm (A474) was measured after 2-18 h in a photo-meter equipped with a 80 µl flush cell. The results of the assay were either assessed as the A474 or as the positive/negative (P/N) ratio, where P is the A474 of the test sample and N that of the negative serum control. In each case the A474 of the PBS control was subtracted from that of the test serum. When routinely applied the absorbance was measured with a Multiskan® photometer.

DAS-blocking ELISA for EIAV-antibody

Test conditions for the DAS-blocking ELISA for EIAV-antibody were as follows:

(i) Plates were coated with an 1:800 dilution of the IgG-fraction of a hyperimmune serum of an EIAV-positive horse (Geronimo, ID-titre 1:4096, kindly provided by Dr. B. Toma, École Nationale Vétérinaire, Maisons Alfort, France) in 50 mM sodium carbonate buffer pH 9.5 for 18 h at 37°C.

(ii) EIA ID-antigen, diluted 1:800 in PBS-Tween, was added and incubated for 3 h at 37°C.

(iii) Test serum, diluted in PBS-Tween supplemented with 50% negative horse serum, was added and incubated for 2 h at 37°C.

(iv) Enzyme-labelled specific antibody (Geronimo IgG-preparation conjugated to HRPO), diluted 1:500 in PBS-Tween supplemented with 4% FCS, was added and incubated for 1 h at 37°C.

(v) The enzyme substrate 5-AS was added.

ID-test for EIAV-antibody

The ID-test using an ether-treated concentrate of the culture super-natant of EMS-cells chronically infected with EIAV was performed essentially as decribed by Coggins and Norcross (1970).

RESULTS

The indirect ELISA for EIAV-antibody

After standardization of the various ELISA-parameters, the specificity of the indirect ELISA for EIAV-antibody was examined by testing horse sera that had not reacted in our routine ID-test. A small number of sera showed P/N values between 1.5 and 5 (Table 1). The reproducible reactivity of these test samples in our ELISA might be caused by sticking of immuno-globuline molecules to the antigen-coated solid phase. In most cases this reactivity could be greatly reduced by incubating the sera in the presence of a low concentration (0.05%) of the mild reducing agent N-Acetyl-L-Cysteine (Nac) (Yolken and Stopa, 1979). At this concentration of Nac, P/N values of weakly positive sera were not significantly lowered. Therefore, incubation of sera in ELISA was performed in the presence of Nac.

Table 1.

Effect of addition of N-Acetyl-L-Cysteine during serum incubation on the non-specific reactivity of horse sera in the indirect ELISA

serum no.[a]	P/N value	
	− Nac	+ Nac[b]
393	3.0	0.7
397	2.9	0.6
398	2.5	0.6
411	1.5	0.5
432	2.5	0.7
448	4.8	3.3
475	4.8	0.5
631	3.1	3.4
26	9.5	9.4
IRS	15.3	14.5

[a] IRS stands for international reference serum; serum 26 was very weak positive by ID; sera 393-631 were selected because of their high non-specific reactivity.

[b] Concentration of N-Acetyl-L-Cysteine was 0.05 per cent.

Examination of 472 horse sera, which were negative by ID, in the ELISA showed that P/N ratios of most sera were lower than two. Only five samples showed P/N values between 2 and 4. Therefore, a P/N value of 5 was chosen as lower limit for positive test samples.

To determine the sensitivity of the indirect ELISA for EIAV-antibody, sera were examined that were negative in ID, sera obtained from natural EIA-cases and from experimentally infected horses. The results were compared with those of the ID-test (Table 2). Fifty-seven sera were scored negative in both tests and 155 positive. One ID-positive sample was negative in ELISA. On the other hand, ELISA detected antibodies in 11 samples which were negative in ID. Five out of these 11 samples were early sera

from experimentally infected horses. Of the remaining 6 samples 5 were
scored positive by ID in Dr. L. Coggins laboratory (New York State College
of Veterinary Medicine, Cornell University, Ithaca).

Table 2.
   Comparison of the indirect ELISA and the ID-test for the
               detection of antibodies against EIAV

number of sera	ID	ELISA[a]
155	+	+
3	±	+
11[b]	−	+
1	+	−
57	−	−

[a]Sera exhibiting a P/N value higher than 5 were scored positive.
[b]Five sera taken early after experimental infection; 5 sera
   scored positive and one serum scored negative by ID in Dr. L.
   Coggins laboratory.

Finally the antibody response to EIA in experimentally infected
horses was measured and compared in ID (data provided by Dr. B. Toma, Maisons
Alfort) and ELISA. Two examples are shown in Figure 1. With both methods a
similar increase of antibody levels was obtained. In one case a weak
response could be measured by ELISA 15 and 20 days p.i. when ID was still
negative (Fig. 1B).

Double antibody sandwich blocking ELISA for EIAV-antibody

   Although, the indirect ELISA seems to be the most obvious enzyme
immunoassay to measure viral antibody, other modifications of this
technique may be suitable as well. If such a system is specific and ex-
hibits similar sensitivity as the indirect method, it may be used as
confirmation test for positive test samples or used instead of the indirect method. For that purpose we developed a double antibody sandwich
(DAS) blocking ELISA. A practical advantage of this approach is that crude
antigen preparations, for example ID-antigen, can be employed.

198

Sensitivity and specificity of the optimized test were compared with
those of ID-test using EIA ID check-test sera. Only samples showing at
least 50 per cent inhibition of conjugate binding were considered positive.
Besides the sera that agreed in both tests, ELISA scored an additional 10
samples positive. These last sera were from EIAV-positive horses showing a
weaker reaction in the ID-test than the international reference serum
(Dr. B. Toma, Maisons Alfort, personal communication).

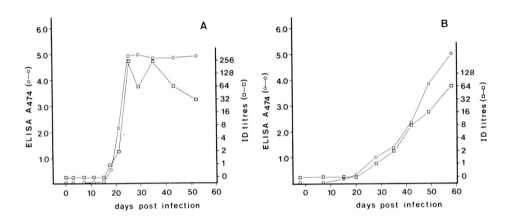

Fig. 1. Antibody response after experimental infection with EIAV.

However, when testing large numbers of ID-negative horse sera it
appeared that some sera exhibited a non-specific inhibition higher than
50 per cent. This could only be reduced by using higher dilutions of
test serum resulting in a significant decrease in sensitivity of the DAS-
blocking assay.

The indirect ELISA for maedi/visna-antibody

The indirect ELISA for MVV-antibody in sheep sera has been routinely
applied in our laboratory over two years and some 30,000 samples have been
tested. So far, our experience indicates that this method is specific and
sensitive and particularly suited for testing of large numbers of sera.

Table 3. Comparison of a DAS-blocking ELISA and the ID-test for the
detection of antibodies against EIAV

number of sera[a]	ID	ELISA DAS-blocking[b]
65	+	+
1[c]	±	+
10[c]	−	+
44	−	−

[a] EIA ID check-test sera.

[b] Sera were scored positive when blocking was higher than 50 per cent at the test dilution 1:4.

[c] Sera from EIA-positive horses exhibiting a weaker reaction in the ID than the international reference serum.

The MVV-ELISA is currently applied in the framework of field experiments on the control of maedi/visna in sheep. Part of this experiment is based on halfyearly testing and culling of reactors and all their progeny. Preliminary results are shown in Table 4.

Table 4.

Field experiment on maedi/visna control.
Results of halfyearly serological testing (ELISA) and
culling of reactors plus all their progeny in 14 commercial
flocks.

	tests					
	1	2	3	4	5	6
pos/tot	138-1095	78-938	17-1088	5-967	0-1135	0-1038
%	(16,7%)	(8,3%)	(1,6%)	(0,5%)	(0%)	(0%)

The percentage of reactors decreases regularly and reaches 0 per cent at the fifth halfyearly test. The sixth and the seventh test, which is almost completed, also yielded no reactors. Experience so far has shown that once a flock has passed two subsequent negative halfyearly tests, the flock will stay negative and thus these flocks are most probably free of maedi/

visna.

Table 5 shows the result of two flocks in which reactors and only their last lamb crop were culled. There is a high level of infection at the start of the experiment and the decrease in percentage of reactors shows a lag at the fourth up to the sixth test. This lag is mainly caused by infected sheep which were born before the start of the experiment and which showed a late antibody response. Recently, the seventh test has been completed and no reactors were found. Consequently, it is concluded that culling of all progeny is necessary for a rapid elimination of MVV infection.

Table 5.

Field experiment on maedi/visna control.
Results of halfyearly serological testing (ELISA) and culling of reactors plus their last lamb crop in 2 commercial flocks.

		tests				
	1	2	3	4	5	6
pos/tot	136-255	38-133	12-159	16-129	14-138	8-98
	(53,3%)	(28,6%)	(7,5%)	(12,4%)	(10,1%)	(8,2%)

DISCUSSION

This report describes an indirect ELISA for the detection of EIAV-antibody. Results obtained with this technique were compared with those of the ID-test, which is generally used for EIA-diagnosis.

Our data demonstrated a higher sensitivity of ELISA in comparison with ID. For instance, we found that sera from EIA-positive horses that produced extremely weak reactions in ID which were not consistently detected, still exhibited ELISA P/N values higher than 8 (Gielkens et al. in preparation). For comparison, in several blind experiments P/N values between 11 and 15 were observed with the very weak positive international reference serum. Using this ELISA, antibodies can be detected directed against the major viral protein p24, but also against one of the low molecular weight proteins p15 (Gielkens and Toma, in preparation). Because of its high sensitivity this ELISA seems to be useful for experimental work.

Besides the usual advantages of this type of enzyme-immunoassays, indirect ELISA-tests also have several disadvantages. Non-specific reactivity of negative sera and high background colouring are often major problems during the developmental stages of the technique. Non-specific reactivity is probably due to sticking of serum proteins, including immunoglobulines, to the protein coated polystyrene surface. The extent of non-specific reactivity varies from serum to serum. Part of this problem may be solved by incubating sera in the presence of a low concentration of the mild reducing agent Nac. In addition, the quality of antigen and anti-species IgG-conjugate employed in the indirect ELISA strongly influence the background colouring of the assay and thus also its sensitivity. Especially the need for a purified EIAV-antigen preparation may be, for the present, a major problem for routine application. Therefore tests should be developed which can be run with crude antigen preparations. An example of this approach is the DAS-blocking ELISA described above.

The MVV ELISA is applied in the framework of field experiments on the control of maedi/visna. Lactogenic transmission is a major route of infection and periods as long as two years may elapse before antibodies can be detected. Therefore, it is recommended to cull ELISA reactors and all their progeny (preceeding years included). The experiments on maedi control already resulted in the launching of an official control and accreditation scheme based on serological testing. Within this scheme it is important to have a sensitive, simple and cheap test for MVV-antibodies. In our hands the MVV-antibody ELISA is the technique of choice because of its sensitivity, specificity, its low cost in labour and ingredients and its possibilities for standardisation and automation.

ACKNOWLEDGEMENTS

We are grateful to Messr. Johan IJzerman and Jan Schaake jr. for their skilful technical assistance. We thank Mr. Nico Huffels for testing many horse sera by ID and Dr. Jan van Oirschot for helpful discussions.

REFERENCES

Briaire, J., Meloen, R.H. and Barteling, S.J., 1979. An enzyme-linked immunosorbent assay (ELISA) for the detection of antibody against Aujeszky's disease virus in pig sera. Zbl. Vet. Med. B., 26, 76-81.
Coggins, L. and Norcross, N.L., 1970. Immunodiffusion reaction in equine infectious anemia. Cornell Vet., 60, 330-335.

202

Ellens, D.J., De Leeuw, P.W., Straver, P.J. and Van Balken, J.A.M., 1978a. Comparison of five diagnostic methods for the detection of rotavirus antigens in calf faeces. Med. Microbiol. Immunol. 166, 157-163

Ellens, D.J., Van Balken, J.A.M. and De Leeuw, P.W., 1978b. Diagnosis of bovine coronavirus infections with hemadsorption-elution-hemagglutination assay (HEMA) and with enzyme-linked immunosorbent assay (ELISA). Proc. Second Int. Symp. on Neonatal Diarrhoea, University of Saskatchewan, Canada, p. 322-329.

Ellens, D.J. and Gielkens, A.L.J., 1980. A simple method for the purification of 5-aminosalicylic acid. Application of the product as substrate in enzyme-linked immunosorbent assay (ELISA). J. Immunol. Methods 37, 325-332.

Engvall, E. and Perlmann, P., 1971. Enzyme-linked immunosorbent assay (ELISA). Quantitative assay of immunoglobulin. Immunochemistry 8, 871-874.

Gielkens, A.L.J., Ressang, A.A., IJzerman, J. and Quak, J., 1981. Test protocol of an enzyme-linked immunosorbent assay (ELISA) for the detection of antibodies against bovine leukosis virus. The Vet. Quarterly 3, 34-37.

Houwers, D.J. and Gielkens, A.L.J., 1979. An ELISA for the detection of maedi/visna antibody. Vet. Rec., 104, 26.

Houwers, D.J., Gielkens, A.L.J. and Schaake, J., 1982. An indirect enzyme-linked immunosorbent assay (ELISA) for the detection of antibodies to maedi/visna virus. Vet. Microbiol., in press.

Ressang, A.A., Gielkens, A.L.J., Quak, J., Mastenbroek, N., Tuppert, C. and De Castro, A., 1978. Studies on bovine leukosis. VI. Enzyme-linked immunosorbent assay for the detection of antibodies to bovine leukosis virus. Ann. Rech. Vét. 9, 663-666.

Ressang, A.A., Gielkens, A.L.J., Quak, J. and Mastenbroek, N., 1981. Studies on bovine leukosis. VII. Further experience with an ELISA for the detection of antibodies to bovine leukosis virus. The Vet. Quarterly, 3, 31-33.

Van Weemen, B.K. and Schuurs, A.H.W.M., 1971. Immunoassay using antigen-enzyme conjugates. FEBS Lett., 15, 232-236.

Voller, A. and Bidwell, D.E., 1975. A simple method for detecting antibodies to rubella. Br. J. exp. Path., 56, 338-339.

Wilson, M.B. and Nakane, P.K., 1978. Recent developments in the periodate method of conjugating horse-radish peroxidase (HRPO) to antibodies. In W. Knapp, K. Holubar and G. Wicks (eds.), Immunofluorescence and related staining techniques. Elsevier/North-Holland Biomed. Press, Amsterdam, p. 215-224.

THE DETECTION OF ANTIBODIES TO MAEDI/VISNA VIRUS IN OVINE SERA: COMPARING THE USE OF AN ENZYME LINKED IMMUNOSORBENT ASSAY AND AN AGAR GEL IMMUNODIFFUSION TEST

M. Dawson

Central Veterinary Laboratory
New Haw, Weybridge
Surrey, KT15 3NB
England

ABSTRACT

A recently developed enzyme linked immunosorbent assay (ELISA) and an established agar gel immunodiffusion test (AGIDT) were compared as serological methods for the detection of antibodies to maedi/visna virus (MVV) in ovine sera.

An initial group of 160 sera were selected from sheep which by their history had had no contact with MVV infected sheep: these were clinically normal sheep and sheep experimentally infected with or vaccinated against a variety of ovine pathogens. All sera were negative in the AGIDT and the upper limit of ELISA readings was 1.5 times that of the reference negative pool.

50 AGIDT seropositive samples were identified in a second group of 210 sera which were taken from a population of animals where recent seroconversion was anticipated. Of these 50 AGIDT positive sera, 31 had ELISA readings equal to or less than twice that of the reference negative, and 13 of these were equal to or less than the upper limit of values recorded for sera in the first group tested. Only 1 serum in this group was recorded positive in the ELISA and negative in the AGIDT, and a further 2 samples produced non specific reactions in the ELISA.

A third group of sera consisted of serial samples taken over a prolonged period from four sheep. ELISA and AGIDT results were in agreement for two of these sheep, but for the other two more sera were conclusively positive in the AGIDT than the ELISA.

This preliminary study demonstrated that currently, in our experience, weak seropositive samples are more confidently identified in the AGIDT than in the ELISA, and that a low percentage of false positive samples may be recorded by the latter technique.

INTRODUCTION

Maedi (= laboured breathing) and visna (= wasting) are Icelandic names which describe two syndromes which may develop in adult sheep and goats following infection with the lentivirus, maedi/visna virus (MVV). Clinical maedi may become apparent following the development of a progressive interstitial pneumonitis and visna is associated with a meningoleucencephalitis. Both diseases are fatal (Dawson, 1980).

Serological evidence of MVV infection in sheep in Great Britain was first detected in the autumn of 1978. MVV was isolated from naturally infected sheep early the following year (Dawson et al, 1979). A complement fixation test (CFT) was used initially for determining the serological status of sheep in flocks under investigation. The CFT proved to be relatively insensitive and inconsistent when compared with the results obtained using an agar gel immunodiffusion test (AGIDT). The AGIDT has now been used routinely in this laboratory for over two years.

Virus persists in the infected host despite the presence of specific antibodies. The demonstration of a serological response in an animal therefore identifies it as a virus carrier. The success of controlling MVV in infected flocks by culling serological reactors is dependant on the early detection of seroconversion in infected sheep. In some cases this may take over two years (Houwers and de Boer, 1981).

Dutch workers developed an enzyme linked immunosorbent assay (ELISA) for the detection of antibodies to MVV. They reported it to be more sensitive than both a CFT and an AGIDT which they had used previously. It was also considered to be more cost and labour efficient and had the additional advantage over the AGIDT of an objective assessment of results (Houwers and Gielkens, 1979; De Boer and Houwers, 1979). An ELISA similar to that used by the Dutch workers has recently been investigated in this laboratory and the results of a preliminary comparative trial with our routine AGIDT are reported here.

MATERIALS AND METHODS

Sera

For the purposes of comparing the AGIDT and the ELISA, the following groups of sera were selected.

Group 1. 160 sera were selected from indigenous British sheep which had had no history of contact with imported sheep or their progeny. The majority of these sera were taken from clinically normal sheep of various breeds including Cluns, Scottish Blackface, Scottish Halfbreds and Dorset Horns. Also included were:-

- sera from 12 sheep experimentally infected with border disease virus.
- sera from 17 sheep experimentally infected with the chlamydial agent of enzootic abortion of ewes.
- sera from 6 sheep vaccinated with a commercial inactivated Salmonella/Pasteurella/E. coli vaccine.

- sera from 2 lambs experimentally infected with both rotavirus and E. coli.
- one serum with precipitating antibodies to bluetongue virus and one serum with precipitating antibodies to contagious pustular dermatitis (contagious ecthyma) virus.

Group 2. A second series of sera were selected from sheep in an infected flock where approximately 50 per cent of adult stock were known to be AGIDT seropositive. These samples were taken from 109 one year old sheep and 101 adult sheep which had been AGIDT seronegative when last tested, six months previously.

Group 3. These sera consisted of serial samples taken from four individual animals. Two of these (10242 and 10272) were sentinel sheep which had been housed with a naturally infected ewe. The third was a lamb (14129) which had been born to a naturally infected ewe and had been housed with her until weaning at approximately 8 weeks of age. The fourth animal was a naturally infected 6 year old ewe (K184) which had been under observation for two and a half years.

All serum samples were stored at $-20^{\circ}C$.

The AGIDT

Antigen preparation and test procedure were modifications of already described methods (Cutlip et al, 1977; Winward et al, 1979).

Monolayers of ovine trachea cells infected with virus strain WLC-1 (kindly provided by Dr. R. C. Cutlip, National Animal Disease Centre, USDA, Ames, Iowa, USA) were maintained in roller vessels for prolonged periods. The culture medium was bicarbonate buffered Eagle's minimal essential medium with Hank's salts, 1 per cent glutamine and 10 per cent foetal bovine serum. Medium was changed at two-weekly intervals and each harvest was concentrated approximately 100-fold by dialysis against polyethylene glycol (molecular weight 2×10^{4}). This concentrated medium constituted the antigen and was stored at $-20^{\circ}C$.

Reference positive serum was raised in two Dorset Horn sheep experimentally infected with virus strain WLC-1. The specificity of these sera was verified with the aid of reference sera supplied by Dr. Cutlip, Dr. D. J. Houwers, Central Veterinary Institute, Lelystad, the Netherlands and Dr. R. Hoff-Jørgensen, State Veterinary Serum Laboratory, Copenhagen, Denmark.

The gel formula was 0.7 - 1% agarose (depending on batch) dissolved in 0.05 M TRIS buffer (pH 7.2) with 8 per cent sodium chloride. The test was performed in 8.5 cm diameter plastic Petri dishes containing 15 ml. of gel. A microhexagonal test pattern was used with alternating large and small peripheral wells around a single central well (Winward et al, 1979). 10 patterns were accommodated in each Petri dish. The central well contained antigen and positive serum was added to each of the three small peripheral wells. Optimal dilution of antigen and positive serum were determined by block titration. Each large peripheral well contained a separate test serum. Plates were incubated at room temperature in a moist chamber and read over reflected light. All sera giving a **positive** or inconclusive result were tested again, if necessary in triplicate.

The ELISA

The assay used was essentially similar to the indirect ELISA developed by Houwers and Gielkens (1979) and described in more detail by Houwers et al. (submitted by publication, 1981).

The major difference was the virus strain used as antigen source, for which WLC-1 infected ovine trachea cultures were used. For antigen production, the culture medium was supplemented with 0.5 per cent foetal bovine serum and harvested at 4-hourly intervals. Antigen was prepared by the differential ultracentrifugation of harvested medium.

The conditions of the various stages of the assay were briefly as follows.

1. Antigen coating: viral antigen was diluted in sodium carbonate buffer (pH 9.5) and 100 ul volumes were added to the wells of flat bottomed microelisa plates (Cooke, M 129 A, Dynatech). Plates were incubated at 37°C for 6 hours and then stored at -20°C.

2. Serum incubation: 5 ul of test sera were added to 100 ul of diluting buffer (0.01M phosphate buffer, 500 mM NaCl, 1 mM EDTA and 0.05 per cent Tween 80). Each serum was incubated in duplicate in both antigen coated and uncoated wells for 1 hour at 37°C. The controls included on each plate consisted of a series of doubling dilutions (1/20 - 1/640) of a reference positive serum taken from a naturally infected sheep, and a single dilution (1/20) of a reference negative serum pool. This pool consisted of 650 AGIDT seronegative samples taken from indigenous British sheep which had not been exposed to MVV.

3. Conjugate incubation: rabbit anti sheep immunoglobulin G conjugated to horseradish peroxidase (Wilson and Nakane, 1978) was diluted

in the same buffer as the test sera with the addition of 4 per cent horse serum. 100 ul was added to each well and plates were incubated for 1 hour at 37°C.

After each of these stages, plates were emptied and subjected to a washing cycle which consisted of five rinses with a solution of 0.05 percent Tween 80 in distilled water.

4. Substrate incubation: Recrystallized 5-amino-salicylic acid (Ellens and Gielkens, 1980) was dissolved in buffer (0.01 M phosphate buffer, 0.1 mM EDTA adjusted to pH 6) at the rate of 1 mg/ml. Immediately before addition to the plates, hydrogen peroxide was added to the substrate solution to a final concentration of 0.005 percent. 100 ul of substrate solution was added to each well and plates were incubated at ambient temperature for 1 hour in the dark.

The optical density (O.D.) of the resulting enzyme/substrate reaction in each well was measured in a multichannel photometer (Multiskan, Flow) operating with a 450 nm wavelength filter.

The results for the test sera were expressed as follows:-

O.D. of test or positive serum ,

O.D. of negative reference pool

or P/N ratio.

Optimal concentrations of antigen and conjugate were determined by checkerboard titration using fixed dilution (1/20) of the reference positive and negative sera.

RESULTS

Group 1 sera

All 160 sera were negative in the AGIDT. In the ELISA, all but 8 sera had P/N values less than 1. The highest P/N value of these 8 was 1.5 (see Fig. 1).

Group 2 sera

50/210 sera were positive in the AGIDT. The ELISA results of these 50 are given in Fig. 1. 13/50 AGIDT seropositive samples had P/N values equal to or less than the upper limit of P/N values (1.5) for group 1 sera. 31/50 AGIDT seropositive samples had P/N values equal to or less than 2. 19 AGIDT seronegative samples recorded P/N values greater than 1. However only one of these had a P/N value substantially higher than 1.5 (see

208

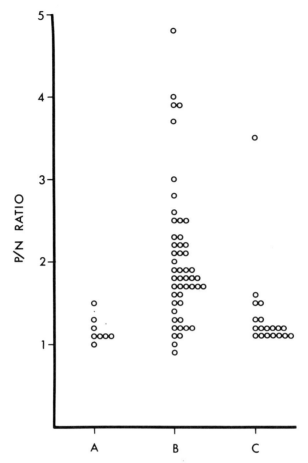

Fig. 1   A. ELISA results of group 1 sera recording P/N values ⩾ 1.
B. ELISA results of the 50 AGIDT positive sera in group 2. C. ELISA
results of AGIDT negative sera in group 2 recording P/N values ⩾ 1.

Fig. 1). An additional two sera, both negative in the AGIDT, produced
substantial colour reactions in the ELISA when incubated in both antigen
coated and uncoated wells.

Group 3 sera

Both sentinel sheep 10242 and 10272 were seropositive in the AGIDT six
months after being placed in contact with a naturally infected ewe. This
status was maintained for all subsequent samples extending to eighteen
months post exposure. These results and the corresponding ELISA results
are given in Fig. 2 (10242) and Fig. 3 (10272). For 10272, the ELISA P/N
value was well above 2 at 6 months post exposure and increased steadily

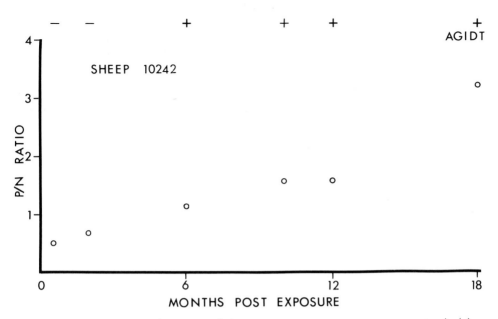

Fig. 2   ELISA P/N values (o) and corresponding AGIDT results (+/-)
for serial samples from sheep 10242.

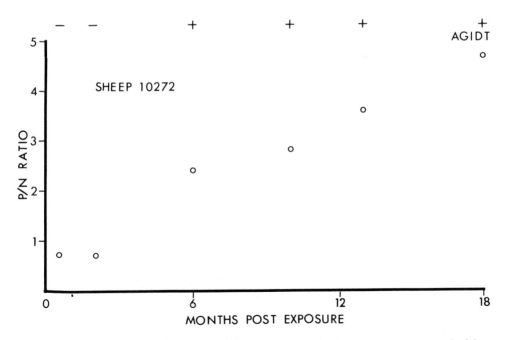

Fig. 3   ELISA P/N values (o) and corresponding AGIDT results (+/-)
for serial samples from sheep 10272.

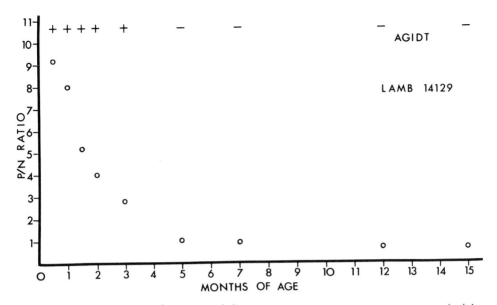

Fig. 4   ELISA P/N values (o) and corresponding AGIDT results (+/-) for serial samples for lamb 14129.

after that. For 10242, however, the P/N value did not rise above 2 until the eighteen month sample.

P/N values for lamb 14129 fell steadily after birth and levelled off at about 1 from five months of age onwards (see Fig. 4). In the AGIDT, serum samples were positive up to 3 months of age and negative from 5 months onwards.

Only three sera were available from K184, the naturally infected ewe. Two of these were taken one month apart early in 1979. Both of these sera have elevated P/N values and were positive in the AGIDT. However, the ELISA reading fell markedly for the third sample but this serum remained positive in the AGIDT (Fig. 5).

DISCUSSION

It is considered that MVV was probably introduced into Great Britain with importations of sheep in the last decade. Serological studies to date indicate that infection is fairly widespread among sheep of imported origin, their progeny and close contacts (unpublished data). Additional evidence to support the contention that native sheep (not exposed to exotic breeds or their progeny) are MVV free was derived from a limited survey of approximately 1400 sera selected from flocks containing many breeds dist-

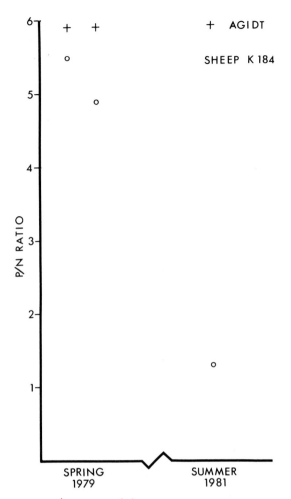

Fig. 5 ELISA P/N values (o) and corresponding AGIDT results (+/-) for serial samples for sheep K184.

ributed throughout Great Britain. No positive samples were found using the AGIDT (Dawson, 1981).

The sera in group 1 could therefore confidently be expected to be free of antibodies to MVV and indeed, all were negative in the AGIDT. These sera were therefore useful for establishing the range of ELISA P/N values for MVV free sheep. As the highest P/N value recorded was 1.5 it would also appear that no cross reactions with antibodies to some other common ovine pathogens were detected in the ELISA.

The sera in group 2 represent a population of sheep in which sero-positive sheep would be emerging. They were selected specifically to test the sensitivities of the two assays. It was considered that these sera would be more suitable for this purpose than sera from experimentally infected sheep, where the kinetics of antibody production may not be typical. Due to the overlap of P/N values for sera from MVV free sheep and AGIDT positive sera (Fig. 1), ELISA results in the P/N value range 1 - 2 must be regarded as inconclusive and sera with P/N values greater than 2 can probably be interpreted as positive. Adopting this system restricts the number of ELISA positive samples to 20/210 whereas 50 AGIDT positive samples were identified.

Applying a P/N cut off value of 2 to the ELISA results of group 3 sera would permit an exact correlation between assays for 10272 and 14129 (Figs. 3 and 4). However, in the case of 10242 (Fig. 2) seroconversion would not be apparent until 18 months post-exposure as determined by ELISA, but it was detected at six months in the AGIDT.

It has generally been considered that following seroconversion, a humoral response probably persists for the animal's natural lifespan (Pálsson, 1976). The results for sheep K184 (Fig. 5) are therefore especially interesting. Again if a cut off P/N value of 2 is adopted, the final sample is apparently inconclusive in the ELISA but remains positive in the AGIDT.

An overall assessment of the sensitivities of the two assays, based on the results from sera in group 2 and 3 would indicate that weak seroposit-ive samples are more confidently identified in the AGIDT. Whereas the specificity of the AGIDT has been satisfactorily established, the two sera in group 2 that produced considerable colour reactions in the ELISA when incubated in the absence of antigen suggests that a low frequency of false positive reactions may be recorded.

These findings are not in agreement with those of the Dutch workers who found their ELISA to be considerably more sensitive than their AGIDT. It should be emphasised that our ELISA is still essentially experimental and can probably be improved. However, a recent comparative study of three immunoassays for MVV antibodies, including the Dutch ELISA and our AGIDT (to be published elsewhere), has indicated a very close correlation between the two techniques, in terms of both sensitivity and specificity. This suggests that the AGIDT in use in this laboratory is more sensitive than the AGIDT previously used in Holland.

ACKNOWLEDGEMENTS

The technical assistance of Mrs. R. H. Newman and Mrs. S. E. N. Drury is gratefully acknowledged. Thanks are also due to Miss M. H. Lucas for useful criticism and Mrs. C. A. Curr for typing the manuscript. I am especially indebted to Dr. D. J. Houwers of the Central Veterinary Institute, Lelystad, for much useful advice on ELISA methodology.

REFERENCES

Cutlip, R. C., Jackson, T. A. and Laird, G. A. 1977. Immunodiffusion Test for Ovine Progressive Pneumonia. Am. J. Vet. Res., 38, 1081.

Dawson, M., Chasey, D., King, A. A., Flowers, M. J., Day, R. H., Lucas, M. H. and Roberts, D. H. 1979. The demonstration of maedi/visna virus in sheep in Great Britain. Vet. Rec., 105, 220.

Dawson, M. 1980. Maedi/visna: A review. Vet. Rec., 106, 212.

Dawson, M. 1981. Maedi/visna in Britain. Vet. Rec., 109, 187.

De Boer, G. F. and Houwers, D. J. 1979. Epizootiology of maedi/visna in sheep. In "Aspects of Slow and Persistent Virus Infections" (Ed. D. A. J. Tyrrell). (ECSC, EEC, EAEC, Brussels-Luxembourg) pp 198 - 220.

Ellens, D. J. and Gielkens, A. L. J. 1980. A simple method for the purification of 5-aminosalicylic acid. Application of the product as substrate in enzyme linked immunosorbent assay (ELISA). J. Immunol. Methods, 37, 325.

Houwers, D. J. and de Boer, G. F. 1981. Maedi/visna in Britain. Vet. Rec. 109, 125.

Houwers, D. J. and Gielkens, A. L. J. 1979. An ELISA for the detection of maedi/visna antibody. Vet. Rec., 104, 611.

Houwers, D. J., Gielkens, A. L. J. and Schaake, J. 1981. An indirect enzyme-linked immunosorbent assay (ELISA) for the detection of antibodies to maedi-visna virus. (Submitted for publication).

Pálsson, P. A. 1976. Maedi and visna in sheep. In "Slow Virus Diseases of Animals and Men" (Ed. R. H. Kimberlin). (North-Holland, Amsterdam, Oxford). pp 17 - 43.

Wilson, N. B. and Nakane, P. K. 1978. Recent developments in the periodate method of conjugating horseradish peroxidase (HRPO) to antibodies. In "Immunofluorescence and related staining techniques". (Ed. W. Knapp, K. Holubar and G. Wick). (Elsevier/North Holland, Amsterdam, New York). pp 215 - 224.

Winward, L. D., Leendertsen, L. and Shen, D. T. 1979. Microimmunodiffusion Test for Diagnosis of Ovine Progressive Pneumonia. Am. J. Vet. Res., 40, 564.

SEMIPURIFIED STRUCTURAL VIRAL PROTEIN FOR THE DETECTION
OF ASF ANTIBODIES BY INDIRECT ELISA TECHNIQUE.

J.M. Sánchez-Vizcaíno, E. Tabarés, E. Salvador and A. Or-
dás.
I.N.I.A. Crida 06. Dpto. de Virología Animal.
Embajadores, 68. Madrid 12. (Spain).

ABSTRACT

A comparative study of soluble ASF antigen and se--
mipurified structural ASF virus protein (VP 73) was ca--
rried out in order to evaluate their use in the detec--
tion of ASF antibodies by Indirect ELISA methods. A total
of 677 field samples were evaluated by ELISA (both antigen) IEOP and IIF. The results of this work prove that
the sensitivity and specificity obtained by ELISA (both
antigen) test are superior to those obtained by IEOP when
the semipurified protein is used as an ELISA antigen the
results offered a 100% correspondence with IIF.

INTRODUCTION

African Swine Fever (ASF) is a viral swine disease,
that presents a similar clinical picture to other hemo--
rrhagic disease of pigs. For this reason a laboratory --
diagnosis have to be done to determine its differentiation. Diagnosis can be made on the basis of the demonstration of infectious virus, viral antigen (hemoadsorption
test, Malmquist and Hay 1960, direct immunofluorescence,
Colgrove 1968, or antibodies produced against the virus,
immunoelectroosmophoresis, Pan et al. 1972, and indirect
immunofluorescence, Sánchez Botija et al. 1970).
Different epidemiological situation like the apea-

rance of low virulent ASF strains in Dominical Republic, Brazil and Spain together with the fact that in countries in which the disease is enzootic, the numbers of carrier animals (apparently healhtly), with specific antibodies - has increased considerably therefore the use of techniques capable of detecting these antibodies is of great impor - tance today.

At the present, the most comun routine techniques used for the detection of ASF antibodies are the IIF and IEOP. None of these techniques, however, enable us to ob- tain high levels of sensitivity anf specificity (IIF) com- bined with mass sample testing (which could be atributed to IEOP). During the past two years an enzyme-linked immu- nosorbent assay (ELISA) test has been developed for the - detection of ASF antibodies in Swine serum (Sánchez-Viz- caíno et al. 1.979), in which high levels of sensitivity and specificity are combined with large scale uses. Howe- ver, some false positive reactions were observed in some particular pig sera when a soluble ASF antigen was used in the indirect ELISA test. Nevertheless the false positive reactions were inferior to those with IEOP (Sánchez-Vizcai- no, 1.980).

In this paper a comparative study of the soluble ASF antigen an a semipurified VP 73 structural ASF protein is carried out in order to evaluate their use for the detec- tion of ASF antibodies. All sera study by this techniques were also test simultaneosly with IEOP and IIF using the latter one as a reference test.

MATERIALS AND METHODS

ANTIGENS

SOLUBLE ANTIGEN PREPARATION

The soluble Antigen was obtained by inoculation of a monolayer MS (Monkey stable) cell line with the ASF vi- rus, strain Spain 75. After infection the cells were ob- served until the cytopathic effect was of 90 to 100% -

(approximately at 48 hours). Then, they were harvested -
and centrifuged at 1.000 g. for 20 minutes. The pellet -
was resuspended in a double volume of PBS pH 7.2, sonicated on ice for 3 minutes at 50 w. and centrifuged at 48000
g. for 45 minutes. The supernatant was used as the soluble
antigen.

SEMIPURIFIED VP 73 PREPARATION

The semipurified VP 73 was obtained by inoculation
of MS cells line with the strain Spain 70 (Tabarés et al
1.981).

MS infected cells were washed with PBS and harves -
ted at 48 h p.i. and then sediment at 650 x g. for 5 minutes. The pellet was washed with 0.34 M sucrose - 5 mM
Tris HCl, pH 8 (3.6 ml per roller bottle or 1.8 ml per -
Rous bottle) for 8 minutes at 0ºC. Cells were lysed by -
addition of Nonidet P40 (NP-40) to a final concentration
of 1 percent (w/v) for 10 minutes at 0ºC with occasional
agitation. 1/7 volume of 64% w/v sucrose - 0.4 M Tris HCl
pH 8 was added and the nucleic were pelleted at 1000 x g.
for 10 minutes at 0ºC. The cytoplasmic fraction was made
in 2 mM EDTA and 50 mM beta-mercaptoethanol. After 15 minutes at 25ºC, the mixture was layered onto 1 ml. 60% w/w
sucrose and about 5 ml. of 20% w/w sucrose in 50 mM Tris
HCl pH 8. Centrifugation of the discontinuous gradient -
was performed with a Beckman SW40 rotor for 1 hour at -
25000 rpm and 4ºC. The material on 60% w/w sucrose was diluted to 3.6 ml. to a final concentration of 0.5 M NaCl -
0.5% w/v NP40 - 2 mM EDTA - 50 mM beta-mercaptoethanol -
50 mM Tris HCl pH 8. After 15 minutes at 25ºC with occasional agitation the preparation was centrifuged at ---
100,000 x g. for 75 minutes at 4ºC and the supernatant -
was taken as VP 73 semipurified preparation. The supernatant of 25000 rpm in SW40 rotor can be used as antigen in
immunoelectroosmophoresis (13).

TEST SERA

A total of 225 positive IIF ASF sera and 452 negative IIF sera from the northeast of Spain were used as a -
test sera.

CONTROL SERA

A pool of 200 positive sera from Portuguese and Spa-
nish field cases was used as the positive reference sera
and, as negative control, a pool of sera from German pigs
was used.

CONJUGATE

A Rabbit IgG peroxydase conjugate anti pig IgG (heavy and light chains) (*) was used as a conjugate.

SUBSTRATE

O. Ohenilediamine (OPD) (**), 0,04 mg/ml. in Citrate buffer pH 5 was used as a substrate.

PLATES SENSITIZED WITH ASF ANTIGEN

One hundred microlitres of the optimum antigen concentration in Carbonate buffer were added to each well.
Then, the plates were incubated at 4ºC overnight, washed
four times and after being shaken and dried, the plates
were ready for use or storage at -20ºC. up to 6 months.

ELISA PROCEDURE

1.- One hundred microlitres of the different diluted sera
samples and controls were added to the wells, two of each,
of the sensitized plates and incubated for 1 hour at 37ºC.
2.- The plates were washed 4 times with washing solution
(saline solution with 0,5 ml/l of tween 20).

(*) Cappel lab. INC. Cochranville, Pa (USA)
(**) Sigma Chemical Company. Saint Louis. Missoury (USA)

3.- One hundred microlitres of conjugate at optimum concentration were added to each well and incubated 1 hour
at room temperature (20-25ºC).

4.- Repeat number 2.

5.- One hundred microlitres of the substrate were added
to each well and incubated 10 minutes a room temperature
(20-25ºC)

6.- The reaction was stopped by the addition of one hundred microlitres of H_2SO_4 3N to each well and incubated
five minutes at room temperature.

7.- The plates were read by Multieskan (*) at 450 nm.

IIF AND IEOP TEST

The indirect immunofluorescence test was done as
described by Sánchez Botija et al. 1.970 and the IEOP -
acording to Pan et al. 1.972 publication.

RESULTS

A total of 225 positive IIF field ASF sera and 452
negative IIF field sera have been analyzed by the indirect
ELISA method using the conventional ASF soluble antigen
as well as the semipurified structural ASF viral protein
(VP 73). All those sera were also tested simultaneosly
with the IEOP anf IIF tests, this latter one was used as
a reference technique.

These 677 field sera tested by IEOP gave 64 false
positive sera and 15 false negative in comparason to IIF.
Resulting in a sensitivity and specificity index of 93%
and 85% respectible (table I).

With the ELISA method using the soluble ASF antigen the false positive sera were 47 and 5 false negative.
Whic gave a sensitivity and specificity index of 97% and
89% respectible (table II).

(*) Multieskan Colorimeter. Flow la. Irvine. Scothland.

When the same sera were tested by ELISA method using the semipurified VP 73, the results presented a perfect - parallelism with IIF. Gave a sensitivity and specificity index of 100% and 100% respectible. (table III).

Table I

Comparative results between IEOP and IIF.

I.I.F.

	+	-		Index
I.E.O.P. +	210	64	274	Sensitivity: 93%
-	15	488	403	Specificity: 85%
			677	

Table II

Comparative results between ELISA (soluble Ag) and IIF.

I.I.F.

	+	-		Index
ELISA (Soluble Ag) +	220	47	267	Sensitivity: 97%
-	5	405	410	Specificity: 89%
			677	

Table III

Comparative results between ELISA (VP73) and IIF.

Index

Sensitivity: 100%

Specificity: 100%

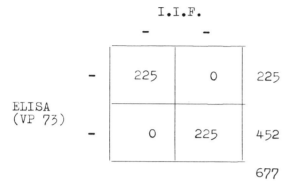

	I.I.F.		
	−	−	
−	225	0	225
−	0	225	452
			677

ELISA (VP 73)

DISCUSSION

The ELISA test described in this paper present a level of sensitivity and specificity of 100% in comparation with IIF, with the advantage of limited cost price, possible automatization and objective reading results which give to ELISA test the possibility of be used for epidemiological studies as well as for the detection of carriers animals.

It is also interesting to mencioned that even though false results do occur when the soluble ASF antigen is − used. These cases are neither numerous and not significant specially when compared with other serological ASF techniques (IEOP) Sánchez-Vizcaíno et al. 1.980. These problem, however, seems to have disappeared when the semipurified protein is used as an antigen in the indirect ELISA method.

The semipurified VP 73 present also the advantage of being easily prepared and produced in large amounts in infected cells. For it from two roller bottles of MS infected cells with 1.52×10^9 FCD_{50} of virus 3.6 ml. of VP 73 semipurified were obtained (Tabarés et al. 1.981) and the optimum dilution to be used in the ELISA method that we found in different badges of protein was between 1:1500 to 1:3000. Also the VP 73 protein present the advantage of non be possible infected which gave the possibility of send to free countries without any danger.

Since a 100% parallelism between ELISA (VP 73 antigen) and IIF exists, and moreover ELISA offers the great possibilities of automatization, and objective reading in contrast to IIF, we believe that the ELISA test described in this paper could be an adecuated method for the screening of large swine population which give us an effective method for the fight against ASF.

REFERENCES

- COLGROVE,G. (1.968). Bull. Epizoot. Dis. Agri. 16, 341
- HAMDY,F.M. and DARDIRY,A.H. (1.979). Vet. Record. 105, (19) 445.
- MALMQUIST,W.A. and HAY,D. (1.960). Am. J. Vet. Res. 21, 104.
- PAN,I.C.,De BOER, C.J. and HESS, W.R. (1.972). Cand. J. Comp. Med. 36, 309.
- SANCHEZ BOTIJA, C., ORDAS, A. and GONZALEZ,J.G. (1.970) Re.Patron. Biol. Animal 14, 159.
- SANCHEZ-VIZCAINO,J.M., MARTIN OTERO,L. and ORDAS,A. (1.979). Laboratorio 67 , 311.
- SANCHEZ-VIZCAINO, J.M. (1.980) EEC, ASF Workshop, December 1.980. Lisbon.

- TABARES, E., FERNANDEZ, M., SALVADOR, E., CARNERO, M.E. and SANCHEZ BOTIJA, C. (1.981). Arch. Virol. (in press).
- WARDLEY, R.C., ABU ELZEIN, E.M.E., CROWTHER, J.R. and WILKINSON, P.J. (1.979). J. Hyg. Camb. <u>83</u> , 363.

SEROLOGICAL DIAGNOSIS OF PSEUDORABIES USING
ENZYME-LINKED IMMUNOSORBENT ASSAY (ELISA)

B. Toma

Chaire des Maladies Contagieuses
Ecole Nationale Vétérinaire d'Alfort
F. 94704 Maisons-Alfort Cedex

ABSTRACT

The ELISA has been perfected for the research of Aujeszky's disease antibodies. Several hundred of sera (antibody kinetics after vaccination or virulent challenge, sera from 46 infected or vaccinated or free of Aujeszky's disease farms) have been comparatively studied using the ELISA and seroneutralisation techniques. The results obtained by the two techniques are very similar. The advantages of ELISA make it perfectly useful for epidemiological surveys and large scale early detection of this disease.

INTRODUCTION

The ELISA has numerous advantages when testing for antibodies, which led many teams to apply it to the diagnosis or early detection of diverse human or animal diseases.

For Aujeszky's disease, the first results were published in 1978 (Moutou et al., 1978). Other teams then disclosed their results (Briaire et al., 1979 ; Bommeli et al., 1980). Now, several laboratories use the ELISA for Aujeszky's disease antibody testing, even if their results have not been published as yet (Toma, 1981).

At the Contagious Diseases Laboratory of the National Veterinary School of Alfort, a first technique was perfected, based on the use of a pig globulin antiserum, labelled by an enzyme (Toma et al., 1979).

This technique was then modified from the antigen preparation point of view and the globulin antiserum was replaced by the A protein labelled by an enzyme.

In the following text, we relate the details of the last technique and results obtained during the comparative study of pig sera using the ELISA and seroneutralisation.

I - MATERIALS AND METHODS

   1) MATERIALS

   - Antigens

A layer of TFP cells in serum-free MEM pyruvate medium was infected by a Aujeszky's disease virus strain. After 24 hours, the cells were unstuck by the joint action of a $4^o/_{oo}$ KCl solution and carefully shaken glass beads. The cell suspension was then centrifuged at 700 g for 10 minutes in an oblique rotor and the sediment washed three times in a KCl solution. The last sediment was resuspended in KCl Triton X 100 ($2^o/_{oo}$) and the cell debris enucleated in Dounce's potter. The mixture is then passed on KCl sucrose (0.25M) for 10 minutes at 700 g. The sediment is resuspended in Tris EDTA (pH 9.6) in 1/50th of the volume of the initial culture medium ; this antigen is stored at -70°C.

A control antigen is prepared in exactly the same way, apart from the inoculation of the virus.

- Sera

Various groups of sera were comparatively studied using the ELISA and seroneutralisation techniques :

. Fifteen pigs were used for antibody kinetics :

3 controls

3 injected once with Alfort 26 strain, then virulent challenge

3 injected twice with Alfort 26 strain, then virulent challenge

1 injected once with Alfort 26 strain

5 injected twice with Alfort 26 strain.

. 487 serum samples from sows and meat pigs were collected from 46 farms which were either free of Aujeszky's disease, infected or vaccinated ;

. The french reference serum (threshold of positivity) at several dilutions has been studied in a blind manner by some european Laboratories (Switzerland, United-Kingdom and France).

- Apparatus

Multiwash (Dynatech)

Multiskan (Dynatech)

- Reagents and plates

. PBS Twen 20 solution 0.05 % : serum diluent

PBS (10 x conc) . . . . .   100 ml

Permuted water . . .   900 ml   pH 7.2

+ 0.05 ml of Tween 20 (Polyoxyethylene sorbitane mono laureate) (Merck)

. PBS Tween 20 solution 0.05 % - Bovine albumin 1 % : diluent of the A
  protein.
  Bovine albumin fraction V Sigma.
. Substrate : orthophenylene diamine   4   mg
  in citrate phosphate buffer pH 5.0   10   ml
  + H_2O_2 10 v . . . .   0.15 ml
. Citrate phosphate buffer solution pH 5.0
  Citric acid 0.1 M   243   ml
  disodium phosphate 0.2 M   257   ml
  permuted water   1000   ml
. M 129 B plates

   2) METHODS
   - ELISA Test
   The wells of the plates are sensitized with 200 microlitres of a viral
antigen suspension for columns n° 1, 3, 5, 7 & 11 and with a control antigen suspension for columns 2, 4, 6, 8, 10 & 12.

   The plate is placed on an antistatic cushion and 200 microlitres of
1/30th diluted sera in PBS Tween 20 at 0.05 % are put in the wells. The
sera are diluted in small rhesus tubes, then redistributed with a multi-
canal pipette with a disposable tip.

   For each serum, a control well and a well containing viral antigen are
used. On each plate, a negative reference serum and a positive reference
serum are placed.

   The plate which is covered by a plastic cover is incubated for 1/2
hour at 37°C on a slow balancing stirrer.

   It is then rinsed with Multiwash apparatus (2 times plot 3) : distilled water/Tween 20 at 0.05 %.

   The protein A-peroxydase is resuspended with 1 ml of distilled water
and then diluted in 79 ml of PBS-Tween 20 containing 1 % bovine albumine.
This amount of reagent is enough for 4 plates.

   200 microlitres of the conjugate solution are put into each well.

   Incubation for one hour at + 37°C with slow balancing.

   Rinsing with the Multiwash apparatus (2 times plot 3) with distilled
water + Tween 20 at 0.05 %.

   The tracer mixture of the enzyme is prepared and then put into the
wells at a rate of 200 microlitres per well, protected from all light

sources. The plates are conserved for 15 minutes at laboratory temperature and protected from light.

At the end of this period, the reaction is stopped by adding 50 microlitres of 2N sulphuric acid to each well.

The results are read with the Multiskan apparatus with 510 nm wave length.

The 0 regulation of the machine is done on an empty plate.

Expression of the results

The O.D. of the serum in the presence of the control cell antigen is subtracted from the O.D. of the same serum in the presence of the viral antigen.

The figure obtained is multiplied by 10. Only one figure is kept after the decimal point.

        Example : O.D. serum with control cell antigen :   0.346
                  O.D. serum with viral antigen :   1.259
                        1.259 - 0.346   =   0.913
                              Index   =   9.1

– Seroneutralisation

The technique has already been published (Toma and Vannier, 1980).

II – RESULTS

The study of several hundred serum of known titre by seroneutralisation led to the retention of the following criteria for the interpretation of the results of the ELISA :

The sera whose index number is lower than 1 are considered as being devoid of Aujeszky's disease antibodies.

The sera whose index number is between 1 and 2 are tested again. If the index obtained is higher than 1, the sera are considered as being positive.

The sera whose index number is higher than 2 are considered as being positive.

The negative reference serum of each plate should give an index number lower than 1.

The positive reference serum should give an index number between 6 and 10.

1) ANTIBODY KINETICS STUDY

Examples of kinetics are given in Figures 1 & 2. Generally speaking, the development of the antibody titres measured by the two techniques is very parallel. After being in contact with the A.D. virus, the response of animals becomes positive with the ELISA technique at the same time or earlier than with seroneutralisation.

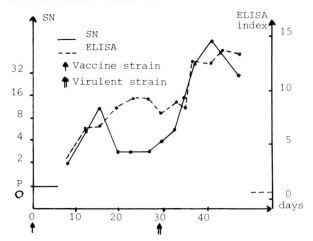

Fig. 1 : Comparative development of antibodies revealed by seroneutralisation or by the ELISA in the serum of a pig injected once with the Alfort 26 strain, and then challenged with a virulent strain.

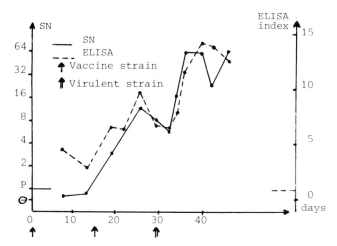

Fig. 2 : Comparative development of antibodies revealed by seroneutralisation or by the ELISA in the serum of a pig injected twice with the Alfort 26 strain, and then challenged with a virulent strain.

2) FIELD SERA STUDY

228

Results can be presented by distinguishing on one hand pig farms free of A.D., and on the other hand, pig farms where the animals are vaccinated or infected by the A.D. virus.

a) Pig Farms free of A.D.

265 samples of sera from sows or meat pigs from 23 pigs farms free of the disease were submitted to the two techniques. All these sera gave a negative response with seroneutralisation. The responses were equally negative with the ELISA technique. The distribution of the ELISA indexes obtained with these 265 serum samples is shown on Figure 3.

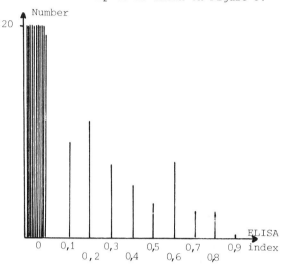

Fig. 3 : Histogram illustrating the distribution of the ELISA indexes for the 265 serum samples from Aujeszky's Disease free pig farms.

b) Pig Farms with Vaccinated or Infected animals

Serum samples of 222 sows and meat pigs from 23 pig farms were studied. Results can be found in Table I.

TABLE I : Comparison of results obtained with the ELISA technique and seroneutralisation of 222 serum samples from infected or vaccinated pig farms.

SERONEUTRALISATION			ELISA		
Positive Response	:	127	Positive Response	:	127
Doubtful Response	:	1	Positive Response	:	1
Negative Response	:	86	Positive Response	:	2
			Negative Response	:	84
Cytotoxic sera	:	8	Positive Response	:	6
			Negative Response	:	2

All the sera which were found to be positive in the seroneutralisation also gave a positive response with the ELISA technique. The ELISA response enabled two serum samples probably possessing a low amount of A.D. antibodies (index numbers 1.8 and 2.2.) to be noted and a response to be supplied for the 8 serum samples which had a cytotoxic action which hindered reading in seroneutralisation.

For the 127 serum samples which had a positive response in seroneutralisation a histogram of the ELISA index distribution can be established (figure 4).

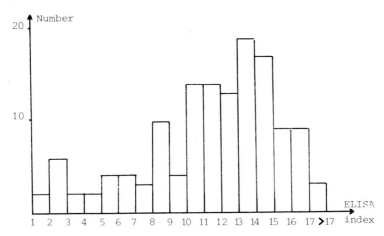

Fig. 4 : Histogram illustrating the distribution of the ELISA indexes for the 127 serum samples which gave a positive response in seroneutralisation.

The results of this comparative study on the sera of sows and of meat pigs either vaccinated or infected are very similar in both the ELISA and in the seroneutralisation. The sera of piglets born of vaccinated sows were also studied. The differences were more numerous due to the low level of antibodies of colostral origin which achieves the limit of sensitivity of one or other of the techniques.

3) STUDY BY SOME EUROPEAN LABORATORIES

The results of this study are reported in the tables II and III.

In the first experience (table II), each dilution was present two times. In this table, we can see that the level of sensitivity is not exactly the same for the four laboratories.

TABLE II : Results of the study by four laboratories of some sera by ELISA (E.) and seroneutralisation (SN).

	Lab. 1		Lab. 2		Lab. 3		Lab. 4	
	E.	SN	E.	SN	E.	SN	E.	SN
French reference serum	+	+	+	+	+	−	+	+
(threshold of positivity)	+	+	+	+	+	−	+	+
1/2	+	+	+	+	±	+	±	+
	+	+	+	+	−	−	+	+
1/4	+	±	+	+	±	−	±	−
	−	±	+	+	−	−	−	−
1/8	−	−	+	−	−	−	−	−
	−	−	+	−	−	−	−	−
1/16	−	−	+	−	−	−	−	−
	−	−	+	−	−	−	−	−
1/32	−	−	−	−	−	−	−	−
	−	−	−	−	−	−	−	−

Sensitivity of Elisa is the best for laboratory 2 and is better than its sensitivity of seroneutralization. For laboratory 3 also, results with Elisa are better than results of seroneutralization. At last, results of laboratories 1 and 4 are very near in seroneutralization and Elisa.

In the second experience (table III) there was only one sample for each dilution of the reference serum. These new results are very similar to the first one and sensitivity of Elisa is a little more important than sensitivity of seroneutralization.

TABLE III : Results of the study by three laboratories of some sera by ELISA (E.) and seroneutralization (SN).

	Lab. 1		Lab. 2		Lab. 3	
	E.	SN	E.	SN	E.	SN
French reference serum (threshold of positivity)	+	+	+	+	+	+
1/2	+	−	+	+	+	tox.
1/4	−	−	+	+	±	−
1/8	−	−	+	−	±	−
1/16	−	−	−	−	−	−

III - DISCUSSION

The ELISA technique which has been perfected possesses a level of sensitivity which is near to that of the seroneutralisation technique used at Alfort. This level of sensitivity could probably be improved even further to reach levels obtained by other research teams. However, as of now, the ELISA is routinely used for the diagnosis and early detection of Aujeszky's disease. Its advantages are undeniable : limited cost price, early responses, partly automatizable implementation and quantitative response with one single dilution. It can readily be used for epidemiological surveys and large scale early detection of disease.

It now remains to realize a comparative study of the ELISA techniques perfected by various teams so that, at a comparable cost, the better one can be selected.

REFERENCES

Briaire, J., Meloen, R.H. and Barteling, S.J. 1979. An enzyme-linked immunosorbent assay (ELISA) for the detection of antibody against Aujeszky's disease virus in pig sera. Zbl. Vet. Med. B, 26, 76-81.
Bommeli, W.R., Kihm, U., Lazarowicz, M. and Steck, F. 1980. Rapid detection of antibodies to infectious bovine rhinotracheitis (IBR) virus by micro enzyme linked immunosorbent assay (micro-ELISA). 2nd International Symposium of Veterinary Laboratory Diagnosticians, 2, 235-239.
Moutou, F., Toma, B. and Fortier, B. 1978. Application of an enzyme linked immunosorbent assay (ELISA) for diagnosis of Aujeszky's disease in swine. Vet. Rec., 103, 264.
Toma, B., Moutou, F. et Fortier, B., 1979. Recherche des anticorps anti-virus de la maladie d'Aujeszky par la technique ELISA. Rec. Méd. Vét., 155 (5), 455-463.
Toma, B. and Vannier, P., 1980. Harmonization attempt between french laboratories involved in the research of neutralizing antibodies against pseudorabies virus or transmissible gastroenteritis virus. 2nd International Symposium of Veterinary Laboratory Diagnosticians, Lucerne, Paper 1.
Toma, B. 1981. Harmonization between European laboratories of seroneutralization of pseudorabies virus. Seminar on Aujeszky's disease, Tübingen.

Acknowledgment : The author thanks Martine Pezron and Micheline Adam for their technical assistance, and IFFA Mérieux for the preparation of the antigen and the A protein.

EVALUATION AND USE OF THE ENZYME-LINKED IMMUNOSORBENT ASSAY

IN THE SEROLOGY OF SWINE VESICULAR DISEASE

C. HAMBLIN and J.R. CROWTHER

Animal Virus Research Institute, Pirbright, Woking, Surrey, England

ABSTRACT

A rapid, qualitative, indirect enzyme-linked immunosorbent assay
(ELISA) has been developed for the detection of antibody against swine
vesicular disease (SVD) virus, using horseradish peroxidase as the enzyme
marker. Although the assay is less sensitive than the serum neutralisation
(SN) test, it is slightly more sensitive than the double immuno-diffusion
(DID) test, which has been used extensively for the surveillance and
confirmation of diagnosis of SVD in this country. No differences were
recorded between visual and optical density readings for individual sera.
The rapidity, relative ease in performance and the lack of sophisticated
technical equipment make this ELISA suitable for field use including the
serological confirmation of diagnosis. Levels of the immunoglobulin classes
raised during infection, merit further work.

INTRODUCTION

Swine vesicular disease (SVD) was first recognised in the United

Kingdom on the 11th December 1972 and has occurred each year with the

exception of 1978 when no new outbreaks were reported or confirmed. It is

a notifiable disease of pigs caused by an enterovirus and is characterised

by mild fever and vesiculation of the feet, skin on the limbs and occasion-

ally the nose, lips and tongue. Mann et al. (1975) reported mild and sub-

clinical infections in some experimentally infected pigs and suggested such

cases undoubtedly occur in the field. Since SVD is very difficult to

distinguish clinically from foot-and-mouth disease, its control is vital

particularly in those countries normally free from vesicular diseases.

The micro-serum neutralisation (SN) test as described by Golding et al.

(1976) has proved useful for the quantitative assay of neutralising antibody

against SVD virus. Although this test is specific and sensitive, it does

make heavy demands on tissue cultures and requires incubation for two to

three days at 37°C before results can be read. The technique is also

relatively laborious for the screening of large numbers of samples. As an

alternative, Pereira et al. (1976) described the use of double immuno-

diffusion (DID) as a qualitative test for SVD antibody. Although less

sensitive than SN, large numbers of sera could be easily examined to give

fairly rapid results. The test does, however, use relatively large amounts of highly concentrated antigens.

Investigations were carried out to establish a rapid indirect enzyme-linked immunosorbent assay (ELISA) suitable for the routine serological confirmation of diagnosis and for the surveillance of SVD in pigs.

MATERIALS AND METHODS

Collection of sera

Diagnostic and epidemiological blood samples taken by venepuncture or at slaughter from pigs on suspected or confirmed SVD affected farms, were despatched to the laboratory by courier or express delivery soon after collection. After separation of the sera and testing by SN and/or DID, the samples were stored at $-20^{\circ}C$ until tested by ELISA.

Experimental animals

A group of five pigs (30 to 40 kg.) were each infected by intradermal inoculation in the junction of the heel and coronary band of three feet with a suspension of original pigs foot epithelium UKG 25/72 SVD virus. The sixth pig was housed in the same room of an isolation unit and exposed to infection by contact with the inoculated donors. Blood samples were taken from each animal at intervals from days 0 to 28 post infection. Sera was separated and stored at $-20^{\circ}C$ until tested by ELISA, DID and SN.

Serum neutralisation tests

Serum neutralisation tests were carried out in microtitre plates with IB-RS-2 cells (de Castro, 1964) using the methods of Golding et al. (1976). Stained monolayers were read after three days incubation at $37^{\circ}C$. Serum titres were expressed as the reciprocal Log_{10} of the final dilution of serum present in the serum/virus mixtures at the 50 per cent end point estimated according to the method of Karber (1931).

Double immuno-diffusion tests

Double immuno-diffusion tests were performed in 1.0 per cent purified agar gels (Oxoid Ltd.) on microscope slides (Pereira et al., 1976). The antigen, strain UKG 25/72, was inactivated with acetylethyleneimine (AEI) and concentrated by a factor of approximately 400.

Enzyme-linked immunosorbent assay

Swine vesicular disease virus, strain UKG 25/72, was prepared in IB-RS-2 cell monolayers. Concentration and purification of the infectious tissue culture fluid was carried out using methods essentially similar to those described by Brown and Cartwright (1963). Whole virus particles (160S) were inactivated with 0.05 per cent AEI for 48 hours at 26°C and this antigen was stored at -70°C in siliconised glass vials until used.

The indirect ELISA was performed in U-bottomed flexible polyvinyl microtitre plates using the methods described by Hamblin and Crowther. (in publication).

Reagents

Coating buffer: 0.05M Carbonate-bicarbonate buffer pH9.6.

Washing buffer: Phosphate buffered saline (PBS).

Diluting buffer: PBS + 0.05 per cent Tween 20 (polyoxyethylene
                     sorbiton monolaurate).

Conjugate: Rabbit anti-swine immunglobulin conjugated to
                     horseradish peroxidase.

Substrate: Orthophenylenediamine.

Stop: 1.25M sulphuric acid.

Briefly this method included the following steps:-

1.   Antigen diluted to 2.5 μg per ml in coating buffer is air dried onto the solid phase of the microtitre plate.

2.   Wash five times with PBS.

3.   A single dilution (sera 1 in 60) of each test sample is added to duplicate wells and the plate incubated for 30 minutes at 37°C with shaking.

4.   Wash five times with PBS.

5.   Conjugate, diluted 1 in 4000, is added to each well and the plate incubated for 15 minutes at 37°C with shaking.

6.   Wash five times with PBS.

7.   Substrate is added at room temperature.

8.   The reaction is stopped with the addition of sulphuric acid.

Controls on each plate included a 28 day post infection positive serum and a previously screened, pooled negative serum from uninfected pigs. Results were read both visually and by spectrophotometry at 492 nm using a Titretek[R] Multiskan (Flow Laboratories, Irvine, Scotland).

RESULTS

Several hundred pig sera without demonstrable neutralising antibody collected from uninfected farms were examined, using the ELISA, to

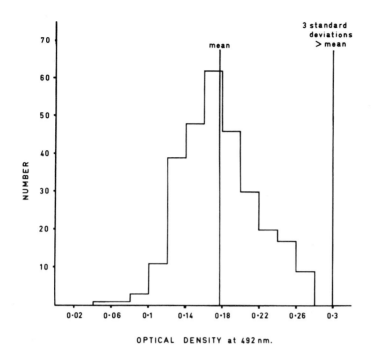

Fig. 1 Distribution of optical density readings recorded in the ELISA for sera, without demonstrable neutralising antibody titres, taken from uninfected farms.

TABLE 1 Serum neutralising antibody responses in sera from a group of pigs experimentally infected with swine vesicular disease virus.

ANIMAL NUMBER	DAYS POST INFECTION									
	0	1	2	3	4	5	7	14	21	28
1	0·9*	⩽0·75	0·9	⩽0·75	1·05	1·65	2·55	2·7	2·85	3·16
2	1·05	0·9	1·2	0·9	1·2	1·5	2·1	2·4	2·4	2·4
3	⩽0·75	⩽0·75	⩽0·75	⩽0·75	1·05	1·8	2·4	2·4	2·25	2·25
4	⩽0·75	⩽0·75	⩽0·75	⩽0·75	1·35	1·95	2·25	2·25	2·25	2·55
5†	⩽0·75	0·9	⩽0·75	⩽0·75	⩽0·75	⩽0·75	1·65	2·55	2·4	2·4
6	⩽0·75	⩽0·75	0·9	⩽0·75	1·05	1·5	2·25	2·55	2·55	2·55

* Reciprocal Log_{10} serum neutralisation titre

† Contact pig

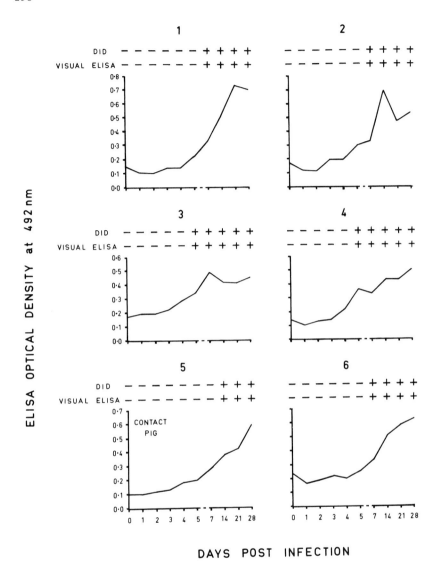

DAYS POST INFECTION

Fig. 2.   Visual and optical density readings recorded by ELISA and DID for sera from pigs following experimental infection.

determine the baseline optical density (OD) for the negative in the animal population.   Fig. 1. shows the results, expressed as a histogram for 287 of these serum samples.   The mean OD for the group was 0.177 with a standard deviation (SD) of 0.041.   A baseline OD of three SD above this mean OD (0.3) was adopted to give 99 per cent confidence in the assessment of positive and negative results.

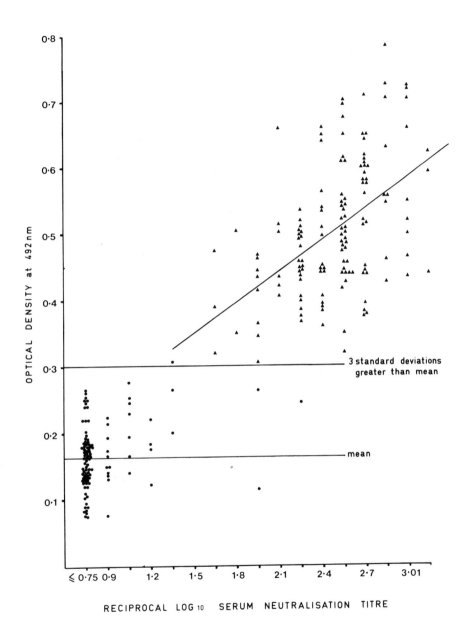

Fig. 3 Detection of antibody to swine vesicular disease in sera from infected and uninfected premises using ELISA and serum neutralisation tests, ● - visually positive by ELISA and ▲ - visually negative by ELISA.

TABLE 2   Comparison between ELISA and double-immuno diffusion for the detection of antibody against swine vesicular disease virus in field samples.

		ENZYME LINKED IMMUNOSORBENT ASSAY	
		POSITIVE	NEGATIVE
DOUBLE	POSITIVE	696	27
IMMUNO			
DIFFUSION	NEGATIVE	69	1928

TABLE 3   Serum neutralising antibody titres in those sera recorded positive by either ELISA or double-immunodiffusion.

	SERUM NEUTRALISATION TITRE															
	≤ 0·75	0·9	1·05	1·2	1·35	1·5	1·65	1·8	1·95	2·1	2·25	2·4	2·55	2·7	2·85	3·01	3·16
ELISA+ DID−	2	0	0	0	0	1	5	3	5	8	14	8	9	7	5	2	1
ELISA− DID+	5	2	0	0	1	1	3	0	4	3	5	1	1	0	0	0	1

Six pigs held in isolation and experimentally infected with SVD virus were bled at intervals from days 0 to 28 and the sera tested by ELISA, DID and SN.   Table 1 shows the neutralising antibody responses recorded for each animal during infection.   Optical densities recorded by ELISA for individual sera were plotted and related to the visual ELISA reading and DID results (Fig. 2).   The mean OD for uninfected pigs assayed in this ELISA was 0.163 and the baseline OD, three SD above the mean, was 0.295.

A total of 244 sera randomly taken from infected and uninfected premises was then examined by ELISA.   Visual and OD readings recorded for the ELISA were compared with those previously reported by SN (Fig. 3).   The mean OD (0.163), SD (0.046) and the baseline OD (0.301) for the sera without demonstrable neutralising antibody were calculated.   The regression line, $y = mx + c$, for those sera accepted as positive in SN (Golding et al., 1976, Hamblin and Crowther, in publication) was calculated to be $y = 0.168x + 0.0817$ where the coefficient of correlation between SN titres and OD readings was 0.517.

The relationship between ELISA and DID results for a further 2720 samples submitted to the laboratory in 228 batches is shown in Table 2. Those sera giving a positive or negative reaction in only one test (69 ELISA and 27 DID) were subsequently tested by SN (Table 3). A small number of these sera without demonstrable SN antibody titres, gave positive reactions in either ELISA or DID tests; however, since some were from farms without disease their significance remains unclear. Results indicate the DID to be slightly less sensitive than ELISA for the detection of antibody, particularly in sera with SN titres equal to or greater than 1.65.

DISCUSSION

Enzyme-linked immunosorbent assays have recently become widely used in the serological diagnosis and surveillance of both human and animal virus diseases (Bishai et al., 1978, Abu Elzein and Crowther, 1978). It is, however, important that the distribution and baseline for the negative in different populations is established before the assay system is routinely used. The baseline OD adopted for the ELISA carried out on large numbers of pig sera submitted from uninfected farms as shown in Fig. 1 gives 99 per cent confidence for the interpretation of positive and negative results. Differing sampling conditions, however, may affect the distribution of the negatives within the animal population. More than 600 sera taken from pigs sent for slaughter from uninfected farms as part of a continuing serological survey for SVD in the north of England have also been tested by ELISA (C. Hamblin, unpublished data). These blood samples were taken in abattoirs and the sera separated under field conditions (J.M. Scudamore, personal communication). Each serum was dispensed, without the addition of antibiotics into pre-labelled plastic bottles, packaged and dispatched to the laboratory. Although the majority of these sera were recorded negative by ELISA, the mean OD for the group and hence the baseline OD, was consistently higher than would be expected for diagnostic or epidemiological samples. Heavy microbial contamination together with the breakdown of serum components caused by prolonged periods at ambient temperatures, could possibly interfere in the ELISA when testing such sera.

Sera taken at intervals for six experimentally infected pigs were tested by ELISA, DID and SN to determine the sensitivity of each system during infection. Although the interpretation of low neutralising antibody titres is difficult in the absence of other information (Golding et al., 1976), developing antibody could be detected in sera from the five animals, challenged with SVD virus, after four days (Table 1). The neutralising antibody response in sera from the sixth pig, a contact, could not be detected until seven days post exposure. The OD readings, plotted in Fig. 2 suggest antibody responses may be detected in sera from individual animals as early as four days after infection. In practice, however, visual ELISA positive and DID positive reactions were only recorded five or more days after infection and where the OD readings exceeded the baseline OD of 0.295. Since no differences were detected between the visual and OD readings above or below the baseline OD, a visual interpretation for ELISA may be considered reliable.

A close agreement between visual, OD readings and SN antibody titres was also demonstrated for random field samples tested by ELISA but there was little correlation between OD levels and corresponding SN titres (Fig. 3). Since only one dilution of serum was used, the amount of antigen coated onto the plate determines the maximum OD obtainable. This would affect the coefficient of correlation but does not totally explain the poor correlation recorded. Therefore, this ELISA is only suitable as a qualitative assay for antibody against SVD. Further work is in progress to determine the nature and ratio of immunoglobulin classes produced during infection as an aid in epizootiological studies of the disease.

The comparison of ELISA and previously reported DID test results carried out on 2720 sera (Tables 2 and 3) show the ELISA to be slightly more sensitive than DID for the detection of antibody against SVD throughout the whole range of antibody titres accepted positive in SN tests. Although negative ELISA or negative DID results were recorded in some sera with positive SN antibody titres, both tests always recorded positive reactions in some sera submitted from each infected premises.

These results together with further details in the original paper by Hamblin and Crowther (in publication) show the ELISA to be a useful test. The assay is suitable for large scale screening of sera for antibody against SVD virus in field laboratories where reagents, including plates already coated with inactivated SVD virus, could be supplied from central diagnostic/research laboratories. Since the SVD viruses isolated in Europe over the last 15 years show high cross reactivity, a single isolate could probably be used as a standard preparation for coating plates. The ELISA described is now routinely used in this laboratory for the serological confirmation of diagnosis of SVD.

ACKNOWLEDGEMENTS

The authors are indebted to J. Mann for the provision of serum samples from serially bled pigs following experimental infection. They also wish to thank I.T. Barnett and M.J. Day for supplying the SN and DID tests from previously reported field samples.

REFERENCES

Abu Elzein, E.M.F. and Crowther, J.R. 1978. Enzyme-linked immunosorbent assay technique in foot-and-mouth disease virus research. J. Hyg. Cambs. 80, 391-399.

Bishai, F.R. and Galli, R. 1978. ELISA for detection of antibodies to Influenza A and B and Parinfluenza Type 1 in sera of patients. J. Clin. Microbiol. 8, 648-656.

Brown, F. and Cartwright, B. 1963. Purification of radioactive foot-and-mouth disease virus. Nature 199, 1168-1170.

De Castro, M.P. 1964. Behaviour of the foot-and-mouth disease virus in cell cultures; susceptibility of the IB-RS-2 cell line, Archos. Inst. biol., S. Paulo 31, 63-78.

Golding, Susan, M., Hedger, R.S., Talbot, P. and Watson, J. 1976. Radial immuno-diffusion and serum neutralisation techniques for the assay of antibodies to swine vesicular disease. Res. in Vet. Sci. 20, 142-147.

Karber, G. 1931. Beitrag zur kollektiven Behandlung pharmakologischer Reihenversuche. Arch. exp. path. pharmak. 162, 480-483.

Mann, J.A., Burrows, R. and Goodridge, D., 1975. Mild and sub-clinical infections with Swine Vesicular Disease virus. Bull. Off. int. Epiz. 88, (1-2), 117-122.

Pereira, H.G., Rowe, L. and Baber, D. 1976. Use of double immuno-diffusion (Ouchterlony) test for the diagnosis of swine vesicular disease. Res. in Vet. Sci. 20, 139-141.

PART VI: APPLICATION OF ELISA TO THE STUDY OF HORMONES

ELISA - THE NUCLEUS OF THE IBR/IPV CONTROL PROGRAMM
IN SWITZERLAND

W. Bommeli[*] and U. Kihm[**]

[*]Diagnostic Laboratories Dr. W. Bommeli, CH-3012 Bern
[**]Federal Vaccine Institute, CH-4025 Basle, Switzerland

Bovine herpesvirus 1 infection in cattle was first reported in Switzerland many years ago. However, the infection was confined to the clinical form of infectious pustular vulvovaginitis (IPV). Prior to the first reports of respiratory IBR in Switzerland, a survey showed that only approx. 0,4 % of the sexually mature female cattle population and 5,1 % of the bulls used for natural mating showed serum antibodies against IPV.

The last IPV reactors were eliminated from the artificial insemination centres in the years between 1971 and 1973. These stations have been free of IBR/IPV since then. Only one case of the respiratory form of IBR was reported in Switzerland before 1977, and the animals of the affected herd were slaughtered.

In late 1977 and early 1978, IBR appeared in the eastern part of Switzerland. It was clearly transferred from infected animals by the aerogenous route. At the same time the incidence of IBR in southern Germany increased. It was assumed that this was caused by cows imported from Austria. Subsequently the disease spread over Switzerland as a result of cattle movement and the introduction of new cattle into herds. Animals mixed in the same transport vehicles were infected and the disease was carried to various susceptible herds. Transport stress may reactivate latent infections with consequent virus shedding. It was therefore frequently possible to trace the original source of infection.

Serologic surveys in 1979 revealed that the virus occured in 0 % to 7 % of the Swiss cattle population depending on region. The low percentage of reactors seemed to justify specific measures against the disease to protect the national herd. Swiss farmers realized the various serious consequences of IBR infection on feed efficiency, milk production and reproduction. The economic importance of the disease to agriculture forced the animal health officials to take decisive action against IBR.

Two different procedures can be used to control IBR:
a) accept the current epidemiologic status of the disease and reduce economic losses by vaccination campaings; or
b) control the disease by management, isolation and eradication procedures.

A general vaccination programm would cost millions yearly. Furthermore, differentiation between vaccinated and infected animals would no longer be possible using serological methods, and any future control programm would thus be hampered.

The low incidence persuaded the Swiss authorities to declare IBR as an notifiable disease. Current animal health regulations should control the disease in different ways. The disease should be contained in the first phase and infected herds culled in the second.

The following measures must be taken:
- vaccination must be prohibited throughout the country
- premises with infected animals must be isolated by quarantine
- bulls with IBR/IPV antibody-titers must be eliminated
- cattle which abort or show respiratory symptoms must be checked for IBR/IPV-antibodies.
- only seronegative animals may be showed at exhibitions and fairs
- only seronegative animals may be moved from one premise to an other
- serological screening programmes should be carried out
- finally the disease is to be eradicated by selective

slaughter, or herd slaughter in areas with low infection rate and intensive cattle breeding.

Fortunately, the IBR virus is less contagious than other viruses like FMD so that enough time is available to prevent further outbreaks.

The Swiss control programm is ambitious and will cost a lot of money during the next years. Several thousand cattle have already been slaughtered and indemnified as part of this animal health programm. The programm has been successful in several regions, and most farmers now agree with and even wish to intensify the measures taken.

The nucleus of the IBR control program is laboratory diagnosis to reveal reactors. The serum neutralisation test is the most commonly used serologic technique for the detection of antibodies against IBR virus.

However, this test presents some disadvantages; it depends on the availability of cell culture facilities in the diagnostic laboratory. The performance of the neutralisation test is time-consuming and results may only be available after days. The presence of non-specific inhibitors in sera interferes in the neutralisation test. In Switzerland only five laboratories are equipped for this test. The capacity of these laboratories was far too low to meet the serodiagnostic requirements of approx. 500'000 tests per year. The micro ELISA which offers the advantages of simplicity and convenience when testing a large number of samples was therefore introduced. At present a dozen regional laboratories perform the micro ELISA to detect IBR antibodies in Switzerland. Most of the laboratories had no previous experience with tests for viral antibodies. The ELISA became so popular and accurate that even laboratories with cell culture facilities changed to the new technique. The usefullness of ELISA for the titration of IBR specific antibodies in milk samples is important for the mass field surveys of entire cattle populations which are just getting under way.

THE ANTIGEN

IBR virus antigens were produced from Colorado strain in secondary cultures of fetal bovine lung or kidney cells in serumfree Eagle's minimal essential medium (Bommeli et al., 1980). Cultures were infected at a ratio of approximately 1 tissue culture infective dose of virus per 5 cells. After 36 to 48 hours of incubation at 37^OC, the cultures showed an extensive cytopathic effect and subsequently were frozen.

The culture material was thawed and centrifuged at 3'000 g for 10 min. at 4^OC. The supernatant fluid constituted the viral antigen and could be used for sensitizing microplates, if the virus titer was at least $10^{7,5}$ TCID/0,1 ml. The clarified antigen derived from infected cell culture fluids proved to be adequately sensitive and specific for detection of antibodies.

Low-titer supernatants were purified and concentrated by differential centrifugation, but we agree with Herring et al (Herring et al., 1980) that an extensive purification generally results in considerable loss of antigen. Control antigens were prepared from uninfected cell cultures in the same manner. It proved to be essential to include uninfected control antigens to check specifity of the reactivity of each test serum. An occasional serum will react as high with uninfected control antigen as with the specific viral antigen.

ELISA

Tests were performed in microtiterplates (Linbro, Flow Laboratories). The uptake capacity of microplates is not crucial as it affects both the virus antigen as well as the control antigen. The optimal dilution of virus and control antigen was estimated by ckeckboard titration. The plates were coated by adding 0,2 ml antigen to each well. After an overnight incubation at 4^OC, unadsorbed antigen was removed and washed away by an automatic washer-aspirator (Titertek Multiwash, Flow Laboratories). All further washes were carried out with this device but could also be executed manually by decanting the reagents followed by two washes with PBS pH 7,4, containing 0,01 % Tween 20. The antigen-sensitized plates could either be used immediately or stored vacuum-packed at 4°C for several weeks. 0,2 ml of the 1:40 diluted sera were added to 4 wells, 2 coated with viral antigen and 2 with control antigen. Control sera included strong and weak positive, and negative sera. After incubating at room temperature in a humid chamber the plates were washed again. A reaction time of 2 hours is necessary for the full development of the antigen - antibody reaction. Incubation time beyond 3 hours resulted in unreproducible data indicating that ELISA is influenced by antibody affinity which is reversible (Butler et al., 1978). However in the routine diagnostic performance of the test, incubation time may be reduced to as little as one hour without significant loss of sensitivity.

After washing, 0,2 ml of the optimally diluted peroxidase labelled rabbit anti-bovine IgG conjugate was added to each well and the plates were incubated at room temperature for 2 hours. Again, if necessary the incubation time could be reduced to one hour. After aspiration of the unreacted conjugate, wells were washed two times with washing fluid.

Conveniently, the solution for serum and enzyme dilution was identical with washing fluid.

The enzyme substrate consisting of 2 mM ABTS (2,2-azino-di-(3-ethyl-benz-thiazoline sulfonic acid (6))) and 2,5 mM H_2O_2 in 0,1 M sodium acetate buffer, pH 4,2 with 0,05 M phosphate was added in a volume of 0,2 ml (Gallati, 1979).

The action of the enzyme was not stopped but the plates were measured after exactly 30 minutes incubation at room temperature with a photometer (Multiscan, Flow Laboratories) at 405 nm and subsequently assessed by visual inspection.

EVALUATION OF ANTIBODY UNITS

The effective absorbance values were calculated by forming the difference between optical density of the sera with viral antigen and control antigen.

Butler et al., 1978 pointed out that ELISAs are influenced by affinity and this means that numerical values given are not a gravimetric measure of antibody in µg or mg. Hence, data obtained with any ELISA should be expressed as "ELISA units" rather than mg/ml. Because an international anti-IBR standard serum is not available, we defined our own standard serum to contain 1'000 units of antibodies against IBR per mililiter.

This standard serum was tested at dilutions of 1:40 = 25 units/ml; 1:80 = 12,5 units/ml and so on in two fold steps up to 1:5'120 = 0,2 units/ml. To obtain the regression curve for the standard serum, linear analysis was computed from the observed absorbance values and the respective units of the diluted standard serum for each trial. The antibody units of unknown sera could then be determined from the individual absorbance values on a computer or on a plotted standard regression curve. This procedure was justifiable because linear analysis of different positive sera all resulted in parallel curves when plotted. Sera were scored positive when the antibody units were equal to or higher than those of the weak positive reference serum.

COMPARISON OF RESULTS USING SERUM NEUTRALISATION TEST AND ELISA

There is a good correlation between results of the serum neutralisation test and ELISA.

A summary of results obtained by using serum neutralisation test and ELISA on 474 serum samples is shown in Table I.

Only 15 samples were not identical with the ELISA and serum neutralisation test. The relative sensitivity and specificity are shown in Table II. The relative sensitivity is the ability of one procedure to give positive results (Thorner and Remein, 1961) when the second procedure gives positive results. The relative specificity is the ability of one procedure to give negative results when the second procedure also gives negative results. Of the various comparisons all were higher than 94 %. These results are in accordance with other reports (Herring et al., 1980; Payment et al., 1979; Zemp and Steck, in press; Solsona et al., 1980).

TABLE I: Comparison of 474 serum samples tested with serum neutralisation test (SNT) and ELISA

SNT	ELISA	
	positive	negative
positive	320	8
negative	7	139

TABLE II: Relative sensitivity and specificity of serum-neutralisationtest and ELISA to detect antibodies to IBR.

	relative sensitivity	relative specificity
SNT versus ELISA	98 %	95 %
ELISA versus SNT	97 %	95 %

It is evident that sera having antibody titers below neutralizing effect can still exhibit low but significant antibody units in ELISA. On the other hand, several virus inhibition factors may simulate a neutralizing effect. Under these considerations, we estimate ELISA to be at least as sensitive as the commonly used neutralisation test for detection of antibodies to IBR. The advantage of ELISA consists in inexpensive equipment and reagents involved, and the rapidity of the procedure. The method is also adaptable to automatization for processing a large numbers of sera.

EXPERIMENTS TO HARMONIZE THE SWISS IBR SERODIAGNOSTIC ACTIVITIES

To be successful in a control program, it is not only important to have a sensitive and reliable diagnosis but also to have coordinated and standardized results in all the national laboratories. To achieve this goal, we distributed sera with various IBR-antibody-titers to all Swiss laboratories on several occasions. One of these attempts to harmonize the laboratories is shown here: 12 weak positive (at the limit of the detection level in the serum neutralization test), 3 strong positive and 5 negative sera were sent to 8 ELISA - laboratories for blind testing. The strong positive and negative sera were correctly recognized by all laboratories. 14 incorrect results were reported with the weak positive sera. Alltogether, an average of 91 % correct results, ranging from 65 % to 100 %, and 9 % incorrect results were reported.

The laboratories doing the serumneutralization test presented only 73 % correct results, and 15 % incorrect results. 12 % of the sera were scored as cytotoxic and therefore the titers could not be determined.

There are two reasons for the low agreement of the serumneutralization tests of different laboratories. The methods are not standardized and different types of cell cultures are used. It should be pointed out that the described experiment for harmonization was very demanding to the laboratories. Low-titer sera, as used in the experiment, occur only in about 10 % of all positive field samples.

One difficulty of ELISA lies with the interpretation of the colour reaction. There are approx. 5 per 1'000 serum samples which react in the range between weak positive and negative. In contrast, the serumneutralization test yields "yes - no" reactions: a serum sample containing less antibodies than necessary for neutralization of the virus dose may cause a negative result.

A great advantage of the ELISA is its applicability to detect antibodies in milk samples (Stuker et al., 1980). Our investigations showed a good correlation between titers in serum and milk. Because of the ease of milk sampling, the examination of milk antibodies is already done routinely. Pooled samples from milk collection plants are useful for screening surveys.

The presented report shows that the ELISA may be a very important tool with many advantages within a disease control programm. However, it should be stressed that neither the ELISA nor an other biologic test will yield 100 % accurate results. The reasons for this fact are manyfold and originate also in human failure at sampling, executing the test and reporting.

It is important that the results are brought into the context of the epidemiologic situation. Most laboratory staff do not have knowledge of the circumstances in the field. Therefore, laboratory results must be interpreted by epidemiologists to achieve maximum benefit in supporting directed actions against a disease.

REFERENCES

Bommeli W.R., Kihm U., Lazarowicz M. and Steck F., 1980: Rapid detection of antibodies to infectious bovine rhinotracheitis (IBR) virus by micro enzyme linked immunosorbent assay (micro ELISA). Proc. 2. Int. Symp. Vet. Lab. Diagnost., 235-239.
Butler J.E., Feldbush T.L., McGivern P.L. and Stewart N., 1978: The enzyme-linked-immunosorbent assay (ELISA): a measure of antibody concentration or affinity ? Immunochemistry 15, 131-136.
Gallati H., 1979: Peroxidase aus Meerrettich: Kinetische Studien sowie Optimierung der Aktivitätsbestimmung mit den Substraten H_2O_2 und 2,3'-Azino-di-(3-ethyl-benz-thiazolin sulfonsäure-(6)) (ABTS). J. Clin. Chem. Clin. Biochem. 17, 1-7.

Herring A.J., Nettleton P.F. and Burrels C., 1980: A micro-enzyme-linked immunosorbent assay for the detection of anti-bodies to infectious bovine rhinotracheitis virus. Vet. Rec. 107, 155-156.

Payment P., Assaf R., Trudel M. and Marois P., 1979: Enzyme-linked immunosorbent assay for serology of infectious bovine rhinotracheitis virus infections. Clin. Microbiol., 10, 633-636.

Solsona M., Perrin B., Perrin M. et Moussa A., 1980: Recher-che des anticorps contre le virus de la rhinotrachéite bovine infectieuse par la méthode ELISA. Bull. Acad. Vet. de France, 53, 215-225.

Stuker G., Haab P. and Giger T., 1980: Nachweis von IBR/IPV-Antikörpern aus der Milch. Schweiz. Arch. Tierheilk., 122, 707-710.

Thorner B.S. and Remein O.R., 1961: Principles and procedures in the evaluation of screening for disease. Public Health Monograph, 67, 24. Public Health Service Publication No. 846. U.S.Department of Health, Education and Welfare.

Zemp K. and Steck F., in press: Vergleichende Untersuchungen mit dem Serumneutralisationstest und der ELISA-Technik zum Nachweis von IBR/IPV-Antikörpern beim Rind. Experimentia, 37.

STUDIES ON AVIAN INFECTIOUS BRONCHITIS VIRUS BY ELISA

J.H. Darbyshire

Houghton Poultry Research Station
Houghton, Huntingdon, Cambs. PE17 2DA.

ABSTRACT

Indirect enzyme-linked immunosorbent assays (ELISA) were used to follow the sequential development of IgG class-specific antibodies to avian infectious bronchitis (IBV) in infected chickens. This method was more sensitive than either neutralisation or haemagglutination-inhibition tests.

In studies on local and humoral immunity in chickens similarly infected, the development of humoral antibodies followed the pattern described previously. Specific anti-viral antibody in the form of IgA and IgG isotypes was demonstrated by ELISA in the tracheal fluids from the seventh day after infection, whereas none could be detected by conventional neutralisation tests. The ELISA tests showed that the IgG isotype appeared to predominate in local antibody to IBV.

INTRODUCTION

The technique of enzyme-linked immunosorbent assay (ELISA) has now been applied to a number of avian virus systems, including reoviruses (Slaght et al., 1978), adenoviruses (Dawson et al., 1980), infectious bursal disease virus (Marquardt et al., 1980) and avian infectious bronchitis virus (IBV) (Mockett and Darbyshire, 1981; Hawkes et al., 1981).

In this laboratory, an indirect ELISA has been used in two studies to detect class-specific antibodies to IBV in infected chickens. In the first, investigations were made of the application of ELISA to follow the sequential development of humoral antibodies in chickens after infection with the Massachusetts M41 strain of IBV (Mockett and Darbyshire, 1981). At the same time, neutralisation and haemagglutination-inhibition (HI) tests were carried out for comparison.

In the second study, ELISA was used in a study of local immunity in the respiratory tract (trachea) of chickens infected with IBV (Hawkes et al., 1981).

MATERIAL AND METHODS

The details of the mode of preparation of the IBV antigens employed in the ELISA tests, and the sources of sera have been given in detail elsewhere (Mockett and Darbyshire, 1981; Hawkes et al., 1981). The ELISA antigen used in the first study was that for the HI tests; virus, in the

form of allantoic fluids of infected embryonated hens' eggs were
concentrated one hundred-fold by ultracentrifugation and then treated for
1 hour at 37°C with phospholipase C. The sera for the tests were
collected from chickens every 3 to 4 days for up to 63 days after
infection with IBV (strain M41).

In the second study, the ELISA antigen was again in the form of
infected allantoic fluids, concentrated and purified by sucrose density
gradient ultracentrifugation (Cavanagh, 1981). Sera were obtained every 3
to 4 days from chickens infected with strain M41. Tracheal fluids were
also collected at the same time for the isolation of infectious virus and
for the demonstration by ELISA of class-specific antibody.

RESULTS

The results of both studies may be found in detail elsewhere, so that
only the more significant findings will be reiterated here.

The indirect ELISA in the first study detected IgG class-specific IBV
antibodies with a high degree of sensitivity, and was more sensitive than
either neutralisation or HI methods (Mockett and Darbyshire, 1981). This
is illustrated by the geometric mean titres (GMT) obtained in each type of
test as shown in Table 1 (data from Mockett and Darbyshire, 1981).

TABLE 1. Sequential serum titres (GMT) to IBV from tests on chickens.

					Days						
	0	3	6	9	14	17	21	28	35	38	63
ELISA	<7.64[a]	8.74	9.46	12.89	13.32	14.01	13.33	13.59	13.39	12.62	12.55
HI	<3.0	<3.0	<3.0	8.52	10.0	10.24	8.46	8.25	8.04	7.68	6.97
SN	<3.0	<3.0	<3.0	3.65	3.70	3.60	3.78	5.53	5.65	6.53	6.64

[a] $\log_2$

When, in addition, sera from 39 commercial hens aged up to 24 weeks
were tested by ELISA at a single dilution of 1 : 200, and their absorbence
values compared with their HI titres, a significant correlation (p <0.01)
was found between both tests.

The second study (Hawkes et al., 1981) concerned the presence of
specific antibody as a defence mechanism in the tracheae and sera of
chickens infected with IBV (M41). The development of humoral antibody
according to ELISA was again similar to the first study, as shown in Table

2 (data from Hawkes et al., 1981).

TABLE 2.   Sequential neutralisation and ELISA titres of sera and
tracheal washes of IBV infected chickens.

Days	Virus recovered[a]	Neutralisation		ELISA					
				Ig		IgG		IgA	
		S^b	T^c	S	T	S	T	S	T
0	-	-	-	<5.6	<3.3	<5.6	<3.3	-	<3.3
3	4.4	-	-	<5.6	<3.3	<5.6	<3.3	-	<3.3
7	2.9	-	-	8.2	4.5	7.3	4.3	-	4.4
10	-	3.1	-	12.3	5.6	11.9	5.9	-	-
13	-	3.3	-	11.5	5.1	11.5	5.5	-	-
17	-	4.5	-	11.1	5.6	11.0	5.1	-	-
20	-	5.7	-	11.5	4.9	11.6	4.8	-	-
24	-	7.0	1.2^d	11.2	5.7	11.3	5.6	-	-
27	-	6.8	3.1^d	11.4	6.5	11.5	6.7	-	-
34	-	6.7	-	10.5	4.2	10.5	4.0	-	-
44	-	6.5	-	10.0	4.6	10.1	4.6	-	-

[a] $\log_{10}$

[b] serum ($\log_2$)

[c] trachea ($\log_2$)

[d] vs 1.0 $\log_{10}CD_{50}$

Specific IgA and IgG isotype antibodies were demonstrated by ELISA in the
tracheal fluids from the seventh day onwards, the IgG isotypes appearing to
predominate. Little significant antibody could be detected in the trachea
by conventional neutralisation tests.

REFERENCES

Cavanagh, D. 1981. Structural polypeptides of coronavirus IBV. J.Gen.Virol.,
    53, 93-103.
Dawson, G.J., Orsi, L.N., Yates, V.J., Chang, P.W. and Pronovost, A.D. 1980.
    An enzyme linked immunosorbent assay for detection of antibodies to
    avian adenovirus and avian adenovirus-associated virus in chickens.
    Avian Dis., 24, 393-402.
Hawkes, R.A., Darbyshire, J.H., Peters, R.W., Mockett, A.P.A. and Cavanagh,
    D. 1981. Avian Path. (to be published).
Marquardt, W.W., Johnson, R.B., Odenwald, W.F. and Schlotthober, B.A. 1980.
    An indirect enzyme-linked immunosorbent assay (ELISA) for measuring
    antibodies in chickens infected with infectious bursal disease virus.
    Avian Dis., 24, 375-385.
Mockett, A.P.A. and Darbyshire, J.H. 1981. Comparative studies with

an enzyme-linked immunosorbent assay (ELISA) for antibodies to avian infectious bronchitis virus. Avian. Path., 10, 1-10.

Slaght, S.S., Young, T.J., van der Heide, L. and Fredrichson, T.N. 1978. An enzyme-linked immunosorbent assay (ELISA) for detecting chicken antireovirus antibody at high sensitivity. Avian. Dis., 22, 802-805.

DETECTION OF ANTIBODY AGAINST PORCINE ROTAVIRUS IN COLOSTRUM AND MILK BY A BLOCKING ELISA TEST

Jon Askaa

Department of veterinary virology and immunology,
The Royal Veterinary and Agricultural University,
Copenhagen, Denmark

ABSTRACT

The content of antibody against rotavirus was followed during the lactation periods in colostrum and milk samples from 7 gilts and sows. Generally high contents were detected in colostrum, but a rapid decrease was seen about day 5. Milk samples collected from one gilt (gilt No. 413) showed a marked increase in the antibody level about day 16, and this high level was almost constant throughout the lactation period.

INTRODUCTION

Rotavirus has been considered to be the cause of or associated with neonatal diarrhoea, 3 week scours and early weaning diarrhoea in pigs in several reports (Rodger et al 1975; Lecce et al 1976; Woode et al 1976; Chacey & Lucas 1977; Bohl et al 1978; Tzipori & Williams 1978; Debouck & Pensaert 1979; Askaa & Bloch 1981. The periods of virus excretion with feces are usually found to range from 2-4 days post infection, but de Leeuw et al (1979) described virus detected in feces in a prolonged period. These authors also found virus in feces from the same piglets both at 3 weeks of age and at 6 weeks.

A rapid decline of antibody in successive colostrum and milk samples after calving and lambing has been described (Woode et al 1975; Ellens et al 1978; Wells et al 1978).

The rotavirus specific antibody in colostrum in sheep and cows has been reported to protect lambs and calves against rotavirus associated diarrhoea and against excretion of rotavirus after challenge (Snodgrass & Wells 1976; Snodgrass et al 1979; Wellemans & van Opdenbosch 1979; Fahey et al 1981). Also administration of bovine colostrum with high contents of antibody against bovine rotavirus has

protected other species e.g. piglets against rotavirus associated diarrhoea (Lecce et al 1976; Bridger & Brown 1979).
The last mentioned authors found that although the bovine
colostrum protected the piglets against development of diarrhoea, virus still propagated in the intestine. Bridger &
Brown suggested that local immunity in the intestine was
developed, protecting the piglets from subsequent illness
in connection with challenge. Recently Corthier & Franz
(1981) reported the contents of antibody against rotavirus
in porcine colostrum as mainly belonging to the IgG fraction and the antibody in milk to the IgA fraction of the
immunoglobulins.

In the present work a blocking ELISA test for demonstration of antibody against porcine rotavirus has been
established. Colostrum and milk samples from 7 gilts and
sows were collected throughout the lactation periods and
examined for contents of antibody against rotavirus.

MATERIALS AND METHODS

Animals: Two swine herds with a previously diagnosed
problem of rotavirus associated diarrhoea were examined.
Two gilts and two sows in one herd and one gilt and two
sows in the other herd were followed throughout the lactation periods.

Demonstration of antibody: Colostrum, milk and serum
were examined for contents of antibody by a blocking ELISA
test according to Yolken et al (1978). Briefly every second
well of polystyrene microtest plates (Nunc[R], Denmark, code
2-62162) was coated with catching antibody (antihuman rotavirus rabbit IgG, Dako-immunoglobulins Ltd., Denmark, code
B 218) in dilution 1:50 with 0.05 mol/l carbonate buffer
(pH 9.6), while the other wells were coated with normal
rabbit IgG (Dako-immunoglobukins Ltd., code X 904) in the
same dilution and the same buffer. After washing of the
plates fecal suspension containing porcine rotavirus antigen was added. The plates were incubated overnight, and
after washing colostrum, milk or serum diluted in washing

buffer supplemented with 0.5% bovine serum albumin (BSA)
was added. For each dilution of a sample two wells coated
with antihuman rotavirus rabbit IgG and two wells coated
with normal rabbit IgG were used. The plates were incubated
for 1 h at 37°C and after washing proxidase conjugated antihuman rotavirus rabbit IgG (Dako-immunoglobulins, code
P 219) diluted 1:500, was added. The plates were incubated
1 h at room temperature. The plates were washed once again,
and after a short rinse in a buffer (pH 5.0) consisting of
34.7 mmol/l citric acid and 66.7 mmol/l Na_2HPO_4, $2H_2O$ the
substrate (40 mg of 1.2-phenylenediamine-dihydrochloride,
Sigma and 20 µl of 30% H_2O_2 per 100 ml) dissolved in the
same buffer, was added. The enzymatic reaction was stopped
after 15 min at room temperature by adding 2N H_2SO_4. The
washing buffer was used as Grauballe et al (1981). At each
addition of catching antibody, antigen, colostrum, milk,
serum dilution, conjugate and substrate 100 µl/well was
used. The absorbance at 492 nm was measured with a Spectron-
ic 21 (Bauch & Lomb) spectrophotometer.

The source of antigen for the blocking ELISA test consists of a pool of feces samples from piglets from which
rotavirus had been detected by EM and ELISA. The pool of
feces samples represents several piglets from several swine
herds. The feces suspension was made by grinding the feces
in Eagles essential medium (Gibco, UK) to make a 20-30%
suspension. After clarification of the feces suspension by
centrifugation at 3000 g for 20 min the supernatant was removed and stored at -80°C until use.

The rotavirus antigen for the blocking ELISA test was
used in a constant dilution giving an optical density at ap-
proximatly 0.8, i.e. a 1:10 dilution of the source of antigen. For dilution washing buffer supplemented with 0.5% BSA.
A titration of the rotavirus antigen was performed in duplicate each time the blocking ELISA test was carried out. The
antigen was diluted from 1:5 to 1:10240 (fig. 2).

Serum, colostrum and milk samples: Antihuman rotavirus
rabbit IgG (Dako-immunoglobulins Ltd., code B 218) and anti-

Fig. 1

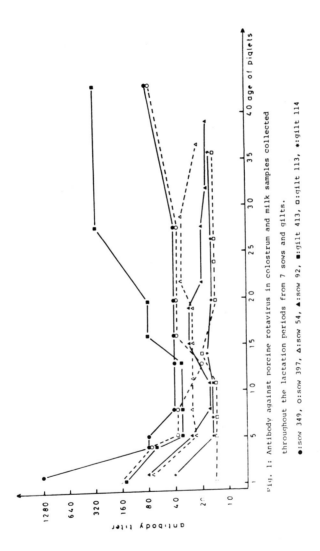

Fig. 1: Antibody against porcine rotavirus in colostrum and milk samples collected throughout the lactation periods from 7 sows and gilts.

●:sow 349, ○:sow 397, △:sow 54, ▲:sow 92, ■:gilt 413, □:gilt 113, *:gilt 114

Fig. 2

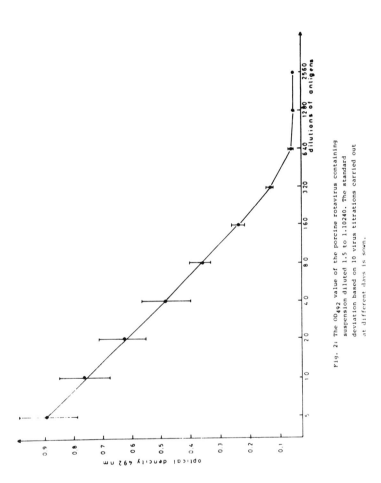

Fig. 2: The OD$_{492}$ value of the porcine rotavirus containing suspension diluted 1.5 to 1.10240. The standard deviation based on 10 virus titrations carried out at different days is sown.

261

Fig. 3

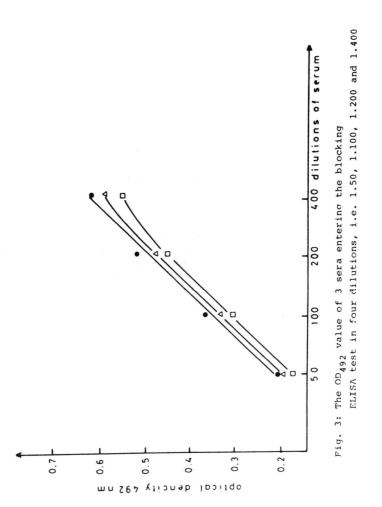

Fig. 3: The OD$_{492}$ value of 3 sera entering the blocking
ELISA test in four dilutions, i.e. 1.50, 1.100, 1.200 and 1.400

porcine rotavirus rabbit IgG (Askaa & Bloch 1981) were used
together with normal rabbit IgG (Dako-immunoglobulins Ltd.,
code X 904) for demonstration of the blocking effect of specific antibodies. These IgG preparations have been tested
in two fold dilution from 1:10 to 1:12800.

In order to test the possibility of using one dilution
for determination of antibody in sera, ten sera from sows
were tested for contents of antibody in dilution 1:50, 1:100,
1:200 and 1:400. A dilution of 1:100 was found to be usable.
Colostrum and milk samples collected from 7 gilts and sows
were also tested in dilution 1:100. The colostrum and milk
samples were collected at the days indicated in fig. 1.

The titer of the colostrum, milk and serum samples was
expressed by the reciprocal value of the antigen dilution
by interpolating the OD value of the sample minus the background value on the antigen titration curve (fig. 2). A
sample was recorded as containing antibody against rotavirus,
if a titer higher than 20 was found. This titer corresponds
to a blocking effect of the sample of half of the given
amount of antigen.

RESULTS

The virus antigen titration curve of the fecal suspension used as antigen source for the blocking ELISA test is
shown in fig. 2, where also the standard deviations based
on ten titrations carried out at different days are shown.

The blocking ELISA test was controlled with dilutions
of the IgG fraction of sera from rabbit hyperimmunized with
human and porcine rotavirus, respectively. As expected the
blocking effect declined proportional to the dilution of
the IgG. It was not possible to demonstrate any blocking effect of the normal rabbit IgG preparation.

Ten sera from sows were tested in the blocking ELISA
test in dilution 1:50, 1:100, 1:200 and 1:400. The OD_{492}
value of three of those are plotted in fig. 3.

The contents of antibodies against rotavirus in colostrum and milk samples from the gilts and sows more closely

followed were generally found to be high in colostrum, but a marked decrease in the antibody contents in milk samples collected at about day 5 was observed. At day 15 of the lactation periods an increase was detected in the milk sample from gilt 413, whereas milk samples from the sows showed only a slight increase (fig. 1). Milk samples from gilt 113 and 114 were mainly constant at a low level throughout the lactation period.

DISCUSSION

The specificity of the blocking ELISA test for the demonstration of antibody against porcine rotavirus remains to be fully evaluated. However, the blocking effect of rabbit anti rotavirus IgG and the non-existing blocking effect of normal rabbit IgG indicate that the test is reliable. Unfortunately until now it has not been possible to find swine sera without contents of antibody against rotavirus. A negative swine serum and the immunoglobulin fraction of positive sera should be included in the evaluation of the test eliminating the presence of non-specific inhibitors in swine serum.

A blocking ELISA test was established rather than using the indirect method (Voller et al 1976, Corthier & Franz 1981). Determination of class-specific antibody will be possible using the indirect assay, but requires the use of enzyme labelled anti-species heavy chain specific immunoglobulins. Preliminary examination has further shown much higher background levels using commercial available conjugates for the indirect assay (Askaa, unpublished observation).

It was concluded from the examination of 10 sera in four dilutions showing a linearity of the blocking effect of the serum dilutions and non-crossing curves shown in fig. 3, that rotavirus specific antibody could be determined in one dilution of serum.

It is generally accepted that antibody in colostrum against rotavirus protects the offspring against rotavirus associated diarrhoea. However, the level of antibody decreases rapidly post partum, and the susceptibility of the young animal increases. In the present examination the antibody levels in colostrum and milk decrease to low titers about day 5, and these levels were nearly constant throughout the lactation periods. Milk samples from gilt 413 showed a marked difference from this general picture. Thus an antibody increase was detected from day 16, and this level was constant the rest of the period.

The examination of the colostrum and milk samples, especially from gilt 413, indicates the possibility of prevention of rotavirus associated diarrhoea by vaccination. The rapid increase of the antibody level may be caused by an antigen stimulation. Thus an elevation of the antibody level has been obtained by vaccination of sheep and cows in the gestation periods with inactivated rotavirus vaccines (Wells & Snodgrass 1978, Snodgrass et al 1979, Wellemans & van Opdenbosch 1979, Fahey et al 1981, Wells et al 1978, Snodgrass et al 1980).

The problems concerning rotavirus infection in swine are different from the infection in lambs and calves in some aspects. The infection causes mainly problems in the neonatal periods in lambs and calves, while the association of rotavirus infection in neonatal diarrhoea and 3 weeks scours may indicate that a vaccination procedure in swine should include both vaccination in the gestation and in the lactation periods. The effect of a vaccination would presumably be dependent on a previous infection of the gilts and sows.

This work was supported by the Danish Agricultural and Veterinary Research Council.

REFERENCES

Askaa, J. & Bloch, B. 1981. Detection of porcine rotavirus by
EM, ELISA and CIET. Acta vet. scand. 22, 32-38.
Bohl, E.H., Kohler, E.M., Saif, L.J., Cross, R.F., Agnes, A.G.,
& Theil, K.W. 1978. Rotavirus as a cause of diarrhea in
pigs. J. Amer. vet. med. Ass. 172, 458-463.
Bridger, J.C. & Brown, J.F. 1979. Protection of piglets from
disease caused by porcine rotavirus by feeding bovine
colostrum. Inserm, 90, 373-376.
Chasey, D. & Lucas, M. 1977. Detection of rotavirus in expe-
rimentally infected piglets. Res. Vet. Sci. 22, 124-125.
Corthier, G. & Franz, J. 1981. Detection of antirotavirus
immunoglobulins A, G and M in swine colostrum, milk and
feces by enzyme-linked immunosorbent assay. Infect.
Immun. 31, 833-836.
Debouck, P. & Pensaert, M. 1979. Experimental infection of
pigs with Belgian isolates of the porcine rotavirus. Zbl.
Vet.-Med. B, 26, 517-526.
Ellens, D.J., de Leeuw, P.W. & Straver, P.J. 1978. The detection of rotavirus specific antibody in colostrum and
milk by ELISA. Ann. Rec. Vet. 9, 337-342.
Fahey, K.J., Snodgrass, D.R., Campbell, I., McDawson, A. &
Burrells, C. 1981. IgG$_1$ antibody in milk protects lambs
against rotavirus diarrhoea. Vet. Immun. Immunpath. 2,
27-33.
Grauballe, P.C., Vestergaard, B.F., Meyling, A. & Genner, J.
1981. Optimized enzyme-linked immunosorbent assay for
detection of human and bovine rotavirus in stools: Comparison with electronmicroscopy, immunoelectro-osmophoresis and fluorescent antibody techniques. J. med. Virol.
7, 29-40.
Lecce, J.G., King, M.W. & Mock, R. 1976. Reovirus-like agent
associated with fatal diarrhea in neonatal pigs. Infect. Immun. 14, 816-825.
Leeuw, de P.W., Ellens, D.J. & Hilbink, F.W. 1979. Rotavirus-
associated diarrhoea in nursing piglets. Inserm, 90,
349-354.
McNulty, M.S., Pearson, G.R., McFerran, J.B., Collins, D.S. &
Allan, G.M. 1976. A reovirus-like agent (rotavirus)
associated with diarrhoea in neonatal pigs. Vet. Microbiol. 1, 55-63.
Rodger, S.M., Craven, J.A. & Williams, I. 1975. Demonstration
of reovirus-like particles in intestinal contents of
piglets with diarrhoea. Aust. vet. J. 51, 536.
Snodgrass, D.R. & Wells, P.W. 1976. Rotavirus infection in
lambs: Studies on passive protection. Arch. Virol. 52,
201-205.
Snodgrass, D.R. & Wells, P.W. 1978, The immunoprophylaxis of
rotavirus infections in lambs. Vet. Rec. 102, 146-148.
Snodgrass, D.R., Fahey, K.J. & Wells, P.W. 1979. Rotavirus
infections in calves from vaccinated and normal calves.
Inserm 90, 365-368.
Snodgrass, D.R., Fahey, K.J., Wells, P.W., Campbell, I. &
hitelaw, A. 1980. Passive immunity in calf rotavirus in-

fections: Maternel vaccination increases and prolongs immunoglobulin G_1 antibody secretion in milk. Infect. Immun. <u>28</u>, 344-349.

Tzipori, S. & Williams, I.H. 1978. Diarrhoea in piglets inoculated with rotavirus. Aust. vet. J. <u>54</u>, 188-192.

Voller, S., Bidwell, D. & Bartlett, A. 1976. Enzyme immunoassays in diagnostic medicine. Bull. WHO, <u>53</u>, 55-65.

Wellemans, G. & van Opdenbosch, E. 1979. Prevention of neonatal diarrhoea by prolongation of secretion of antibodies in the milk at a high level. Inserm. <u>90</u>, 369-372.

Wells, P.W. & Snodgrass, D.R. 1978. The effect of vaccination on titres of antibody to rotavirus in colostrum and milk. Ann. Rec. Vet. <u>9</u>, 265-267.

Wells, P.W. Snodgrass, D.R., Herring, J.A. & Dawson, A.M. 1978. Antibody titres to lamb rotavirus in colostrum and milk of vaccinated ewes. Vet. Rec. <u>103</u>, 46-48.

Woode, G.N., Jones, J. & Bridger, J. 1975. Levels of antibodies against neonatal calf diarrhoea virus. Vet. Rec. <u>97</u>, 148-149.

Woode, G.N., Bridger, J., Hall, G.A., Jones, J.M. & Jackson, G. 1976. The isolation of reovirus-like agents (rotaviruses) from acute gastroenteritis of piglets. J. med. Microbiol. <u>9</u>, 203-209.

Yolken, R.H., Wyatt, R.G. & Barbour, B.A. 1978. Measurement of rotavirus antibody by an enzyme-linked immunosorbent assay block-assay. J. clin. Microbiol. <u>8</u>, 283-287.

IMPROVED ELISA FOR THE DETECTION OF BLUETONGUE ANTIBODIES

O.J.B.Hübschle

Federal Research Institute for Animal Virus Diseases
P.O.Box 1149, 7400 Tübingen, Fed.Rep.Germany

ABSTRACT
    A comparative study employing two different antigen preparations for the detection of Bluetongue antibodies with the ELISA was performed. Partially purified Bluetongue virus (BTV) and a Bluetongue core preparation obtained by enzymatic digestion were tested as antigen. Whereas both antigen preparations are suitable for the ELISA, core preparations did enhance the specificity of the test as negative serum values were greatly reduced in comparison to partially purified antigen.

INTRODUCTION

    Bluetongue virus infections in ruminants have greatly increased in recent years inflicting areas which have been unaffected with the disease to date. In order to recognise the spread of infection either the isolation of the virus or the demonstration of antibodies are required. For countries unaffected with the disease one method of control is the monitoring of seroconversion to Bluetongue disease. When faced with the task to set up a serological test for the detection of Bluetongue virus we attempted to adapt the ELISA test for Bluetongue virus (BTV) serology. As with all serological tests, their quality depends heavily on the antigen used. In the case of BTV one particular characteristic is its strong affinity to cellular material. In a previous paper (Hübschle et al., 1981) we reported upon the performance of partially purified BTV antigen in the ELISA. The present communication deals with an improved BTV antigen applied in the ELISA.

MATERIALS AND METHODS

    Production of BTV in cell cultures has been reported before (Hübschle et al., 1981); in short plaque purified BTV serotype 10 was used to infect BHK cells seeded on roller bottles at a multiplicity of infection of 0.1. Upon appearance of the cytopathic effect cultures were harvested and further treated as indicated on the flow chart below.

Purification scheme for Bluetongue - ELISA antigen

Infectious cell material

Disruption of cells in 2mM Tris pH,8.8

3 x Freon extraction (1/3 vol. Freon + 1/10 vol. Sephadex G 200) combined supernatants 25 000 rpm 150 min. (SW 27) through a 1/7 vol. 40% sucrose cushion with 3 mg/ml tween 80

Pellet obtained is dissolved in 1 mM EGTA pH,8.8 (SW 27)

Gradient sedimentation on a 20-40% sucrose gradient in 2mM Tris pH,8.8 25 000 rpm 55 min. (SW 27)

Virus band ($\pm$26%) dilution 1:5

Pelleting 25 000 rpm 45 min.

Determination OD_{260} 1 OD_{260} = 0,2 mg/ml Bluetongue virus

Core preparation

0.6 mg and 80 µg chymotrypsin in 0.1 M Tris -Hcl pH,8.0 with 0.6 M $MgCl_2$ 37°C 30 min. (van Dijk et al.)

Separation of subviral particles via centrifugation through 40% sucrose cushion.

The performance of the ELISA was done according to established procedures. The antigen concentration used to coat individual wells was 500 ng and incubation took place at 4°C overnight. Commercially available Horse Radish Peroxidase conjugated to antibovine or antisheep immunoglobulins G were purchased from Cappel Laboratories. BTV positive sera were obtained from experimental cases whereas negative serum samples were obtained from local sheep and cattle with no history of previous exposure to BTV.

RESULTS

A wide fluctuation of absorbance readings for negative serum samples were observed with BHK derived antigen which has been purified in a conventional way. This is clearly demonstrated in Fig.1. Using enzymatically digested BTV antigen very uniform negative serum absorbance line was observed (Fig.2). In addition the specificity of the ELISA was greatly enhanced as indicated by the larger absorbance ratios between negative and positive serum samples.

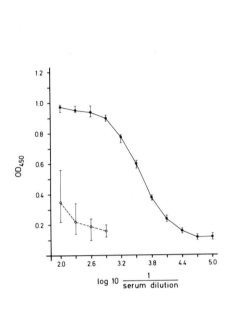

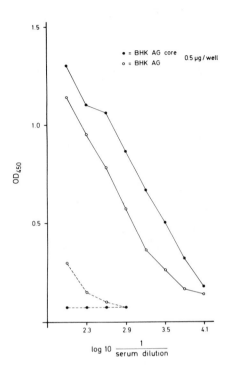

Fig. 1

Fig. 2

SCHEME BTV

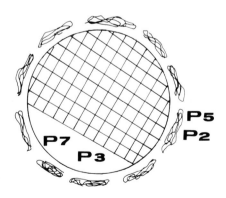

Fig. 3

The enzymatically purified antigen assayed was shown to be devoid of protein 2 and protein 5 in PAGE. Furthermore an additional indication that the outer protein shell had been removed was obtained in the haem-agglutination test. Whereas partially purified BTV did haemagglutinate sheep red blood cells, the core antigen used did not cause any haemagglutination.

CONCLUSIONS

The removal of the outer protein shell of BTV as initially described by van Dijk and Husmans (1980) greatly enhanced the ELISA of BTV. This is in accordance with the designation of protein 7 as the common protein shared by all 20 serotypes which is to be located in the core unit of Blue-tongue virus (Fig.3). The increased sensitivity obtained by the removal of protein 2 and 5 indicated that neither protein played a determing role with regard to group specificity as discussed by Jochim et al. (1981) for type 5. However it would appear that both proteins present on the complete virion are responsible for the strong membrane affinity which itself creates high background values for BTV negative sera. Though the preparation of the antigen is somewhat laborious on it would appear that the results presented supports the application of BTV core antigen in the ELISA.

REFERENCES

Hübschle, O.J.B., Matheka, H.D. and Lorenz, R.J. 1981. Encyme-linked immu-nosorbent assay for the detection of Bluetongue virus antibodies. Amer.J.vet.Res., 42, 61-65.

Jochim, M.M and Jones, J.C. 1980. Evaluation of a hemolysis-gel test for detection of quantitation of antibodies to Bluetongue virus. Amer.J. vet.Res., 41, 595-599.

Van Dijk, Alberdina, A. and Husmans, H. 1980. The in vitro activation and further characterisation of the Bluetonngue virus associated trans-criptase. Virology, 347-356.

THE USE OF ENZYME IMMUNOASSAY FOR THE MEASUREMENT OF HORMONES WITH
PARTICULAR REFERENCE TO THE DETERMINATION OF PROGESTERONE IN
UNEXTRACTED WHOLE MILK

M.J. Sauer, A.D. Cookson, B.J. MacDonald, J.A. Foulkes

Ministry of Agriculture, Fisheries and Food, Cattle Breeding Centre,
Church Lane, Shinfield, Reading, RG2 9BZ, United Kingdom

ABSTRACT

Prior to the development of enzymeimmunoassay (EIA) techniques, radioimmunoassays or radioreceptor assays were the most practical means by which hormone concentrations could be measured in large numbers of samples. EIA requires only simple colorimetry for quantitation and avoids the use of radioisotopes and associated counting equipment.

EIA's have been developed for various trophic, thyroid and steroid hormones during the past six year. These developments should enable veterinary laboratories to monitor abnormal hormone secretion in various disorders. Periodic assessment of progesterone levels can provide considerable information regarding the reproductive status of an animal. Milk would be the sample of choice in many domestic species.

The use of EIA for the determination of hormones in biological fluids and the methods by which hapten-enzyme conjugate may be formed are reviewed and factors influencing EIA sensitivity discussed. The development of a simple microtitre plate EIA for progesterone in unextracted whole milk is described.

INTRODUCTION

Enzyme immunoassay (EIA) or enzyme linked immunosorbent assay (ELISA) techniques have been the subject of continuous intensive development since their use was first reported (Engvall and Perlmann, 1971; Van Weeman and Schuurs, 1971). In the veterinary field, however, the application of EIA has remained almost totally restricted to the investigation and detection of infectious diseases. This is reflected in the scope of topics reported at this meeting. Other areas of application should surely include residue determinations in tissues and body fluids (anabolic steroids, antibiotics etc.) in order to police legislation relating to meat inspection and testing for drugs in racing.

The measurement of hormones associated with growth, development and reproductive function have obvious value in the livestock industry and the use of EIA procedures for their determination would enable their routine assessment to become a practical proposition.

The hormone EIA's which are listed in Table 1 and the procedures which we shall later describe are quantitative, competitive immunoassay procedures analagous with radioimmunoassay (RIA). This paper will not

TABLE 1. Application of EIA to the determination of hormones

Hormone	Enzyme Label	Conjugation Method	Hetero/Homo-logy	Body Fluid Assayed	Direct Addition or Extraction	Separation Technique	Detection Limit (pg/tube)	Author
Cortisol	β-Gal	MA	homo	plasma	E	DA, DASPc	100	Comoglio & Celada, 1976
	AP	CDI	hetero (b)	serum	D	DA	1000	Kobayashi et al, 1978
	β-Gal	MA	homo	plasma	E	DA	10	Monji & Castro, 1979a
	β-Gal	MBae	hetero (b)	plasma	D	DA	200	Ogihara et al, 1977
	AP	CDI	homo	plasma	D	DA	100	
Oestradiol	β-Gal	CDI	hetero(b)+(s)	–	–	DA	25	Abuknesha & Exley, 1978
	HRP	Glut*	homo	serum	E	SPct	10	Sadeh et al, 1979
	HRP	MA	homo & hetero (b) & (s)	–	–	DA	–	Van Weeman & Schuurs, 1975
Oestriol	HRP	MA	homo	urine	D	PEG	140	Korhonen et al, 1980
	AP	CDI	homo	serum	D	DA	10	Otsuki et al, 1979
Oestrogens (total)	HRP	MA	homo	serum	D	DASPc	30	Bosch et al, 1978a
	HRP	MA	homo	plasma	D	PEG	30	Osterman et al, 1979
Progesterone	HRP	MA	homo	milk (b)	E	SPc	30	Arnstadt & Cleere, 1981
	β-Gal	CDI	homo	–	–	DA	15	Dray et al, 1975
	β-Gal	NHSae	hetero (b)	–	–	DASPgb	20	Gros et al, 1978
	β-Gal		homo	serum (p)	E	DA	25	Johnen et al, 1980
	HRP	MA	homo	plasma	E	SPso	125	Joyce et al, 1977a
	HRP	MA	homo	plasma	E	DA	10	Joyce et al, 1978
	HRP	MA	homo	plasma (b)	E	DASPc	50	Kamonpatana, 1979
	β-Gal	CDI	homo	serum (b)	E	DA	25	Nakao, 1980
	β-Gal	CDI	homo	serum (b)	E	DA	12	Nakao & Kawata, 1980
	β-Gal	CDI	homo	cream (b)	D	DA	55	Patricot et al, 1978
	β-Gal	CDI	homo	plasma	D	DASPgb, SPmt, SPc	5	Sauer et al, 1981
	β-Gal	NHSae	homo	milk (b)	D		20	
	β-Gal	CDI	homo	serum (e)	E	SPct	93	Seeger et al, 1979
Prostaglandin F$_{2a}$	AP	MA	homo	urine	E	DA	180	Hayashi et al, 1981
Testosterone	HRP	MA	hetero (s) + (b)	serum	E	SPct		Bosch et al, 1978b
	β-Gal	NHSae	hetero (b+s) + homo	–	–	DA		Hosada et al, 1979, 1980
	HRP	MA	homo	–	–	SPc	50	Rajkowski et al, 1977
	GA	CDI	homo	serum	E	DA	250	Tateishi et al, 1977

Hormone	Enzyme	Conj. Meth.	Procedure	Body Fluid	Direct Addition or Extraction	Separation Technique	Sensitivity	Reference
Triiodothyronine	HRP		homo	plasma, saliva	E	SPc	4	Turkes et al, 1979
	HRP	-	homo	plasma, saliva	E	SPc	0.5	Turkes et al, 1980
Thyroxine	β-Gal	PDM*1	-	-	-	DASPc	16	Gnemmi et al, 1978
	HRP	NHSae	homo	serum	D	SPct	25	Albert et al, 1978
	β-Gluc AP	Glut	hetero (b)	serum	D	DA	250	Miyai et al, 1978
	HRP	NHSae	homo	serum	D	SPct	400	Albert et al, 1978
	β-Gal	MBae	hetero (b)	serum	-	DA	1000	Monji et al, 1979b
HCG	β-Gal	MCAE	-	urine	D	SPrbc	2.5mIU/ml	Hamada et al, 1978
	β-Gal	MBS	-	plasma	D	DA	0.4mIU/ml	Kitagawa et al, 1979
	β-Gal	MCAE	-	plasma	D	SPsr	1mIU/ml	Tomada et al, 1978
	HRP	Glut	-	-	D	DASPc	0.4mIU/ml	Van Weeman & Schuurs, 1971
Insulin	GA	Glut	-	-	-	SPs	1μU/tube	Ishikawa, 1973
	β-Gal	PDM	-	-	D	SPs	1μU/tube	Kato et al, 1975b
	β-Gal	PDM	-	serum	D	SPsr	5μIU/ml	Kato et al, 1979
	β-Gal	MBS	-	-	-	DA	0.5μU	Kitagawa & Aikawa, 1975
LH	AP	PAC	-	urine, serum	D	SPgb	100mIU/ml	Saxena et al, 1979
PMSG	AP	Glut*	-	-	-	SPmt	0.01IU/ml	Marion et al, 1978
HPL	AP + HRP	Periodate	-	plasma	D	DA	0.1μg/ml	Williams, D.G., 1978
Thyrotropin	AP	Glut	-	serum	D	DA	10μU/ml	Miyai et al, 1976
	GO	Periodate	-	serum	D	DA	1.5μU/ml	Albert et al, 1978

ABBREVIATIONS

Hormone - hCG human chorionic gonadotrophin; LH luteinizing hormone; PMSG, pregnant mare serum gonadotrophin; hPL, human placenta lactogen. Enzyme - β-Gal, β-galactosidase; AP, alkaline phosphate; HRP horse raddish peroxidase; GA, glucoamylase; GO, glucose oxidase; β-Gluc, β-glucosidase; *enzyme conjugated to antibody ('sandwich' technique or *1 immunoenzymometric assay). Conj. Meth. - MCAE & MBS, N-hydroxysuccinimide esters of N-(4-carboxyphenylmethyl)-maleimide & maleimido benzoic acid respectively (heterobifunctional reagents). Glut, gluturaldehyde; PDM, N,N'-o-phenylelemaleimide (homobifunctional reagent); PAC, photo affinity coupling; MA, mixed anhydride; CDI, water soluble carbodiimide; MBae, maleimido benzoate active ester; NHSae, N-hydroxysuccinimide active ester. Procedure - Homo, homologous assay (hapten linkage to immunogen is same as linkage to enzyme); hetero, heterologous assay (linkage differs, either in bridge (b) or site (s) of conjugation). Body Fluid - Species is human except where indicated; bovine (b), equine (e) or porcine (p). Direct Addition or Extraction - D, direct addition; E, hapten extracted prior to assay. Separation Technique - SP, solid phase antibody; DA, double antibody; DASP, double antibody solid phase; PEG, polyethylene glycol precipitation; rbc, red blood cells; sr, silicone rods; c, cellulose; s, sephadex; gb, glass balls; mt, microtitre plate; ct, coated tube; so, sepharose.

consider the relative merits of the different methods by which enzymes can be employed as labels in EIA nor the merits of various enzymes used since these areas have been adequately reviewed by others (O'Sullivan et al, 1979; Oellerich, 1980; Scharpe et al, 1976; Schuurs and Van Weeman, 1977). Attention will, however, be paid to the methods by which enzyme-immunogen conjugates may be made.

Table 1 illustrates hormones for which EIA's have been developed. It can be seen that interest in this procedure has remained largely confined to the human clinical sphere. Progesterone is an exception and is the only hormone to have been assayed in a number of species as well as in several body fluids. This is perhaps because the patterns of progesterone secretion provide a wealth of information on aspects of reproductive performance such as the occurrence of cyclical activity or ovulation, differential diagnosis of luteal or ovarian cysts and pregnancy diagnosis.

The sensitivity of EIA is in many cases comparable with that achieved using RIA although many of the hapten EIA procedures have involved extraction of the analyte before assay (Table 1). Where cross-reacting substances are likely to be present in the test sample, purification by means of extraction or even chromotography may be necessary: this obviously applies equally to RIA. If high specificity is not required, however, prior extraction of sample may not be essential for the EIA provided the conjugates used are of suitable purity and do not contain a substantial proportion of unconjugated enzyme or steroid, or conjugated but denatured enzyme since this may affect the sensitivity of the assay. We believe, therefore, that particularly where quantitative, direct-addition assays are to be performed the mode of preparation of the conjugate is of the utmost importance.

PREPARATION OF PROTEIN-ENZYME CONJUGATES

A number of conventional procedures are available for the conjugation of enzymes to proteins and these include the one-step (Avrameas, 1969) and two-step (Avrameas and Ternynck, 1971) gluteraldehyde methods, the periodate method (Nakane and Kawaoi, 1974) and the use of homobifunctional reagents such as N,N'-o-phenylenedimaleimide (Kato et al, 1975a). These methods have been reviewed by Kennedy et al (1976) and others at this symposium (Doel and Collen, 1981).

The nature of these reactions makes co-conjugation of either enzyme to enzyme or protein to protein almost inevitable. For this reason, the development of heterobifunctional reagents represents a major advance for production of enzyme-protein conjugates since they eliminate the possibility of co-conjugation of enzyme or protein.

Protein-enzyme conjugation using heterobifunctional reagents

A number of heterobifunctional reagents have recently been developed which, as the name implies, contain two differing reactive groups. The reagents reported up to now have reactivity towards sulphydryl groups at one end and towards amino groups at the other (fig. 1). Thus, in the first instance, if the reagent is reacted with a protein (or enzyme) which does not contain available sulphydryl groups no polymerzation can occur: if excess reagent is then removed (ie. by gel filtration or dialysis) the other protein may then be added in order that conjugation may proceed. If the second protein does not normally contain available sulphydryl residues it may be possible either to introduce them by chemical means (mercaptoimidation or mercapto-succinylation (Traut et al, 1973; Kato et al, 1975b) or by reduction of existing disulphide bridges (Kato et al, 1975a).

m-Maleimidobenzoyl-N-hydroxy   N-succinimidyl 3-(2-pyridyl
          succinimide   dithio) propionate

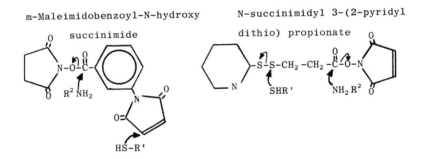

Fig. 1   Conjugation using heterobifunctional reagents. R' and R^2 can be protein or hapten moieties.

Bifunctional compounds which have been employed in the preparation of protein-enzyme conjugates include m-maleimidobenzoyl-N-hydroxysuccinimide (MBS) for conjugation of enzymes with insulin (Kitagawa and Aikawa, 1976) and donkey anti-sheep IgG Fc fragment (O'Sullivan et al, 1978a), N-hydroxy-succinimide esters of N-(4-carboxycyclohexylmethyl)-maleimide and N-(4-carboxyphenylmethyl)-Maleimide for conjugation with protein hormones (Hamada et al, 1978; Ishikawa et al, 1978) and N-succinimidyl 3-(2-pyridyl dithio) propionate (SPDP) for conjugation with protein A (Pain, D. and Surolia, A.).

PREPARATION OF HAPTEN-ENZYME CONJUGATES

The preparation of enzyme-hapten conjugates for EIA has generally involved use of the standard mixed anhydride or carbodiimide procedures originally developed for linking haptens to protein carriers such as BSA for use in raising hapten antisera (fig. 2). In essence, the procedures give rise to the formation of peptide bonds between an acid group on the hapten or hapten derivative and lysine ϵ-amino groups on the enzyme.

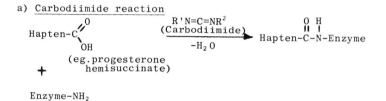

a) <u>Carbodiimide reaction</u>

b) <u>Mixed anhydride reaction.</u>

Fig. 2   Summary of carbodiimide and mixed anhydride reactions.

The carbodiimide method

The basic water-soluble carbodiimide procedure has been use by a number of workers for producing enzyme-hapten conjugates (Table 1) but is losing favour since it inevitably results in co-conjugation of enzyme molecules. This is because it is not possible with currently available carbodiimide reagents to conjugate enzyme to hapten without the continued presence of excess carbodiimides since the intermediate o-acylurea is unstable (Kurzer and Douraghi-Zadeh, 1967).

The mixed anhydride procedure

This procedure eliminates the possibility of co-conjugation of enzyme since the generation of the intermediate mixed anhydride is only possible under anhydrous conditions (fig. 2). When aqueous enzyme solution is added for conjugation enzyme carboxylic acid groups cannot themselves form anhydrides and the enzyme-mixed anhydride reaction prevails.

Although a within laboratory comparison of the different methods of conjugation has not been reported, it has been argued that the mixed anhydride procedure may not be so efficient as procedures utilising hapten "active esters" described later.

Homobifunctional reagents

Homobifunctional reagents such as dimethyl adipimate (fig. 3) may also be used for coupling haptens to enzymes (Al-Bassam et al, 1978; O'Sullivan et al, 1978b) but reaction conditions must be carefully selected to minimize the inevitable co-conjugation of either enzyme or hapten.

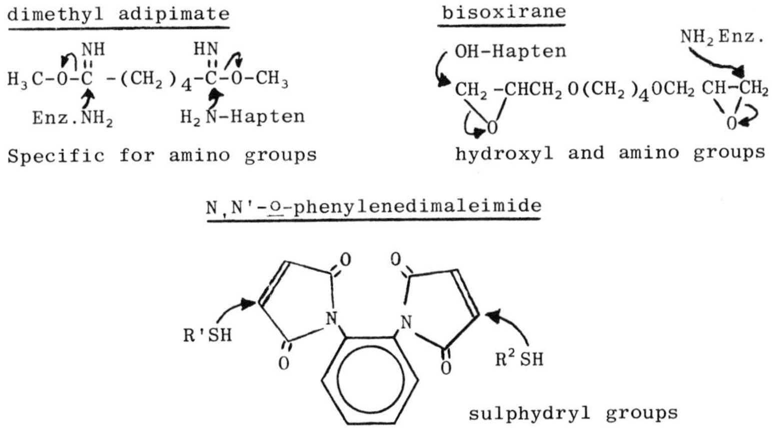

Fig. 3   Conjugation using homobifunctional reagents. R' and R^2 can be protein or hapten moieties.

Heterobifunctional reagents

Heterobifunctional reagents may similarly be used for conjugating haptens essentially without the hazards of co-conjugation (fig. 1). They have not found general application in the hapten hormone field largely because derivatives containing amino or sulphydryl groups are not generally available or easily synthesised.

Heterobifunctional reagents have, however, found application in coupling certain drugs to enzymes: MBS has been used for coupling β-gal-actosidase to Viomycin (Kitagawa et al, 1976) and N-(3-maleimidopropionyl glycyloxy) succinimide for coupling Viomycin, Gentamycin (Kitagawa et al, 1978a) and Ampicillin (Kitagawa et al, 1978b) to β-galactosidase.

"Active ester" derivatives of haptens

The synthesis of reactive esters of haptens or hapten derivatives provides the basis for what may be the most convenient and efficient means of producing enzyme-hapten conjugates (fig. 4). These esters may be isolated and purified and thus used directly for conjugation with the enzyme under aqueous conditions and neutral pH. This eliminates the possibility of co-conjugation and enzyme denaturation (fig. 4). N-hydroxy-succinimide and p-nitrophenyl esters will readily react with primary, unhindered amino groups such as the ε-amino groups of lysine to form a peptide bond:such reactions have been used for conjugating progesterone

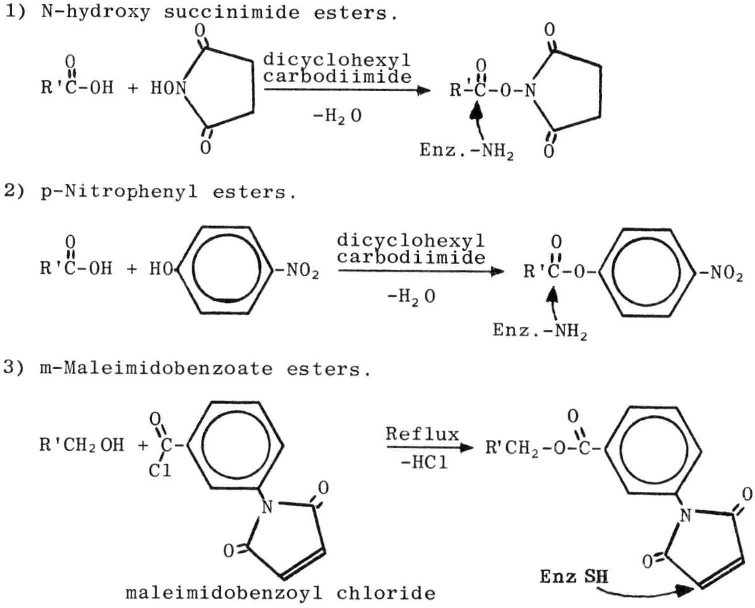

1) N-hydroxy succinimide esters.

2) p-Nitrophenyl esters.

3) m-Maleimidobenzoate esters.

maleimidobenzoyl chloride

Fig. 4   Active ester derivatives of haptens. R' represents the hapten portion.

11-hemisuccinate (Sauer et al, 1981) and testosterone derivatives (Hosada et al, 1979; 1980) to β-galactosidase and for conjugating oestrone sulphate 6-hemisuccinate to BSA (Nambara et al, 1980). Gros et al, (1978) have also used N-hydroxysuccinimide esters to link progesterone 11-hemisuccinate and progesterone 11-hemimaleate to β-galactosidase but without prior purification or isolation of the active ester (carbodiimide may therefore have been present when the enzyme was added). Monji and Castro (1979a) have isolated and purified m-Maleimidobenzoate esters of cortisol and cortisol derivatives which they subsequently used to enable direct conjugation with the free sulphydryl residues of β-galactosidase in buffer at pH 7.0. These reports indicate that these active esters react with enzyme or protein in a near stoichiometric manner and result in only minimal loss of enzyme activity.

Typical procedure for coupling haptens to enzymes using N-hydroxysuccinimide esters

The formation of the N-hydroxysuccinimide ester of 11 ∝ -hydroxyprogesterone 11-hemisuccinate (Sauer et al, 1981) provides a typical example of the means by which N-hydroxysuccinimide esters of carboxylated haptens or hapten derivatives may generally be made (fig. 5).

A slight molar excess (10-20%) of N-hydroxysuccinimide and dicyclohexylcarbodiimide was added to progesterone 11-hemisuccinate (43mg) and dissolved in a minimum volume of dry dioxane. The mixture was stirred at 25°C for 30 mins and the insoluble by-product dicyclohexylurea removed by washing through a sintered glass funnel. The clear filtrate was dried under a stream of nitrogen and the residue dissolved in a minimum volume of dichloromethane at 35°C. Addition of cold diethyl ether allowed crystallization of the N-hydroxysuccinimide ester.

Progesterone-β-galactosidase conjugates were subsequently produced as described (Sauer et al, 1981) by addition of a suitable molar excess of the active ester (in a minimum volume of dry dimethylformamide) to β-galactosidase* in 0.1M phosphate buffered saline, pH 7.0. The reaction was performed at room temperature with stirring for one hour before "exhaustive" dialysis against three changes of 3 litres of 0.1M phosphate-buffered saline containing sodium azide (0.1% w/v) at pH 7.0. Conjugates were then subjected to gel filtration (Sephadex G25) prior to assessment and subsequent use for EIA. The importance of extensive dialysis and gel filtration for

* see appendix

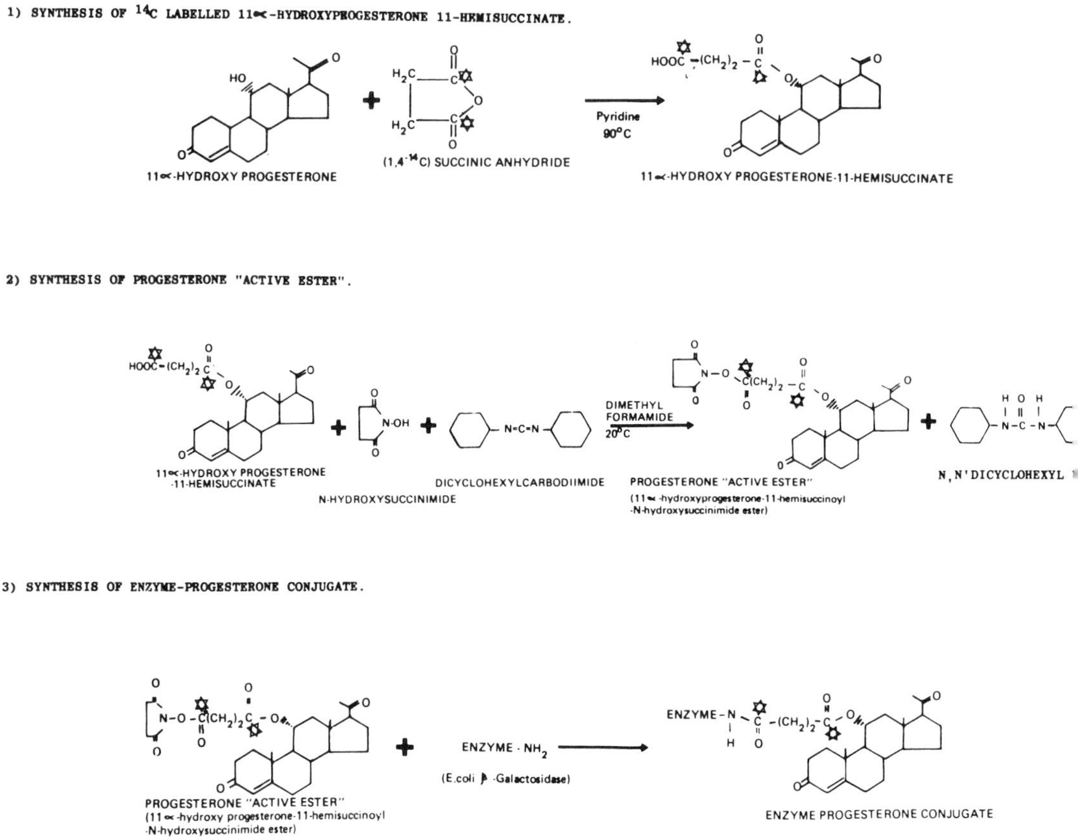

1) SYNTHESIS OF ^{14}C LABELLED 11α-HYDROXYPROGESTERONE 11-HEMISUCCINATE.

11α-HYDROXY PROGESTERONE   (1,4-^{14}C) SUCCINIC ANHYDRIDE   11α-HYDROXY PROGESTERONE-11-HEMISUCCINATE

2) SYNTHESIS OF PROGESTERONE "ACTIVE ESTER".

11α-HYDROXY PROGESTERONE-11-HEMISUCCINATE   N-HYDROXYSUCCINIMIDE   DICYCLOHEXYLCARBODIIMIDE   PROGESTERONE "ACTIVE ESTER" (11α-hydroxyprogesterone-11-hemisuccinoyl -N-hydroxysuccinimide ester)   N,N'DICYCLOHEXYL

3) SYNTHESIS OF ENZYME-PROGESTERONE CONJUGATE.

PROGESTERONE "ACTIVE ESTER" (11α-hydroxy progesterone-11-hemisuccinoyl -N-hydroxysuccinimide ester)   ENZYME · NH$_2$ (E.coli β-Galactosidase)   ENZYME PROGESTERONE CONJUGATE

Fig. 5   Formation of β-galactosidase-progesterone conjugates by the N-hydroxysuccinimide ester method.

the removal of unconjugated progesterone cannot be over-stressed: it is essential if a high degree of assay sensitivity is to be achieved. Even after dialysis against four changes of buffer (over 5 days), and gel filtration followed by a final dialysis, we have still been able to detect immunoreactive material in the dialysate. By this stage, however, the quantity present would not be sufficient to interfere with the EIA at the conjugate dilution employed.

Several methods have been employed to assess the number of hapten molecules conjugated per enzyme and these include spectrophotometric methods (Erlanger et al, 1957), or analysis of free amino groups on the enzyme subsequent to conjugation (Fields, 1971). The most direct and perhaps least misleading approach is through the use of radioactively-labelled hapten (Abuknesha and Exley, 1978; Comoglio and Celada, 1976; Sauer et al, 1981).

Using the latter method of assessment the N-hydroxysuccinimide ester method of conjugation was shown to be highly efficient, particularly at lower molar ratios (Table 2). Incorporation approaching the theoretical maximum of 116 progesterone molecules per enzyme can be achieved (there being 116 lysine residues per β-galactosidase molecule; Craven et al, 1965) although high molar incorporation was found to result in loss of enzyme activity (Sauer et al, 1981). Determination of steroid incorporation by binding inhibition

TABLE 2   Molar incorporation of progesterone into β-galactosidase and enzyme activity of the resulting conjugates.

Molar ratio progesterone: enzyme in conjugation reaction mixture	Enzyme activity of conjugates (% of original activity)	Molar ratio of progesterone to enzyme:	
		Radioactivity determination	Radioimmunoassay
0	103.4	0	0.01
2	104.4	2.0	0.02
20	111.1	7.9	0.15
100	91.6	48.6	0.27
200	82.4	87.7	0.34
500	62.6	104.4	1.16
2000	22.6	107.0	0.83

tests detected substantially lower molar incorporation (see Table 2), indicating that the actual molar steroid incorporation may have little bearing on the sensitivity of an assay except where it can be shown that all conjugated steroid is immunologically apparent as well as physically detectable.

METHODS OF SEPARATION OF FREE FROM BOUND ENZYME CONJUGATE

The EIA's described in this paper (termed heterogenous EIA's) require separation of free from bound enzyme label following the immunoreaction in order to quantitate the unlabelled hapten or protein. Separation techniques which have been employed are generally methods adapted from RIA procedures. These include polyethylene glycol precipitation, double antibody precipitation, double antibody solid phase and solid phase primary antibody techniques (Table 1). The use of dextran-coated charcoal for separation is probably the most widely used technique for hapten RIA but since absorption is based on the large difference in molecular weight (of the order of 200 fold) between free label and that bound to antibody it cannot be applied to EIA.

Where possible the use of solid phase antibodies (preferably primary antibodies) gives rise to the most convenient form of separation. Where particulate solid phases are used it has been necessary to employ a centrifugation stage. To avoid a centrifugation step, methods have been developed enabling magnetic solid phases to be prepared: materials used include polyacrylamide-agarose beads (Guesdon and Avrameas, 1977), ferric oxide particles (Hersch and Yaverbaum, 1975; Nye et al, 1976), cellulose (Anderson, 1978) and plastic coated steel balls (Smith and Gehle, 1977).

Using polystyrene test-tubes or polyvinyl or polystyrene microtitre plates coated with primary antibody, separation of free from bound enzyme-conjugate is achieved simply by pouring off the free fraction. The quantity of enzyme label bound may be simply determined by addition of substrate following an initial washing to remove residual free enzyme conjugate.

In this laboratory we have largely used solid phase separation techniques, including primary antibody linked to microgranular cellulose. We now use microtitre plates in a progesterone enzymeimmunoassay (Sauer et al, 1981) in what we believe is the first reported use of such plates in a hapten EIA. This procedure combines a convenient, simple and less tedious method with rapid assay and end-point determination - particularly when used in conjunction with an automatic plate reader such as the "twin beam" Dynatech MR 580.

MICROTITRE PLATE ENZYMEIMMUNOASSAY FOR PROGESTERONE

For the majority of quantitative coated test-tube or microtitre plate immunoassays it is essential to isolate the γ-globulin fraction of the antiserum prior to coating of tubes or microtitre plate wells. This enables significant antibody binding to be achieved at reasonable antibody dilution.

Antibody purification

We have used BSA-absorbed (Thorneycroft et al, 1970) goat antiprogesterone serum (G711/12) raised against 11$\propto$-hydroxyprogesterone 11-hemisuccinate-BSA for our assay. Adequate purification was achieved by treating the antiserum with 4 volumes of 0.4% Rivanol; this precipitates the majority of serum proteins leaving globulins in solution (Horejsi and Smetana, 1956). Thorneycroft et al, (1970) indicated the importance of pH in this purification procedure and our results underline the point. The indications are that it is essential to establish not only the pH for the precipitation but also the volume of 0.4% Rivanol to be added, since these optima may vary from species to species. Goat antiserum was treated with 4 volumes of

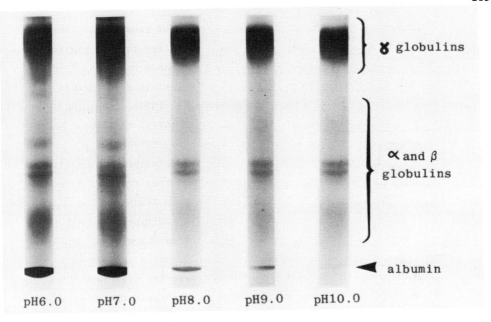

Fig. 6   The effect of pH on the precipitation of serum proteins by Rivanol.

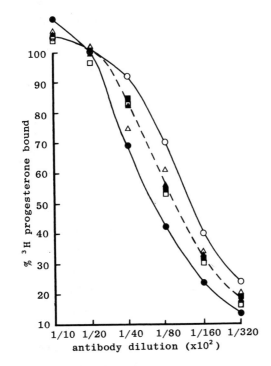

Fig. 7   Effect of pH on recovery of anti-progesterone γ-globulin from serum treated with Rivanol (pH 6.0, □-□; pH 7.0, ▲-▲; pH 8.0, △-△; pH 9.0, ■-■: pH 10.0, ●-●; untreated serum, ○-○).

buffered 0.4% Rivanol (0.1M phosphate or tris buffer, pH 6-10) for 15
minutes at room temperature and then centrifuged. Rivanol was removed by
Sephadex G-25 column chromatography (eluting with 0.005M phosphate buffer,
pH 7.0) and the protein fraction freeze-dried and re-dissolved in deionized
water to give a volume of 10 x that of the original serum. Polyacrylamide
gel electrophoresis (fig. 6) and subsequent assessment of antibody titre
(fig. 7) indicated that pH 9.0 was optimal and resulted in removal of the
majority of other serum proteins. Antiserum treated in this way was subsequently used for binding to microtitre plates. When dilution curves
obtained with the original antiserum were compared with those following
treatment at pH 6-9, a small but similar drop in binding was seen consistent with experimental losses. At pH 10, however, a further more substantial
drop in binding was found, indicating a loss of γ-globulins by treatment
at this pH (fig. 7).

Adsorption of antibodies to microtitre plate wells

We have used Dynatech 96-well flat-bottomed polyvinyl plates (M29A)
and found that these gave more consistent binding than did the use of their
polystyrene equivalent reported previously (Sauer et al, 1981). Binding of
^{3}H progesterone to the wells was used to assess the extent to which the
anti-progesterone γ-globulin was adsorbed. At temperatures of 25, 30, 35
and 40°C binding of γ-globulin was virtually complete by one hour (fig. 8A).
We eventually chose a 3hr incubation at 40°C to ensure good standardization.

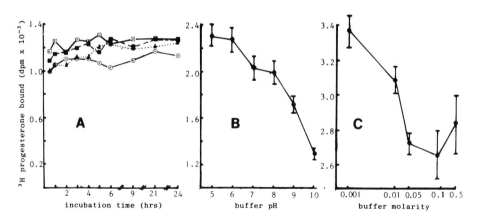

Fig. 8   Effect of A, incubation duration and temperature (25°C, ⊙-⊙;
30°C, ▲-▲; 35°C, ■-■; 40°C, ▣-▣); B, pH and C, buffer molarity on adsorption of antibody onto microtitre plate wells. Values are mean of 4
determinations (A) or 8 determinations (B and C) ± 2 SEM.

The pH of the coating buffer had a considerable influence on binding of γ-globulin to the wells, maximum binding being achieved at pH 5.0 (Fig. 8B). The influence of acetate buffer concentrations at pH 5.0 on binding of antibody to the wells is shown in fig. 8C. Buffer solutions were prepared in water which had undergone a primary deionization, glass distillation and further deionization prior to use. The highest binding levels were achieved using 1mM buffer.

Later studies therefore used standard adsorption conditions: γ-globulin diluted in 1mM acetate buffer pH 5.0 (0.2ml), was added to each well and incubated at 40°C for 3 hrs. The plates were then inverted and sharply tapped to eject the residual antibody. The wells were washed once with 0.1M phosphate buffer (pH 7.0) containing sodium chloride (0.9% w/v), sodium azide (0.1% w/v) and 0.1% (w/v) gelatin (PAS-gelatin buffer) and then incubated overnight at 4°C with the same buffer (250µℓ). Plates were stored in this condition at 4°C and further washed with PAS-gelatin buffer immediately prior to use for EIA.

Enzymeimmunoassay procedure

This assay procedure was developed to enable the determination of progesterone in milk by direct addition of whole milk to the assay system. Experiments to determine optimum conditions with regards antibody and enzyme conjugate dilutions were therefore carried out in the presence of whole milk. Progesterone-β-galactosidase conjugate prepared using a 20 fold molar excess of steroid was used in subsequent EIA procedures unless otherwise indicated.

Standards were prepared by the dissolution of progesterone in whole milk (containing a minimum of endogenous progesterone) from a cow at oestrus. These standards (10µℓ), or whole milk from test animals (10µℓ) were added to each well of an antibody-coated microtitre plate followed by 200µℓ of progesterone-enzyme conjugate suitably diluted in PAS-gelatin buffer. After a three hour incubation period at 40°C the wells were emptied and washed three times as above. The amount of enzyme conjugate bound was determined by addition of freshly prepared substrate, o-nitrophenyl β-D-galactopyranoside (3mg ml^{-1}), in PAS-gelatin buffer containing 0.01M magnesium chloride and 0.1M mercaptoethanol. Following an incubation period of 1 hr at 45°C the optical density (OD) at 405nm was measured directly through the wells using a Dynatech MR580 automatic plate reader.

Selection of antibody and enzyme conjugate dilutions

A 1 hr period was chosen for incubating enzyme and substrate to mini-mise time differences associated with substrate addition to the first and last well. This also enabled economical use to be made of antibody and conjugate. The antibody dilution at which wells were coated and the conju-gate dilution used in the EIA procedure were determined on an empirical basis; account was taken of the optical density achieved following binding in the absence of competing progesterone (Bo value) since this dictates the OD range measured in the standard curve.

Conjugate and antibody dilutions giving rise to acceptable standard curves were compared in order to assess their influence on the limits of detection. It can be seen from figs. 9A and 9B that neither parameter had

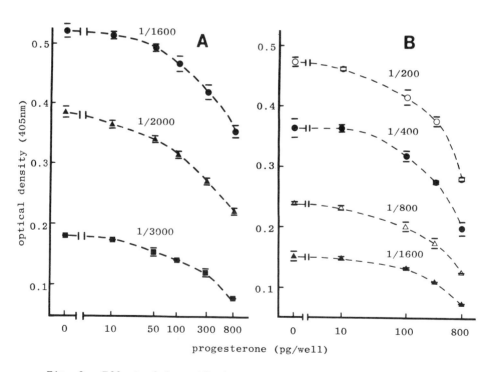

Fig. 9   Effect of A, antibody dilution (at 1/400 conjugate dilution) and B, conjugate dilution (at 1/200 antibody dilution) on the sensiti-vity of EIA standard curves. Values are mean of 4 determinations ± 2 SEM.

a dramatic effect over the ranges tried. In some respects this may not be surprising. The range of antibody dilutions indicated in fig. 9A would result in a quantity of antibody bound to the wells, which, if used in RIA would bind a maximum of 1pg of ^{3}H progesterone in the absence of competing steroid. Further reduction in the quantity of antibody bound to the wells would be unlikely to result in a substantial increase in sensitivity under the immunoassay conditions adopted here; the theoretical arguements applied to RIA by Ekins (1974) would suggest that by using such small quantities of antibody the system may already be operating around the limits of sensitivity for the assay. At a 1/2000 antibody dilution (fig. 9A) a significant difference in binding of conjugate was shown between 0 and 10pg (p $<$ 0.05). No significant difference in the limit of detection was found between standard curves using the different conjugate dilutions.

In subsequent assays of progesterone in test milk samples each well was coated with anti-progesterone γ-globulin (1/2000 dilution $\equiv$ 0.6μg/well) and conjugate (1/400 dilution; 135ng in 200$\mu\ell$ PAS-gelatin buffer $\equiv$ 6pg of immunoreactive progesterone) added to 10$\mu\ell$ of milk.

Comparative RIA systems

A microtitre plate RIA and a liquid phase RIA were developed to compare whole milk progesterone concentrations determined by RIA and EIA.

The microtitre plate RIA was carried out in essentially the same manner as the EIA procedure except that the plates were coated with γ-globulin at 1/200 dilution. Following removal of the free steroid by washing as before, bound label was measured by cutting up the plates and counting individual wells in Toluene Scintillator (7ml, Packard).

The liquid phase RIA was carried out as follows:-

Whole milk standard (10$\mu\ell$; 0-300pg progesterone) was pipetted into polystyrene test tubes and ^{3}H progesterone in PAS-gelatin buffer (100uℓ, 4,000 dpm $\equiv$ 6pg progesterone) and progesterone antiserum (200$\mu\ell$ G711/12 at 1/30,000 dilution in PAS-gelatin buffer) added. The tubes were mixed and incubated for 1 hr at room temperature and then overnight at 4°C. Free ^{3}H progesterone was separated from bound by the addition of dextran-coated charcoal suspension (500$\mu\ell$, 2.5mg charcoal; "Separex", Steranti, UK) in PAS-gelatin buffer at 4°C. After 6 mins at 4°C tubes were centrifuged at 4,000g (10 min) and the supernatant poured off into scintillation vials and counted following extraction into Toluene Scintillator (7ml).

288

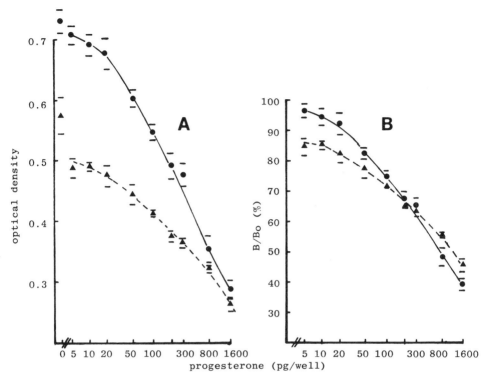

Fig. 10   Comparison of EIA standard curves using standards prepared
in buffer (●-●) or milk (▲-▲). Values are mean of 4 determinations ±
2 SEM. For ease of comparison results are expressed in terms of optical
density (A) and B/B_O (B).

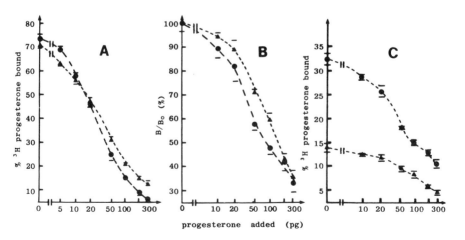

Fig. 11   Comparison of liquid phase (A) and microtitre plate (B and C)
RIA standard curves using standards prepared in buffer (●-●) or milk
(▲-▲). Values are mean of 4 determinations ± 2 SEM. For ease of
comparison microtitre plate results are expressed in terms of B/B_O (B)
and % bound (C).

The application of EIA to the determination of milk progesterone

Fig. 10 shows a typical comparison between EIA standard curves prepared in the presence and absence of milk. It is apparent that milk caused a considerable drop in enzyme conjugate binding (21%), but even so the sensitivity of the curve was still 10pg/well at the 95% confidence limit. A similar drop in binding was noted for the microtitre plate RIA (fig. 11B). These EIA standard curves were not as sensitive as we have reported in a previous publication (Sauer et al, 1981); this may be due to the presence of slightly higher levels of endogenous progesterone in the "oestrus milk" sample used to prepare the standards. The milk used for these standards had been stored for about 5 months at 4°C in the presence of 0.1% sodium azide. Storage of the milk in this way had a minimal effect on progesterone concentrations when assayed by liquid phase RIA but may influence the stability of certain milk proteins over a period of several months: this may in turn influence conjugate binding to the antibody.

During November and December 1980, representative milk samples were

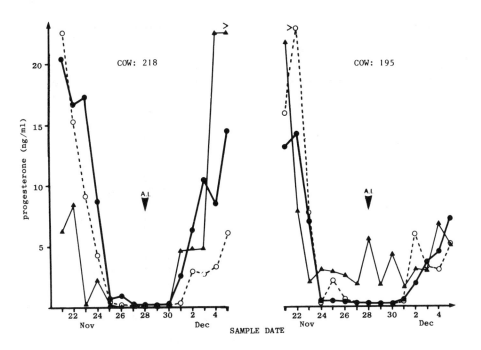

Fig. 12   Comparison of progesterone concentrations in milk samples collected around the oestrus period. Samples were assayed by microtitre plate EIA (▲-▲) and RIA (O---O) and by liquid phase RIA (●-●). Values are mean of 4 determinations.

taken from the milk collection jars of two cows at the morning milking. Aliquots (1ml) were stored at 4°C in the presence of 0.1% sodium azide. The samples were assayed within three months by liquid phase RIA and subsequently by liquid phase RIA, microtitre plate RIA and microtitre plate EIA in August 1981. Results from samples collected around the oestrus period at which artificial insemination (AI) was carried out are illustrated in fig. 12.

A correspondence can be seen when comparing profiles obtained by the three methods. The long period of storage may have influenced the EIA results since protein precipitation occured in some of the samples. Such changes in milk constituents may conceivably have a greater influence on the binding of enzyme conjugate in the EIA system than the RIA system. A comparison of milk samples assayed after three months with those assayed after eight months revealed only minimal changes in progesterone concentration when examined by liquid phase RIA. A study of progesterone concentrations in fresh whole milk is currently being undertaken to resolve the differences observed between the EIA and RIA systems.

Clinical value of milk progesterone determinations in fertility control

Progesterone concentrations in milk have been shown to correlate closely with the growth and secretary function of the corpus luteum (Hoffmann et al, 1976; Laing and Heap, 1971; Pope et al, 1976): luteal function in cattle may therefore be conveniently monitored through determination of progesterone concentrations in milk rather than plasma, allowing sampling by lay personnel.

Analysis of progesterone in milk samples has been used for the investigation of a number of physiological conditions. These include pregnancy diagnosis, enabling early re-submission of non-pregnant cows for service (Laing and Heap, 1971), confirmation of cyclic activity (Günzler et al, 1979; Lamming and Bulman, 1976), accurate differential diagnosis of ovarian cysts (Hoffmann et al, 1976) and the confirmation and prediction of oestrus (Ball and Jackson, 1979; Günzler et al, 1979). The latter application is of particular interest to the artificial insemination industry since it is now well established that in large herds the detection of oestrus can be a major problem (McCaughey and Cooper, 1980; Oltner and Edqvist, 1981) and can result in a considerable extension of the calving to conception interval. The economic losses involved can be considerable since a missed oestrus period will result in a delay of 21 days before subsequent AI and each day lost has been estimated to cost of the order of £1.50 in lost production.

Failure to detect oestrus can be a particular problem during the early post-partum period when "silent" oestrus periods may occur. Whether failure to detect oestrus is due to "silent" heat or management problems, a quick and simple progesterone test could circumvent the necessity for oestrus observation. Ball and Jackson (1979) used progesterone levels (measured by RIA) as the basis for determining when cattle should be inseminated. Subsequent conception rates of animals in which oestrus was not observed demonstrated the value of this approach. The potential of a suitable on-farm milk progesterone test in this respect is obvious. The microtitre plate EIA currently offers the quickest and most convenient means for determining progesterone concentrations directly in whole milk. The use of enzyme rather then isotopic labels offers the opportunity for further development of "dip-stick" techniques for use by stockmen.

PRELIMINARY APPLICATION OF DIRECT EIA OF SERUM SAMPLES

In heifers and non-lactating cows it is obviously not possible to obtain a milk sample. Similarly, in other species such as the pig, sheep and horse, progesterone estimations would need to be carried out on blood samples under most circumstances, although saliva might be suitable. Preliminary findings suggest that the microtitre plate procedure may be equally applicable to the assay of serum samples. Fig. 13 shows standard curves obtained using essentially the same conditions described for the direct assay of milk. Serum samples ($10\mu\ell$) were taken from animals in which endogenous levels of progesterone should have been minimal. RIA standard curves are also shown for comparison (fig. 14). The results appear particularly promising in the pig since plasma progesterone concentrations during the oestrus cycle cover a similar range to those in bovine milk. The large depression in binding observed with the RIA standard curve in the presence of prepubertal pig serum (fig. 13) could have arisen from the presence of endogenous progesterone or steroid binding globulins.

FACTORS INFLUENCING EIA SENSITIVITY

Discussions regarding the limits of sensitivity that may be achieved by hapten EIA have largely evolved from the development of steroid enzyme immunoassays. Two main factors have been considered important (given that the conjugative procedure is efficient and does not result in enzyme denaturation) namely,

    i) the number of steroid molecules incorporated per molecule of enzyme and

292

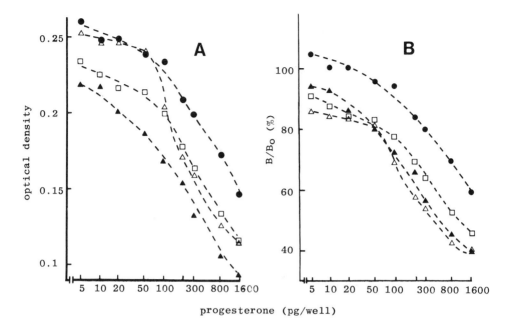

Fig. 13 Comparison of EIA standard curves in the presence of serum ($10\mu\ell$) from pre-pubertal gilt (●-●), pre-pubertal heifer (▲-▲), castrate ram (△-△) and gelding (□-□). Values are mean of 4 determinations. For ease of comparison results are expressed in terms of optical density (A) and B/B_0 (B).

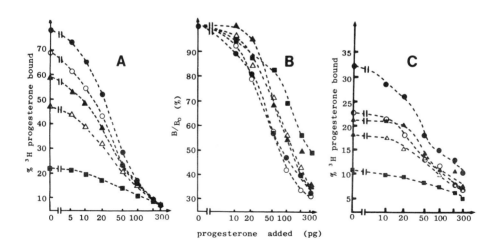

Fig. 14 Comparison of liquid phase (A) and microtitre plate (B and C) RIA standard curves without serum (●-●) and in the presence of serum ($10\mu\ell$) from pre-pubertal gilt (■-■), pre-pubertal heifer (▲-▲), castrate ram (○-○) and gelding (△-△). Values are mean of 4 determinations. For ease of comparison results are expressed in terms of % bound (A and C) and B/B_0 (B).

ii) the affinity of the antibody for the hapten relative to its affinity
for the congugate.

i) The steroid: enzyme incoporation ratio aspect has been stressed by a
number of workers (Exley and Abuknesha, 1977; Joyce et al, 1977b). It has
been suggested, either on theoretical grounds (Exley and Abuknesha, 1977)
or on the basis of experimental findings (Joyce et al, 1977a); Hosada et al,
1980), that the ratio of steroid : enzyme should be of the order of 1 : 1
for optimal sensitivity to be achieved. The findings of Joyce et al (1977b)
indicated that with oestradiol - horse radish peroxidase conjugate, reducing
the incorporation ratio from 11 : 1 to 2.6 : 1 gave rise to a 30% increase in
sensitivity. No explanation was given as to how, by reducing the ratio by a
further small degree (from 2.6 : 1 to 2.1 : 1) they achieved an increase in
sensitivity of 70%. Their results indicate rather that the assay system was
not optimised for particular conjugates. This is reinforced by their further
observations that using an optimised double antibody separation technique
rather than solid phase primary antibody, a 50 fold increase in sensitivity
was achieved, considerably more than that realised by alteration in steroid
incorporation ratios. More recent publications by this group (Joyce et al,
1978; Turkes et al, 1979) better reflect the high degree of sensitivity
which can be attained by using a heterologous EIA under optimum conditions.
The work of Hosada et al (1980) does not enable conclusions to be drawn
regarding the limits of detection achievable using conjugates with different
steroid : enzyme ratios, particularly since they have not determined the
degree of steroid incorporation in their enzyme conjugates.

The actual number of hapten molecules conjugated to an enzyme may be
at least a magnitude higher than those which are accessible to antibody
binding sites (Comoglio and Celada, 1975; Hayashi et al, 1981; Kominami
et al, 1980; Sauer et al, 1981). Since only conjugated hapten molecules
which are not sterically hindered are likely to be of immunological significance it is our view that for hapten EIA systems the total number of
haptens incorporated may have little bearing on the absolute sensitivity of
the system (the sensitivity will be appreciably reduced, however, when, as
a result of very high steroid incorporation, a large proportion of the conjugated steroids are immunoreactive). Despite their arguements to the cont-
rary, this view is supported by the data of the Riad-Fahmy group. For their
progesterone and testosterone EIA systems they have indicated that 20 - 50ng
of steroid-horse radish peroxidase conjugate (1.2 : 1 steroid : enzyme

incorporation ratio) proved optimal (Turkes et al, 1979 and 1980). Theoretical considerations argue against the possibility of realising the high degree of sensitivity which they have achieved (Joyce et al, 1978; Turkes et al, 1979) were all the steroid in this quantity of conjugate immunologically apparent: 20 - 50ng of conjugate is approximately equivalent to 200 - 500pg of steroid, assuming a molecular weight for HRP of 40,000. Further, it has not been our experience that optimal sensitivity can be achieved using β-galactosidase-progesterone conjugates which contain of the order of one steroid molecule per molecule of β-galactosidase. It can be seen by comparison of figs. 15A and 15B that such low incorporation requires the use of considerably more conjugate per assay in order to achieve an acceptable degree of conjugate binding in the absence of competing steroid. Note that in fig. 15B the 5, 10 and 20pg standards cannot be distinguished from the B_O value. In practise, where steric hinderance of conjugated hapten occurs it will be necessary to employ a conjugate with appreciably more hapten incorporated since only a fraction of these will be immunoreactive (Table 2).

ii) It is widely accepted that in an homologous hapten EIA system the affinity of binding of enzyme conjugate to antibody is higher than that for native hapten since the same hapten derivative is used in forming the immunogen as is used for conjugating hapten to enzyme. This phonomenon was originally investigated for oestrogens by Van Weeman and Schuurs (1975) who argued that by employing 'site' or 'bridge' heterology more sensitive assays could be achieved. It can now be seen that similar improvements in sensitivity can be achieved by the use of more refined conjugation and separation techniques. In a practical sense, however, antibody avidity dictates that, for an homologous hapten-enzyme conjugate, very high concentrations of hapten are required in order to reduce enzyme label binding to blank values (10 - 100 times those required to reduce ^{3}H label binding in a comparable RIA system to blank levels) even though the sensitivity achieved may still be very high (compare figs. 10 and 11).

A number of workers have investigated aspects of bridge and site heterology in order to increase the sensitivity of steroid EIA's but with varying degrees of success (Van Weeman and Schuurs, 1975; Joyce et al, 1977b; Exley and Abuknesha, 1977; Dawson et al, 1979; Hosada et al, 1980). Different methods of assessing sensitivity have, however, made it difficult to compare their findings. Although increases in sensitivity have been achieved in some instances (Dawson et al, 1979; Van Weeman and Schuurs, 1975) they may be accompanied by loss of specificity (Hosada et al, 1980)

The data of Dray and co-workers (Dray et al, 1975; Gros et al, 1978)

appear conflicting. They indicate in one instance (Gros <u>et al</u>, 1978) that
it is necessary to use bridge heterology (hemimaleate rather than hemisuccinate) to achieve similar dose response curves when comparing binding of
tritium and enzyme-labelled progesterone whereas in a previous publication
(Dray <u>et al</u>, 1975) an almost identical response was achieved using an homologous system. We have found that such comparisons can be misleading since

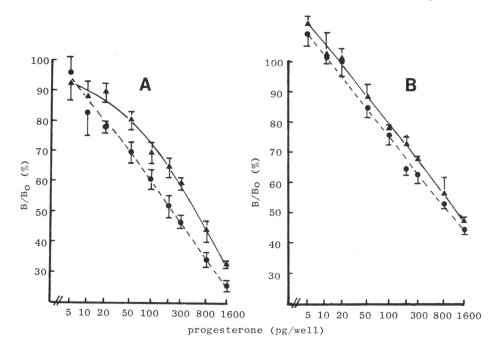

progesterone (pg/well)

Fig. 15   Comparison of EIA standard curves (in the absence of milk)
using progesterone hemisuccinate (▲-▲) or progesterone hemimaleate
(●-●) conjugates prepared with a molar ratio of progesterone
derivative: β-galactosidase of 25 : 1 (A) or 2.5 : 1 (B). Results are
mean of 4 determinations ± 2 SEM. For A, B_O values ± 2 SEM for the
hemisuccinate (23ng conjugate/well) and hemimaleate (21ng/well) conjugates were 0.920 ± 0.055 OD and 0.784 ± 0.010 OD respectively. For B,
B_O values ± 2 SEM for the hemisuccinate (54ng conjugate/well) and
hemimaleate (57ng conjugate/well) conjugates were 0.460 ± 0.015 OD
and 0.331 ± 0.011 OD respectively.

it cannot be assumed that assay conditions which are optimal for one conjugate are also optimal for the other or that conjugation efficiency is the
same when using different hapten derivatives. We have compared β-galactosidase
conjugates of progesterone hemimaleate (heterologous) and progesterone hemisuccinate (homologous); under the same conditions it was apparent, using
conjugates prepared with a 25 : 1 molar steroid excess that greater sensitiv-

ity was achieved using the hemimaleate conjugate (fig. 15A). Standard curves obtained using conjugates formed with a 2.5:1 steroid excess, however, showed no significant difference in sensitivity (fig. 15B).

SUMMARY

The fragmentary nature of the information which has been derived from investigations of heterology and the extent of hapten conjugation on the performance of EIA's is such that it is impossible to draw hard and fast conclusions about their influence on assay sensitivity. In general, where heterology has been introduced to effect increases in sensitivity little attention has been given to the degree of hapten incorporation achieved under these conditions (Van Weeman and Schuurs, 1975; Hosada et al, 1980). Increases or decreases in sensitivity under these circumstances may partly be attributed to differing degrees of steroid incorporation. Further, it has proved possible to achieve equally sensitive EIA's using homologous systems (Sauer et al, 1981; Turkes et al, 1979; Dray et al, 1975) as was previously thought possible only by using heterology (Joyce et al, 1977; Van Weeman and Schuurs, 1975). Closer attention to the elimination of free hapten following conjugation may have contributed to these improvements.

To our knowledge no studies have been performed under suitably comparable conditions to furnish evidence that for hapten assays an actual incorporation ratio of approximately 1 hapten per enzyme molecule does indeed result in standard curves of the greatest sensitivity. This arguement has a theoretical attraction which cannot be ignored but it does not take into account the extent to which incorporated haptens are sterically available for antibody binding. In future it would seem pertinent, when evaluating the influence of heterology on the sensitivity of EIA standard curves to consider concurrently the relationship between the total number of haptens incorporated into the enzyme and the number of haptens which are immunoreactive.

Acknowledgements

We wish to thank Dr G.S. Pope of the National Institute for Research in Dairying for his continued advice and criticism and for the generous provision of progesterone antiserum used for this work. The skilful technical assistance of Mr Paul O'Neill is gratefully acknowledged.

Appendix

It is only recently that the Sigma Chemical Company have indicated in their catalogue that the grade IV E. Coli β-galactosidase used in these studies is standardized by the addition of BSA. Since this would clearly be conjugated by the progesterone active ester and subsequently interfere with the assay, we now use the grade VIII product.

REFERENCES

Abuknesha, R. & Exley, D. 1978. Design and development of oestradiol -17β Enzyme-Immunoassay. In "Enzyme Immunoassay of Hormone and Drugs" (Ed. S.B. Pal) (Walter de Gruyter, Berlin) pp. 139-152.

Al-Bassam, M.N., O'Sullivan, M.J., Gremi, E., Bridges, J.W. & Marks, V. 1978. Nortryptiline enzyme-immunoassay. In "Enzyme Labelled Immunoassay of Hormones and Drugs" (Ed. S.B. Pal) (Walter de Gruyter, Berlin) pp. 375-386.

Albert, W.H.W., Kleinhammer, G., Linke, R., Tanswell, P. & Staehler, F. 1978. Enzyme immuno assays for invitro diagnosis of thyroid function. In " Enzyme Labelled Immunoassay of Hormone and Drugs" (Ed. S.B. Pal) (Walter de Gruyter, Berlin) pp. 153-174.

Anderson, M.J. 1978. Continuous flow radioimmunoassay - a completely automated continuous flow radioimmunoassay system. Med. Lab. Sci. 35, (2) 173-185.

Arnstadt, K.I. & Cleere, W.F. 1981. Enzymeimmunoassay for determination of progesterone in milk from cows. J. Reprod. Fert. 62, 173-180.

Avrameas, S. 1969. Coupling of enzymes to proteins with glutaraldehyde. Immunochemistry 6, 43-52.

Avrameas, S. & Ternynck, T. 1971. Peroxidase-labelled antibody and Fab conjugates with enhanced intracellular penetration. Immunochemistry 8, 1175-1179.

Ball, P.J.H. & Jackson, N.W. 1979. The fertility of dairy cows inseminated on the basis of milk progesterone measurements. Br. Vet. J. 135, 537-540.

Bosch, A.M.G., Dijkhuizen, D.M., Schuurs, A.H.W.M. & Van Weeman, B.K. 1978a. Enzyme-immunoassay for total oestrogens in pregnancy plasma or serum. Clin. Chim. Acta 89, 59-70.

Bosch, A.M.G., Stevens, W.H.J.M., Vanwijngaarden, C.J. & Schuurs, A.H.W.M. 1978b. Solid phase enzyme-immunoassay (EIA) of testosterone. Z. Anal. Chem. 290, 98.

Comoglio, S. & Celada, F. 1976. An immuno-enzymatic assay of cortisol using E. Coli B-galactosidase as label. J. Immunol. Meth. 10, 161-170.

Craven, G.R., Steers, E. & Anfinsen, C.B. 1965. Purification, composition and molecular weight of the β-galactosidase of Escherichia Coli K12. J. Biol. Chem. 240, 2468-2477.

Dawson, E.C., Anneke, M.G. & Van Weeman, B.K. 1979. Enzyme immunoassay for steroids. Res. Steroids 8, 139-146.

Doel, T.R. & Collen, T. 1981. Chemical cross-linking and the preparation of conjugates for ELISA. In ELISA - its role in veterinary research and diagnosis (Ed. J.R. Crowther & R.C. Wardley)

Dray, F. Andrieu, J-M. & Renaud, F. 1975. Enzyme immunoassay of progesterone at the picogram level using β-galactosidase as label. Biochim. Biophys. Acta 403, 131-138.

Engvall, E. & Perlmann, P. 1971. Enzyme-linked immunosorbent assay (ELISA). Quantitative assay of immunoglobulin G. Immunochemistry 8, 871-874.

Erlanger, B.F., Borek, F., Beiser, S.M. & Lieberman, S. 1954. 1. Preparation and conjugation of bovine serum albumin with testosterone and with cortisone. J. Biol. Chem. 228, 713-727.

Exley, D. & Abuknesha, R. 1977. The preparation and purification of a β-D-galactosidase-oestradiol-17β conjugate for enzyme immunoassay. FEBS Lett. 79, 301-304.

Fields, R. 1971. The measurement of amino groups in proteins and peptides. Biochem. J. 124, 581-590.

298

Gnemmi, E. O'Sullivan, M.J., Chieregatti, G., Simmons, M., Simmons, A., Bridges, J.W. & Marks, V. 1978. A sensitive immunoenzymometric assay (IEMA) to quantitate hormones. In "Enzyme labelled Immunoassay of Hormones and Drugs". (Ed. S.B. Pal) (Walter de Gruyter, Berlin) pp. 29-41.

Gros, C., Flecheux, D. & Dray, F. 1978. Dosage immuno-enzymatique des stéroides. Ann. Biol. Clin. 36, 393-396.

Guesdon, J.L. & Avrameas, S. 1977. Magnetic solid phase enzyme-immunoassay. Immunochemistry 14, 443-447.

Günzler, O., Rattenberger, E., Görlach, A., Hahn, R., Höcke, P., Claus, R. & Karg, H. 1979. Milk progesterone determination as applied to the confirmation of oestrus, the detection of cycling and as an aid to veterinarian and biotechnical measures in cows. Br. Vet. J. 135, 541-549.

Hamada, K., Tomada, S., Sugawa, T. & Takahashi, K.P. 1978. Simultaneous competitive enzyme immunoassay for human choriomic gonadstrophin. Endocrinol. Jpn. 25, 515-517.

Hayashi, Y. Yano, T. & Yamamoto, S. 1981. Enzyme immunoassay of prostaglandin F_2 . Biochim. Biophys. Acta 663, 661-668.

Hersch, L.S. & Yaverbaum, S. 1975. Magnetic solid-phase radioimmunoassay. Clin. Chim. Acta 63, 69-72.

Hoffman, B., Günzler, O., Hamburger, R. & Schmidt, W. 1976. Milk progesterone as a parameter for fertility control in cattle; methodological approaches and present status of application in Germany. Br. Vet. J. 132, 469-476.

Harejsi, J. & Smetana, E. 1956. The isolation of gamma globulin from blood serum by Rivanol. Acta Med. Scand. 155, 65-70.

Hosada, H., Sakai, Y., Yoshida, H. & Nambara, T. 1979. Enzyme labelling of steroids by the activated ester method. Chem. Pharm. Bull. 27, 2147-2150.

Hosada, H., Yoshida, H., Sakai, Y., Miyairi, S. & Nambara, T. 1980. Sensitivity and specificity in enzymeimmunoassay of testosterone. Chem. Pharm. Bull. 28, 3035-3123.

Ishikawa, E. 1973. Enzymeimmunoassay of insulin by fluorimetry of the insulin-glucoamylase complex. J. Biochem. 73, 1319-1321.

Ishikawa, E., Yamada, Y. Hamaguchi, Y., Yoshitake, S., Shiomi, K., Ota, T., Yamamoto, Y. & Tanaka, K. 1978. Enzyme-labelling with maleimides and its application to the immunoassay of peptide hormones. In "Enzyme-linked Immunoassay of Hormones and Drugs". (Ed. S.B. Pal) (Walter de Gruyter, Berlin) pp. 43-57.

Johmen, M., Nakao, T., Tsunoda, K. & Kawata, K. 1980. Enzyme immunoassay of progesterone in swine serum. Jpn. J. Anim. Reprod. 26, 77-78.

Joyce, B.G., Read, G.F. & Fahmy, D.R. 1977a. Specific enzymeimmunoassay for progesterone in human plasma. Steroids 29, 761-770.

Joyce, B.G., Read, G.F. & Riad-Fahmy, D. 1977b. Enzyme immunoassay for progesterone and oestradiol. A study of factors influencing sensitivity. In "Radioimmunoassay and Related Procedures in Medicine" Vol. 1. (International Atomic Energy Agency, Vienna) pp. 289-295.

Joyce, B.G., Wilson D.W., Read, G.F. & Riad-Fahmy, D. 1978. An improved enzyme immunoassay for progesterone in human plasma. Clin. Chem. 24, 2099-2102.

Kamonpatana, M., Van de Wiel, D.F.M., Koops, W., Leenanuruksa, D., Ngramsuriyaroj, C. & Usanakornkul, S. 1979. Oestrus control and early pregnancy diagnosis in the swamp buffalo: comparison of enzymeimmunoassay and radioimmunoassay for plasma progesterone. Theriogenol. 11, 399-409.

Kato, K., Hamaguchi, Y., Fukui, H. & Ishikawa, E. 1975a. Enzyme-linked immunoassay. II. A simple method for synthesis of the rabbit antibody-β-D-galactosidase complex and its general applicability. J. Biochem 78, 423-425.

Kato, K., Hamaguchi, Y., Fukui, H. & Ishikawa, E. 1975b. Enzyme-linked immunoassay. I. Novel method for synthesis of the insulin-β-D-galactosidase conjugate and its applicability for insulin assay. J. Biochem. 78, 235-237.

Kato, K., Umeda, Y., Suyuki, F., Hayashi, D. & Kosaka, A. 1979. Evaluation of solid phase enzyme immunoassay for insulin in human serum. Clin. Chem. 25, 1306-1308.

Kennedy, J.H., Kricka, L.J. & Wilding, P. 1976. Protein - protein coupling reactions and the applications of protein conjugates. Clin. Chem. Acta 70, 1-31.

Kikutani, M., Ischiguro, M., Kitagawa, T., Imamura, S. & Miura, S. 1979. Enzyme immunoassay of human chorionic gonadotrophin employing β-galactosidase as label. J. Clin. Endocrinol. Metab. 47, 980-984.

Kitagawa, T. & Aikawa, T. 1976. Enzyme coupled immunoassay of insulin using a novel coupling reagent. J. Biochem. 79, 233-236.

Kitagawa, T., Fujitake, T. & Taniyama, H. 1976. Enzyme-coupled immunoassay of Viomycin. J. Antibiot. 29, 1343-1345.

Kitagawa, T., Kanamura, T., Kato, H., Yano, S. & Asanuma, Y. 1978a. Novel EIA of three antibiotics. New methods for preparation of antisera to the antibiotics and for enzyme labelling using a combination of two heterobifunctional reagents. In "Enzyme-linked Immunoassay of Hormones and Drugs" (Ed. S.B. Pal) (Walter de Gruyter, Berlin) pp. 59-66.

Kitagawa, T., Kanamura, T., Wakamatsu, H., Kato, H., Yano, S. & Asanuma, Y. 1978b. A novel method for the preparation of an antiserum to penicillin and its application for novel enzyme immunoassay of penicillin. J. Biochem. 84, 491-494.

Kobayashi, Y., Ogihara, T., Amitani, K., Watanabe, F., Kiguchi, T., Ninomiya, I. & Kumahara, Y. 1978. Enzyme immunoassay for cortisol in serum using cortisol 21-amine. Steroids 32, 137-144.

Kominami, G., Fujisaka, I., Yamauchi, A. & Kono, M. 1980. A sensitive enzyme immunoassay for plasma cortisol. Clin. Chim. Acta 103, 381-391.

Korhonen, M.K., Juntunen, K.O. & Stenman, U-H. 1980. Enzyme immunoassay of estriol in pregnancy urine. Clin. Chem. 26, 1829-1831.

Kurzer, F.- Douraghi-Zadeh, K. 1967. Advances in the chemistry of carbodiimides. Chem. Rev. 67, 107-151.

Laing, J.A. & Heap, R.B. 1981. The concentration of progesterone in the milk of cows during the reproductive cycle. Br. Vet. J. 127, xix-xxii.

Lamming, G.E. & Bulman, D.C. 1976. The use of milk progesterone radioimmunoassay in the diagnosis and treatment of subfertility in dairy cows. Br. Vet. J. 132, 507-517.

Marion, S.L., Estergreen, V.L. & Reeves, J.J. 1978. Dtermination of pregnant mare serum gonadotrophin by an enzyme-linked immunoassay. In "Enzyme-labelled Immunoassay of Hormones and Drugs" (Ed. S.B. Pal) (Walter de Gruyter, Berlin) pp. 277-285.

McCaughey, W.J. & Cooper, R.J. 1980. An assessment by progesterone assay of the accuracy of oestrus detection in dairy cows. Vet. Rec. 107, 508-510.

Miyai, K., Ishibashi, K. & Kumahara, Y. 1976. Enzyme-linked immunoassay of thyrotropin. Clin. Chim. Acta 67, 263-268.

Miyai, K., Ishibashi, K., Ogihara, T., Nishi, K., Kawashima, M. & Kumahara, Y. 1978. Evaluation of enzyme-immunoassay of hormones for clinical applications. In "Enzyme-labelled Immunoassay of Hormones and Drugs" (Ed. S.B. Pal) (Walter de Gruyter, Berlin) pp. 287-310.

Monji, N. & Castro, A. 1979a. An enzyme immunoassay for cortisol using a novel meta-maleimide derivative of cortisol coupled with β-galactosidase. J. Appl. Biochem. 1, 311-317.

Monji, N., Malkus, H. & Castro, A. 1979b. Maleimide derivative of hapten for coupling to enzyme: a new method in enzyme immunoassay. Biochem. Biophys. Res. Commun. 85, 671-677.

Nakao, T. 1980. Practical procedure for enzyme immunoassay for progesterone in bovine serum. Acta Endocrinol. Copenhagen 93, 223-227.

Nakao, T. & Kawata, K. 1980. Enzyme immunoassay of progesterone in bovine serum and milk and its application in monitoring the luteinization of ovarian follicular cysts after hormone treatments. In "XI Int. Cong. Dis. Cattle" Vol II. (Ed. E. Mayer) (Bregman Press, Haifa) pp. 916-933.

Nambara, T., Shimada, K. & Ohta, H. 1980. Preparation of specific antiserum to estrone sulphate. J. Steroid Biochem. 13, 1075-1079.

Nakane, P.K. & Kawaoi, A. 1974. Peroxidase-labelled antibody. A new method of conjugation. J. Histochem. Cytohistochem. 22, 1084-1091.

Nye, L., Forrest, G.C., Greenwood, H., Gardner, J.S., Jay, R., Roberts, J. R. & Landon, J. 1976. Solid-phase, magnetic particle radioimmunoassay. Clin. Chim. Acta 69, 387-396.

O'Sullivan, M.J., Gnemmi, E., Morris, D., Chieregatti, G., Simmons, M., Simmonds, A.D., Bridges, J.W. & Marks, V. 1978a. A simple method for the preparation of enzyme-antibody conjugates. FEBS Lett. 95, 311-313.

O'Sullivan, M.J., Gnemmi, E., Morris, D., Al-Bassam, M.N., Simmons, M., Bridges, J.W. & Marks, V. 1978b. An enzyme-immunoassay for Tri-dod-thyronine. In "Enzyme-labelled Immunoassay of Hormones and Drugs" (Ed. S.B. Pal) (Walter de Gruyter, Berlin) pp. 301-310.

O'Sullivan, M.J., Bridges J.W. & Marks, V. 1979. Enzyme immunoassay: A review. Ann. Clin. Biochem. 16, 221-240.

Oellerich, M. 1980. Enzyme immunoassays in clinical chemistry: present status and trends. J. Clin. Chem. Clin. Biochem. 18, 197-208.

Ogihara, T., Miyai, K., Ishibashi, K. & Kumahara, Y. 1977. Enzyme-labelled immunoassay for plasma cortisol. J. Clin. Endocrinol. Metab. 44, 91-95.

Oltner, R. & Edqvist, L.E. 1981. Progesterone in defatted milk: its relation to insemination and pregnancy in normal cows as compared with cows on problem farms and individual problem animals. Br. Vet. J. 137, 78-87.

Österman, T.M., Juntunen, K.O., Gothoni, G.D. 1979. Enzyme immunoassay of estrogen-like substances in plasma, polythene glycol as precipitant. Clin. Chem. 25, 716-718.

Otsuki, Y., Yamaji, K., Tanizawa, O., Fujita, M., Kurachi, K., Ishibashi, K. & Miyai, K. 1979. Enzyme-immunoassay for estriol. Endocrinol. Jpn. 26, 687-691.

Pain, D. & Surolia, A. 1981. Preparation of protein A-peroxidase moncon-jugate using a heterobifunctional reagent and its use in enzyme immunoassays. J. Immunol. Meth. 40, 219-230.

Patricot, M.C., Poggi, B. & Revol, A. 1978. Dosage immunoenzymatique de la progesterone plasmatique au cours de la grossesse. Pharm. Biol. 12, 523-525.

Pope, G.S., Majzlik, I., Ball, P.J.H. & Leaver, J.D. 1976. Use of progest-erone concentrations in plasma and milk on the diagnosis of pregnancy in domestic cattle. Br. Vet. J. 132, 497-506.

Rajkowski, K.M., Cittanova, N., Urios, P. & Jayle, M.F. 1977. An enzyme-linked immunoassay of testosterone. Steroids 30, 129-137.

Sadeh, D., Sela, E. & Hexter, C.S. 1979. Novel enzymeimmunoassay for 17β estradiol. J. Immunol. Meth. 28, 125-131.

Sauer, M.J., Foulkes, J.A. & Cookson, A.D. 1981. Direct enzymeimmunoassay of progesterone in bovine milk. Steroids, 38, 45-53.

Saxena, B.B., Post, K.G., Roy, A.K., Khan, F.S. & Rathnam, P. 1979. Development of a solid phase centrifugation-free enzymeimmunoassay for LH for ovulation detection. In "Psychoneuroendocrinology in Reproduction. An interdisciplinary approach. Developments in Endocrinology" Vol 5. (Eds. L. Zichella & P. Pancheri) (Elsevier North Holland Biomed Press, Amsterdam) pp. 277-288.

Scharpé, S.L., Cooreman, W.M., Blomme, W.J. & Laekeman, G.M. 1976. Quantitative enzyme immunoassay: current status. Clin. Chem. 22, 733-738.

Schuurs, A.H.W.M. & Van Weeman, B.K. 1977. Enzyme-immunoassay. Clin. Chim. Acta 81, 1-40.

Seeger, K., Thurow, H., Haede, W. & Knappe, E. 1979. An Enzyme immunoassay (EIA) for progesterone in horse plasma. J. Immunol. Meth. 28, 211-217.

Smith, K.O. & Gehle, W.D. 1977. Magnetic transfer devices for use in solid-phase radioimmunoassays and enzyme-linked immunosorbent assays. J. Infect. Dis., Suppl. 136, S319-S336.

Tateishi, K., Yamamoto, H., Ogihara, T. & Hayashi, C. 1977. Enzyme immunoassay of serum testosterone. Steroids 30, 25-32.

Thorneycroft, I.H., Tillson, S.A., Abraham, G.E., Scaramuzzi, R.J. & Caldwell, B.V. 1970. Preparation and purification of antibodies to steroids. In "Immunologic methods in steroid determination" (Eds. F.G. Penn & B.V. Caldwell) (Meredith Corporation, New York) pp. 63-86.

Tomodo, S., Hamada, K. & Sugawa, T. 1978. Competitive enzyme immunoassay of hCG, silicone rod as solid phase. Acta Obstet. Gynaec. Jpn. 30, 1620-1621.

Traut, R.R., Bollen, A., Sun, T-T., Hershey, J.W.B., Sunberg, J. & Pierce, L.R. 1973 Methyl 4-mercaptobutyrimidate as a cleavable cross-linking reagent and its application to the E. Coli 30s ribosome. Biochemistry 12, 3266-3273.

Turkes, A., Turkes, A.O., Joyce, B.G., Read, G.F. & Riad-Fahmy, D. 1979. A sensitive solid phase enzymeimmunoassay for testosterone in plasma and saliva. Steroids 33, 347-359.

Turkes, A.O., Turkes, A., Joyce, B.G. & Riad-Fahmy, D. 1980. A sensitive enzymeimmunoassay with a fluorimetric end point for the determination of testosterone in female plasma and saliva. Steroids 35, 89-101.

Van Weeman, B.K. & Schuurs, A.H.W.M. 1971. Immunoassay using antigen-enzyme conjugates. FEBS Lett. 15, 232-236.

Van Weeman, B.K. & Schuurs, A.H.W.M. 1975. The influence of heterologous combinations of antiserum and enzyme-labelled estrogen on the characteristics of estrogen enzyme-immunoassays. Immunochemistry 12, 667-670.

Williams, D.G. 1978. Enzyme immunoassay for human placental lactogen suitable for use in a routine hospital laboratory. In "Enzyme-labelled Immunoassay of Hormones and Drugs" (Ed. S.B. Pal) (Walter de Gruyter, Berlin) pp. 129-136.

PART VII: REPORT ON PACIA SYSTEM

PARTICLE COUNTING IMMUNOASSAY (P A C I A)

- ITS RELEVANCE TO VETERINARY MEDICINE

H.W. Holy and Vera Reicher

Technicon International Division
Geneva, Switzerland

ABSTRACT

The Technicon[TM] PACIA System is a new fully automated non-isotopic immunoassay system for the determination of antigens, antibodies, haptens and immune complexes.

After briefly describing the underlying principles, the system and the range of assays, the paper details work done in the determination of bovine leukosis virus antibodies. After establishing feasibility of the assay and adjusting the sensitivity so as to obtain yes/no decisions without false positives or negatives, 100 serum samples were tested at different dilutions and correctly identified at a 1:20 dilution, except for one sample which was only identified at a 1:10 dilution.

Further work is in progress to exploit the advantage of the technique, including its great sensitivity for other veterinary applications such as the determination of other antibodies as well as infectious antigens (e.g. brucellosis) and animal immune complexes; the determination of progesterone in milk is also being developed.

INTRODUCTION

In any programme for animal disease eradication or control, large serial runs are routinely made using a single assay. Given the need for large serial runs, the only economic and overall effective method is through automation. The acceptance of automation some 20 years ago by clinical chemistry has led to its meteoric rise in importance.

However, the extreme specificity required by veterinary diagnosis has, to date, excluded automation used by biochemistry or haematology. Attention has been increasingly focussed on "work rationalisation" using immunoassay. The profession has been extremely reluctant to accept radioisotopes. For these reasons we have developed the Technicon PACIA System - Particle Counting Immunoassay. The method is fully automated and completely non-isotopic running at 60 samples/hour and producing its results in 40 minutes of dwell time. Hence we believe that the same advantages of automation enjoyed by clinical chemistry are now available to veterinary medicine: minimum operator involvement, objective reporting, inter-laboratory comparability and finally overall economy.

PRINCIPLE

Antigens and antibodies

The sample is mixed with antibody coated latex particles. Sample antigen agglutinates some of the particles, so that the unagglutinated fraction decreases.

An optical cell counter is set to read only particles whose diameters lie between 0.6 μ and 1.0 μ and therefore counts only the non-agglutinated latex particles. The concentration of antigen in the sample is inversely proportional to the particle concentration (Fig. 1).

Antibodies are determined similarly using their agglutinating activity on latex particles coated with antigen.

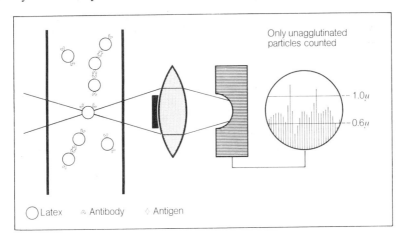

Fig. 1   Antigen determination

Haptens

Haptens are determined by agglutination inhibition. Sample containing free hapten is mixed with excess specific antibody. Hapten covalently coated on to latex particles is added, and antibody not coupled to free hapten forms a complex with the latex-hapten. Rheumatoid factor, or similar macromolecule, is used to agglutinate this complex. The concentration of unagglutinated latex is then directly proportional to the concentration of hapten in the sample (Fig. 2).

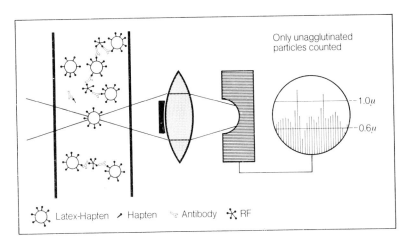

Fig. 2   Hapten determination

Immune complexes

Rheumatoid factor (RF) and some other macromolecules agglutinate both latex coated with human IgG and immune complexes. When a limited amount of rheumatoid factor is added to a mixture of latex IgG and immune complexes in serum, the concentration of unagglutinated particles is directly proportional to the concentration of immune complexes in the sample (Fig. 3).

In the PACIA immune complex application, several agglutinations may be used to detect different varieties of immune complexes.

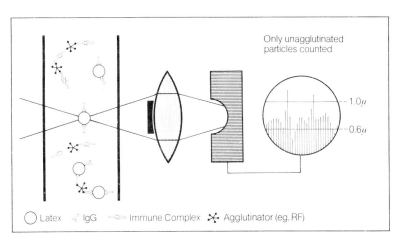

Fig. 3   Immune complex determination

EQUIPMENT

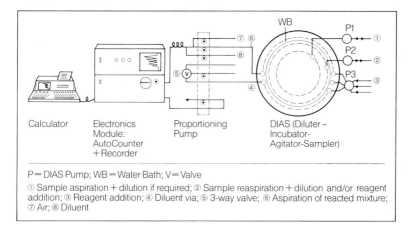

Fig. 4   Schematic of Technicon PACIA System with
          simplified flow diagram

The Technicon PACIA System consists of 4 elements together with a
Hewlett Packard HP85 calculator.

DIAS (Diluter-Incubator-Agitator-Sampler)

This module is used for all aspects of the agglutination reaction
including sampling, reagent additions, mixing, incubation time and temperature and first dilution of agglutinates.

Proportioning pump

The reacted sample is aspirated from DIAS into the continuous flow
manifold where it is segmented, further diluted and fed to the optical
particle counter.

Electronics module

In addition to the Technicon AutoCounter[TM] optical particle counter
the module includes a recorder and the necessary controls.

Microcomputer

All operational parameters of DIAS are controlled and performance is
monitored with signals for malfunction.

Data handling is fully automatic.

HP85 calculator

Requirements for the assays (e.g. cycle rate, incubation time and temperature, sample and reagent additions, number of standards etc.) are entered using the keyboard which is also used for system commands.

A printout of results is provided.

PROCEDURE

Reaction (Fig. 4)

Sample (50–200 µl) is placed in cups in the innermost row of holes in the sampler tray; reaction tubes are inserted in two outer rows. The system command "Start" causes a pre-determined amount of sample to be aspirated via Probe 1 by clockwise rotation of a DIAS peristaltic metering pump. Probe 1 moves to the second row of tubes, the pump reverses rotation, dispensing sample and continues rotation to add a diluent or first reagent. A second metering pump transfers diluted sample to the outer row of reaction tubes with further dilution or reagent addition.

Under continuous vortex mixing at 37°C, the reaction tube is indexed once/minute until it arrives at Station 3 where the latex and other reagents are added through a third metering pump.

The final station is positioned so as to allow sufficient incubation time before the reaction mixture is again diluted and an aliquot is aspirated by a proportioning pump for final dilution and detection.

The analytical steps for all PACIA assays are very similar.

Detection

The stream of liquid containing agglutinated particles flows at the rate of 2 ml/min through an optical flowcell of 150 x 150 micron cross-section. When no particles flow, light from the source is blocked to the photomultiplier by a dark spot on the focusing lens.

The passage of a particle through the light beam scatters the light past the dark spot on to the photomultiplier.

The amount of scatter and hence light striking the photomultiplier is proportional to the size of the scattering particle. Thresholds are selected to count only particles between 0.6 µ and 1.0 µ, thus rejecting noise and agglutinated particles.

INTERPRETATION

The unagglutinated particle concentration for each sample is registered as an analogue signal on the recorder in the form of a peak.

By means of the microcomputer, the analogue signals are converted to digital data. Data from the standards are stored to provide a standard curve according to a sophisticated curve fitting programme which includes safeguards against outliers.

The peak heights from samples are automatically picked and the concentration is calculated from this curve in units chosen by the user.

The HP85 calculator draws the standard curve and calculates the concentration for each sample. The printout also includes peak heights as shown on the recorder (Fig. 5). The operator can use any other method of data reduction he prefers. Peak shape provides a continuous guide on how well the system functions, i.e. function monitoring.

DATE =26.11.81

ASSAY- HLF

UNITS=NG/ML

STANDARDIZATION

BEST CURVE = SPLIT MULTI-VAR.REGR.

STANDARD	PEAK HEIGHT		STANDARD (CALC.)
10	95.5	95.5	10
20	93.0	93.0	20
50	85.5	85.5	50
100	74.0	74.0	100
200	58.0	58.0	200
500	34.0	34.0	500
1000	22.5	22.5	1000

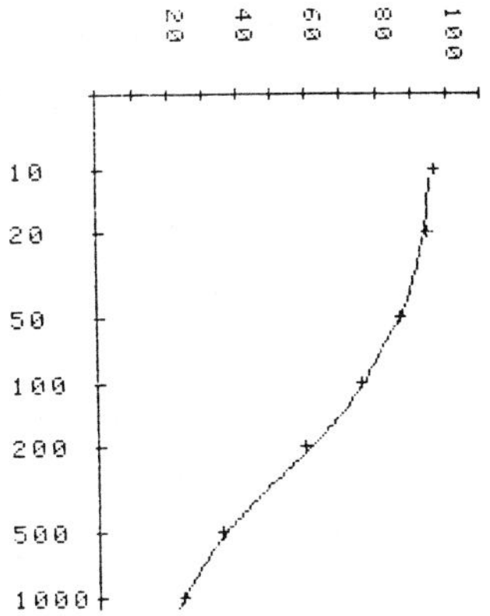

TEST RESULTS

SAMPLE NO. 1
PK.HT. =49.5
CONC. =268.4

SAMPLE NO. 2
PK.HT. =92.5
CONC. =22

SAMPLE NO. 3
PK.HT. =66.0
CONC. =146.9

SAMPLE NO. 4
PK.HT. =67.0
CONC. =140.7

SAMPLE NO. 5
PK.HT. =93.5
CONC. =18

SAMPLE NO. 6
PK.HT. =92.5
CONC. =22

Fig. 5 Technicon PACIA printout

RANGE OF P A C I A ASSAYS

Much of the research on the PACIA system to date has concentrated on defining the limits of its applicability. Tables 1 and 2 list the assays whose feasibility has been established; Table 1 covers completed assays and Table 2 includes assays which are either under development or part of research projects.

TABLE 1   PACIA system performance.

Method	Intra CV%		Inter CV%		Recovery %		Correlation y (PACIA) = x (RIA) + 2
	Level	Value	Level	Value	Level	Value	
A F P (ng/ml)	13.5	7.4	48	6.1	46	93.5	y = 4.4 + 1.00x
	39.0	2.6	144	9.6	133	97.4	n = 127
	125.0	2.4	275	8.0	186	98.4	r = 0.99
	255.0	2.0	469	6.4	–	–	
Ferritin (µg/L)	25	4.0	28	6.0	10	100.2	y = 93.8 + 1.07x
	78	2.6	55	5.8	100	103.0	n = 91
	260	3.8	175	7.3	1000	93.0	r = 0.98
	420	11.9	338	7.7	–	–	
I g E (IU/ml)	12.5	12.0	30.5	12.8	–	–	y = 0.95x – 7.50
	62.0	13.0	132.2	9.9	–	–	n = 99
	115.0	4.3	192.0	8.5	–	–	r = 0.985
	372.0	5.4	311.0	8.9	–	–	
	1275.0	5.9	965.0	11.1	467	101.9	
T4 (µg/l)	39.9	4.3	21.8	10.0	28*	97	y = 0.13 + 0.89x
	83.9	3.7	92.0	11.3	66*	98	n = 96
	304.0	4.4	222.3	8.7	–	–	r = 0.96
Digoxin (µg/L)	0.96	12.5	0.75	8.4	0.70	116.0	y = 0.37 + 0.68x
	1.10	10.9	1.49	8.9	1.42	100.0	n = 109
	1.25	12.0	2.92	5.8	1.65	98.9	r = 0.943
	2.97	4.4	–	–	2.9	102.3	
	–	–	–	–	5.8	99.8	

* added to normal sera

TABLE 2   PACIA   assays - feasibility study.

Analyte	Sensitivity	Analyte	Sensitivity
IgM (low level)	22 µg/L	β_2 microglobulin	10 µg/L
IgA	5 µg/L	Lactoferrin	1 µg/L
IgG	5 µg/L	Insulin	1 ng/L (1 pg/ml)
C3	25 µg/L	Growth Hormone	5 µg/L
T3	0.2 µg/L	Myoglobulin	1 µg/L
TBG	1 µg/L	Measles antibody	Yes/No decision
TSH	1 µg/L	Herpes antigen & antibody	Yes/No decision
HPL	1 µg/L		
CEA	1 µg/L	Streptococcal antigen & antibody	Yes/No decision
Progesterone	10 µg/L	Brucellosis antigen	Yes/No decision
Cortisol	10 µg/L	BLV antibody	Yes/No decision

P A C I A   SYSTEM FOR THE DETERMINATION OF BOVINE LEUKOSIS VIRUS ANTIBODY

In summary: The method uses latex (0.8 µ diameter) to whose surface
is covalently bonded bovine leukosis virus antigen. When mixed with bovine
serum, the antigen attached to the surface of the latex combines with the
antibodies, if they are present. If the antibodies are IgG, however,
agglutination is very weak owing to the relatively small size of this
immunoglobulin.

To enhance the agglutination reaction, IgM rheumatoid factor (RF) is
added to the serum-latex mixture. RF with a valence of 10 and a molecular
weight of 1,000,000 then agglutinates the latex through the IgG, attaching
itself to the F(c) chain. The concentration of free latex particles is
inversely proportional to the concentration of antibody in the serum.

REAGENTS

Antigen - Behringwerke (Marburg, Germany) Rinderleukose-Antigen 01PW14 -
          as supplied for their bovine leukosis immunodiffusion assay kit.
GBS   - Glycine Buffered Saline
          0.1M glycine and 0.17M NaCl adjusted to pH 9.2 with 1M HCl.
GBS-bSA - GBS containing 0.1% bovine serum albumin (bSA).

<u>Latex coated with antigen (Lx-Ag)</u> - Antigen covalently coupled to latex
(Sindic et al.,1981).

<u>Rheumatoid Factor (RF)</u> - Plasma of patients with high titre of RF diluted
1:50 in saline.

SAMPLES

One negative and one positive control serum together with 4 positive
and 4 negative test sera were the gift of Dr. R. Hoff/Jørgensen, State
Serum Laboratory, Copenhagen, Denmark.

A further series of 50 positive and 50 negative test sera were the
gift of Dr. D.H. Roberts, Ministry of Agriculture Fisheries and Food,
Central Veterinary Laboratory, Weybridge, Surrey, England.

Unless otherwise stated, all samples were manually diluted 1:20 in
GBS-bSA before analysis.

RESULTS

The sensitivity of the PACIA system is directly dependent on the
antigen loading on the latex particles. A series of loadings were tested
against positive control sera and one was chosen which yielded a positive
response at a 1:40 dilution but no positive response at the same dilution
with negative controls (Fig. 6).

The positive samples and 4 negative samples were subsequently run
at varying dilutions and at 1:20 all showed positive results where required
and all were negative with the appropriate samples (Fig. 7).

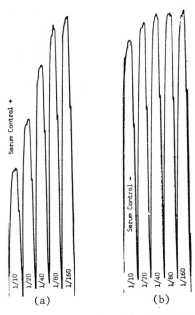

Fig. 6   Selection of latex-antigen for PACIA bovine leukosis
         antibody assay.
         (a) Results using chosen latex reagent with positive
             control serum at different dilutions.
         (b) Results using chosen latex reagent with negative
             control serum at different solutions.

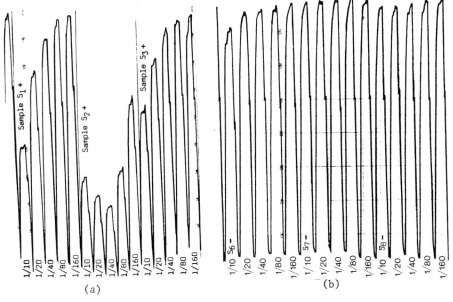

Fig. 7   Results of PACIA assay for bovine leukosis virus antibodies.
         (a) Recorder trace for positive sera at different dilutions.
         (b) Recorder trace for negative sera at different dilutions.

The 100 serum samples were then run. The 50 negatives were correctly identified and 49 of the 50 positives were also correctly identified. One positive was missed at a 1:20 dilution but was subsequently identified at a 1:10 dilution (Fig. 8).

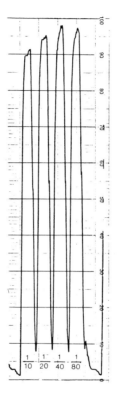

Fig. 8   Recorder trace for weakly positive bovine leukosis virus test serum assayed for antibodies by the PACIA system. At the 1:10 dilution the sample is correctly identified.

DISCUSSION

One of the major difficulties in using the PACIA technique is the extreme sensitivity of the assay. Concentrations as low as 10^{-15} molar are readily detectable. Hence, thresholds must be set for each assay based on a series of accepted positive or negative samples, preferably hovering about the decision point.

We are currently attempting to exploit this sensitivity to determine brucellosis antigen to detect cows which are infected but fail to make antibodies. Initial results are promising.

Obviously, too, since RF is shown to be an effective agglutinator for bovine leukosis virus antigen bound to antibody, it will also agglutinate bovine immune complexes. Considerable effort is now being expended in this direction: the measurement of immune complexes as a sensitive indicator of animal health.

The measurement of progesterone in milk using the hapten assay above described is now under development.

CONCLUSION

The PACIA method has already been shown to be adequate for the determination of low concentration of proteins such as Ferritin (Limet et al., 1982), Alpha-Fetoprotein (Collet-Cassart et al., 1981a), IgE (Magnusson et al., 1981) and Digoxin (Collet-Cassart et al., 1981b). Several publications have shown the effectiveness of PACIA in the determination of circulating immune complexes (Cambiaso et al., 1978; Cambiaso et al., 1979; Masson et al., 1981). We have now shown that the system can also be used for the determination of bovine leukosis antibodies in veterinary medicine.

As a fully automated system using non-isotopic techniques and running at 60 samples/hour with a through time of 40 minutes, we feel the system could have an important place in future disease eradication or control programmes.

REFERENCES

Cambiaso, C.L., Riccomi, H., Sindic, C. and Masson, P.L. 1978. Particle counting immunoassay (PACIA) II. Automated determination of circulating immune complexes by inhibition of the agglutinating activity of rheumatoid sera. J. Immunological Methods, 23, 29-50.

Cambiaso, C.L., Sindic, C. and Masson, P.L. 1979. Particle counting immunoassay (PACIA) III. Automated determination of circulating immune complexes by inhibition of an agglutinating factor of mouse serum. J. Immunological Methods, 28, 13-23.

Collet-Cassart, D., Magnusson, C.G.M., Ratcliffe, J.G., Cambiaso, C.L. and Masson, P.L. 1981. Automated particle-counting immunoassay for alpha-fetoprotein. Clin. Chem., 27, 64-67.

314

Collet-Cassart, D., Magnusson, C.G.M., Cambiaso, C.L., Lesne, M. and
    Masson, P.L. 1981. Automated particle counting immunoassay (PACIA)
    for digoxin. Clin. Chem., 27, 1205-1209.
Limet, J.N., Collet-Cassart, D., Magnusson, C.G.M., Sauvage, P.,
    Cambiaso, C.L. and Masson, P.L. 1982 (in press). Particle counting
    immunoassay (PACIA) for ferritin. J. Clin. Chem. Clin. Biochem., 20.
Magnusson C.G.M., Collet-Cassart, D., Merrett, T.G. and Masson, P.L. 1981.
    An automated particle counting immunoassay (PACIA) for serum IgE.
Masson, P.L., Cambiaso, C.L., Collet-Cassart, D., Magnusson, C.G.M.,
    Richards, C.B. and Sindic, C.J.M. 1981. Particle counting immunoassay
    (PACIA). In,"Immunochemical Techniques, Methods in Enzymology"(Ed.
    Langone,J.J. and Vanvunakis, H.).(Academic Press) 74, 106-139.
Sindic C.J.M., Chalon, M.P., Cambiaso, C.L., Collet-Cassart, D. and
    Masson, P.L. 1981. Particle counting immunoassay (PACIA) VI. The
    determination of rabbit IgG antibodies against myelin basic protein
    using IgM rheumatoid factor. Molecular Immunology, 18 (4) 293-299.
    1981

LIST OF AUTHORS

BELGIUM

P. Callebaut

Laboratory of Virology,
Faculty of Veterinary Medicine,
State University of Gent,
Casinoplein 24, B-9000, Gent.

M. Pensaert

Laboratory of Virology,
Faculty of Veterinary Medicine,
State University of Gent,
Casinoplein 24, B-9000, Gent.

DENMARK

J. Askaa

Department of Veterinary Virology
and Immunology,
The Royal Veterinary and
Agricultural University,
Copenhagen.

P. Have

State Veterinary Institute
for Virus Research,
Lindholm DK-4771,
Kalvehave.

R. Hoff-Jorgensen

State Veterinary Serum Lab.,
Bülowsuej 27,
1830 Copenhagen V.

A. Meyling

State Veterinary Serum Lab.,
Bülowsuej 27,
1830 Copenhagen V.

FRANCE

B. Toma

Chaire des Maladies Contagieuses
Ecole Nationale Vétérinaire
D'Alford,
F.94704 Maisons-Alfort,
Cedex.

GERMANY (FEDERAL REPUBLIC)

O.J.B. Hübschle

Federal Research Institute for
Animal Virus Diseases,
P.O. Box 1149,
7400, Tübingen.

NETHERLANDS

A.L.J. Gielkens

Central Veterinary Institute,
Department of Virology,
8221, R.A. Lelystad.

D.J. Houwers

Central Veterinary Institute,
Department of Virology,
8221, R.A. Lelystad.

SPAIN

J.M. Sánchez-Vizcaíno   I.N.I.A., Crida 06,
Dept. de Virologia Animal
Embajadures, 68, Madrid.

A. Ordás   I.N.I.A., Crida 06,
Dept de Virologia Animal
Embajadures, 68, Madrid.

E. Tabarés   I.N.I.A., Crida 06,
Dept de Virologia Animal
Embajadures, 68, Madrid.

E. Salvador   I.N.I.A., Crida 06,
Dept de Virologia Animal
Embajadures, 68, Madrid.

SWITZERLAND

W. Bommeli   Diagnostic Laboratories,
CH-3012, Bern.

H. Fey   Veterinary Bacteriological
Institute,
University of Bern,
Bern.

U. Kihm   Office Vétérinaire Federal
Institut Vacciral,
Hasel Hageranstrausse 74,
4000 Basel 25.

H.W. Holy   Technicon International Division,
Geneva.

V. Reicher   Technicon International Division,
Geneva.

UNITED KINGDOM

J. Anderson   Animal Virus Research Institute,
Pirbright, Woking, Surrey.

P. Barnett   Wellcome Foundation Ltd.,
Wellcome Foot-and-Mouth Disease
Laboratory,
Ash Road, Pirbright, Woking.

C. Burrells   Moredon Institute (ADRA),
408 Gilmerton Road,
Edinburgh, **EH17 7JH.**

T. Collen   Animal Virus Research Institute,
Pirbright, Woking, Surrey.

A.D. Cookson   Ministry of Agriculture, Fisheries
and Food,
Cattle Breeding Centre,
Church Lane, Shinfield,
Reading, RG2 98Z

J.R. Crowther	Animal Virus Research Institute, Pirbright, Woking, Surrey.
J.H. Darbyshire	Houghton Poultry Research Station, Houghton, Huntingdon, Cambs. PE17 3DA.
A. Dawson	Moredon Institute (ADRA), 408 Gilmerton Road, Edinburgh, EH17 7JH.
M. Dawson	Central Veterinary Laboratories, New Haw, Weybridge, Surrey, KT15 3NB.
T. Doel	Animal Virus Research Institute, Pirbright, Woking, Surrey.
W. Donachie	Moredon Institute (ADRA), 408 Gilmerton Road, Edinburgh, E4 3DA.
W.P.H. Duffus	University of Cambridge, Department of Clinical Veterinary Medicine, Madingly Road, Cambridge, CB3 OES.
J. Eynon	Institute for Research on Animal Diseases, Compton, Newbury.
J.A. Foulkes	Ministry of Agriculture, Fisheries and Food, Cattle Breeding Centre, Church Lane, Shinfield, Reading, RG2 9BZ.
R.N. Gourlay	Institute for Research on Animal Diseases, Compton, Newbury.
C. Hamblin	Animal Virus Research Institute, Pirbright, Woking, Surrey.
J.S. Harrison	Centre for Tropical Veterinary Medicine, Easter Bush, Roslin, Midlothian, Scotland.
A.J. Herring	Moredon Institute (ADRA), 408 Gilmerton Road, Edinburgh, EH17 7JH.
J.A. Herring	Moredon Institute (ADRA), 408 Gilmerton Road, Edinburgh, EH17 7JH.
P.J. Hingley	Wellcome Foundation Ltd., Wellcome Foot-and-Mouth Disease Laboratory, Ash Road, Pirbright, Woking, Surrey.

C.J. Howard	Institute for Research on Animal Diseases, Compton, Newbury.
G.E. Jones	Moredon Institute (ADRA), 408 Gilmerton Road, Edinburgh, EH17 7JH.
G.L. Kampfner	I.C.I. Pharmaceuticals Division, Macclesfield, Cheshire.
G.T. Layton	I.C.I. Pharmaceuticals Division, Macclesfield, Cheshire.
D.A. Lammas	University of Cambridge, Department of Clinical Veterinary Medicine, Madingly Road, Cambridge, CB3 OES.
B.J. McDonald	Ministry of Agriculture, Fisheries and Food, Cattle Breeding Centre, Church Lane, Shinfield, Reading RG2 9BZ.
B. Morris	University of Surrey, Department of Biochemistry, Guildford, Surrey, GU2 5XH.
P. Nettleton	Moredon Institute (ADRA), 408 Gilmerton Road, Edinburgh EH17 7JH
G. Oldham	Institute for Research on Animal Diseases, Compton, Newbury.
E.J. Ouldridge	Wellcome Foundation Ltd., Wellcome Foot-and-Mouth Disease Laboratory, Ash Road, Pirbright, Woking.
J.H. Platt	I.C.I. Pharmaceuticals Division, Macclesfield, Cheshire.
D. Reynolds	Institute for Research on Animal Diseases, Compton, Newbury.
L.W. Rowe	Animal Virus Research Institute, Pirbright, Woking, Surrey.
M.M. Rweyamamu	Wellcome Foundation Ltd., Wellcome Foot-and-Mouth Disease Laboratory, Ash Road, Pirbright, Woking.
M.J. Sauer	Ministry of Agriculture, Fisheries and Food, Cattle Breeding Centre, Church Lane, Shinfield, Reading RG2 9BZ.

J.M. Sharp

Moredon Institute (ADRA),
408 Gilmerton Road,
Edinburgh, EH17 7JH.

I. Sinclair

Central Veterinary Laboratories,
New Haw,
Weybridge, Surrey, KY15 3NB.

A. Smithyman

I.C.I. Pharmaceuticals Division,
Macclesfield, Cheshire.

L.H. Thomas

Institute for Research on Animal
Diseases,
Compton, Surrey.

A.J. Townsend

University of Cambridge,
Department of Clinical Veterinary
Medicine,
Madingly Road,
Cambridge, CB3 OES.